A Global History of Medicine

T0177579

A Global History
of Medicine

Edited by
MARK JACKSON

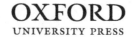
OXFORD
UNIVERSITY PRESS

OXFORD

UNIVERSITY PRESS

Great Clarendon Street, Oxford, OX2 6DP,
United Kingdom

Oxford University Press is a department of the University of Oxford.
It furthers the University's objective of excellence in research, scholarship,
and education by publishing worldwide. Oxford is a registered trade mark of
Oxford University Press in the UK and in certain other countries

© Oxford University Press 2018

The chapters in the main body of the text of this book were published in an
earlier form in *The Oxford Handbook of the History of Medicine*, 2011

The moral rights of the author have been asserted

First Edition published in 2018

Published in the United States of America by Oxford University Press
198 Madison Avenue, New York, NY 10016, United States of America

British Library Cataloguing in Publication Data
Data available

Library of Congress Control Number: 2017955707

ISBN 978–0–19–880318–8

Printed in Great Britain by
Clays Ltd, St Ives plc

For Kevin
One of the few to remain loyal

Acknowledgements

This book owes its existence to a number of people and circumstances. The chapters included here were originally published in 2011 as the second section of *The Oxford Handbook of the History of Medicine*. The suggestion that they might work together in a more focused volume on the global history of medicine came from Cathryn Steele at Oxford University Press. The timing was apposite: I had just completed a large edited volume on the history of disease and was incubating my next book on the midlife crisis, leaving me with a suitable temporal window within which to concentrate on bringing the chapters together as *A Global History of Medicine*. I am grateful to Cathryn for her initial proposition and for her support through the reassuringly smooth and swift process of production. Of course, the volume would not have materialized without the commitment, knowledge, and skill of the contributors, who have provided up-to-date revisions of the text and further readings with their customary combination of promptness and generosity. It has been, as ever, a pleasure to work with them.

When I was languishing in south London thirty years ago, having left medicine and waiting to start a PhD in medico-legal history, it would have been difficult to imagine that I would now be married with three (nearly) grown-up children and a career that has challenged and fulfilled me in equal measure. And yet, at the age of fifty-eight, here I am with a family filling my heart. Siobhán, Ciara, Riordan and Conall constitute my world, my health, my history. Without their love and support, neither my life nor my work would possess meaning or momentum. This book is theirs as much as it is mine.

Contents

List of contributors

Sanjoy Bhattacharya is Professor of the History of Medicine and Director of the Centre for Global Health Histories at the University of York, UK. Sanjoy's work explores the history of global and international health programmes in South Asia and beyond: his current research deals with the eradication of smallpox in Bangladesh and Afghanistan. Sanjoy leads the World Health Organization's Global Health Histories initiative and has an active interest in global health policy assessment: he is involved in assessing the social determinants of vaccine-preventable diseases in the developing and less developed world. Sanjoy is editor of both the journal *Medical History* and a new monograph series *Global Health Histories*, and he co-edits, with Dr. Niels Brimnes and Dr. Nitin Sinha, *New Perspectives in South Asian History*, a series of monographs published by Orient Blackswan India Ltd.

Anne-Emanuelle Birn is Professor of Critical Development Studies and Global Health at the University of Toronto. She is the author of numerous books and articles on the history of public health in Latin America, international health policy and politics, and women and international health, including: *Marriage of Convenience: Rockefeller International Health and Revolutionary Mexico* (University of Rochester Press, 2006); *Comrades in Health: US Health Internationalists, Abroad and at Home*, co-edited with Theodore Brown (Rutgers University Press, 2013); and lead author of the *Textbook of Global Health*, 3rd and 4th editions (Oxford University Press, 2009; 2017).

Linda Bryder is Professor of History at the University of Auckland and Fellow of the Royal Society of New Zealand and holds an Honorary Chair at the London School of Hygiene and Tropical Medicine. She has published widely in the history of public health in the twentieth century, including: *Below the Magic Mountain: A Social History of Tuberculosis in Twentieth-century Britain* (1988); *A Voice for Mothers: The Plunket Society and Infant Welfare, 1907–2000* (2003); *Women's Bodies and Medical Science: An Inquiry into Cervical Cancer* (2010); *Western Maternity and Medicine, 1880–1990*, edited with Janet Greenlees,

(2013); and *The Rise and Fall of National Women's Hospital: A History* (2014). She is currently on the editorial board of *Medical History* and *Health and History* and is a member of the Council of the Australian and New Zealand Society of the History of Medicine.

Harold J. Cook is John F. Nickoll Professor of History at Brown University. He has previously taught and held administrative positions at Harvard, the University of Wisconsin-Madison, and the Wellcome Trust Centre for the History of Medicine at UCL. He publishes mainly on medicine in early modern Europe, particularly with attention to England and the Netherlands and with an interest in understanding how the scientific revolution was shaped by the medical community. He helped to pioneer the method of studying the medical marketplace and has published an award-winning book on medicine, science, and commerce entitled *Matters of Exchange: Commerce, Medicine, and Science in the Dutch Golden Age* (Yale University Press, 2007).

Hormoz Ebrahimnejad is a Lecturer in History at the School of Humanities, University of Southampton. His doctoral research focused on power structures in eighteenth- and nineteenth-century Iran and his work in the history of medicine continues to explore the relationship between medicine and power, the impact of institutions on scientific developments, the emergence of the medical profession and hospital institutions, and their relationship with medical knowledge in both the medieval and modern periods. His publications include: *Medicine, Public Health and the Qâjâr State: Patterns of Medical Modernization in Nineteenth-Century Iran* (2004); and *The Development of Modern Medicine in Non-Western Countries: Historical Perspectives* (ed., 2008). He is currently working on the transition from traditional to modern medicine in nineteenth- and twentieth-century Iran.

Mark Harrison is Professor of the History of Medicine and Director of the Wellcome Unit for the History of Medicine at the University of Oxford. He is the author of many books and articles on the history of disease, medicine, and colonialism, including: *Public Health in British India* (1994); *Climates and Constitutions* (1999); with Sanjoy Bhattacharya and Michael Worboys, *Fractured States: Smallpox, Public Health and Vaccination Policy 1800–1947* (2006); *The Medical War: British Military Medicine in the First World War* (2010)—winner of the Templer Medal Book Prize;

Medicine in the Age of Commerce and Empire: Britain and its Tropical Colonies, 1660–1830 (2010); and *Contagion: How Commerce Has Spread Disease* (2013). With Biswamoy Pati, he is editor of *Health, Medicine and Empire: Perspectives on Colonial India* (2001) and *The Social History of Health and Medicine in British India* (2009), and with Margaret Jones and Helen Sweet, of *From Western Medicine to Global Medicine: The Hospital Beyond the West* (2009).

Mark Jackson is Professor of the History of Medicine and Director of the Wellcome Centre for Cultures and Environments of Health at the University of Exeter. He has served as Chair of the Wellcome Trust History of Medicine and Research Resources funding committees, as Senior Academic Advisor (Medical Humanities) to the Wellcome Trust, and as a member of the History sub-panel for REF 2014. He has taught modules in the history of medicine and the history and philosophy of science for over thirty years at undergraduate and postgraduate levels to both medical and history students, and has been involved in teaching medical history to GCSE and A level students. His books include *Newborn Child Murder* (1996); *The Borderland of Imbecility* (2000); *Infanticide: Historical Perspectives on Child Murder and Concealment 1550–2000,* (ed., 2002); *Allergy: The History of a Modern Malady* (2006); *Health and the Modern Home* (ed., 2007); *Asthma: The Biography* (2009); *The Oxford Handbook of the History of Medicine* (2011); *The Age of Stress: Science and the Search for Stability* (2012); *Stress in Post-War Britain, 1945–85* (ed., 2015); and *The Routledge History of Disease* (ed., 2016). He is currently writing a book on the history of the midlife crisis.

Vivienne Lo is Director of the China Centre for Health and Humanity at UCL. She has been teaching the history of Asian medicine and classical Chinese medicine at BSc and MA level in UCL since 2002. Her research concerns the social and cultural origins of acupuncture and therapeutic exercise. She translates and analyses manuscript material from early and medieval China and the transmission of scientific knowledge along the so-called Silk Roads through to the modern Chinese medical diaspora. She is the editor with Christopher Cullen of *Mediaeval Chinese Medicine* (2005), and with Waltraud Ernst of the journal *Asian Medicine: Tradition and Modernity*. Forthcoming publications include: *Potent Flavours: A History of Nutrition in China* (Reaktion Press, 2017); and with M. S. B. Stanley-Baker (eds), *Routledge Handbook of Chinese Medicine* (Routledge, 2017).

Edmund Ramsden is a Wellcome Trust University Award Lecturer at Queen Mary University of London. His current research is focused on the involvement of social and behavioural scientists in architecture, planning, and design in the post-war United States, so as to improve mental health and social well-being, particularly in relation to institutional environments and public housing. Other key areas of research include the history of experimental psychiatry and psychology in relation to neuroses, emotional disorders, addiction, and suicide; the history of eugenics, population science, and policy; social survey methods in relation to health, growth, and intelligence; and the role of animals in science and medicine. He is the editor, with David Cantor, of *Stress, Shock and Adaptation in the Twentieth Century* (University of Rochester Press, 2014).

Lyn Schumaker completed her PhD in history and sociology of science, technology, and medicine at the University of Pennsylvania in 1994, with previous training in anthropology and African history at Michigan State University. Her book, *Africanizing Anthropology: Fieldwork, Networks, and the Making of Cultural Knowledge in Central Africa*, was published in 2001 by Duke University Press. She worked at the Wellcome Unit for the History of Medicine at Manchester, 1994–2009, receiving a Wellcome Trust University Award in 1999 for research in the history of indigenous, mission, and mining medicine on Zambia's colonial Copperbelt. Her work situates anti-retroviral therapy in the history of Western pharmaceuticals and indigenous medicines in Zambia as well as exploring African perspectives on privately funded medical philanthropy, such as the Bill and Melinda Gates Foundation's funding of malaria, tuberculosis, and HIV/AIDS research and mining magnate A. Chester Beatty's funding of early malaria research.

Michael Stanley-Baker is a practitioner and historian of Chinese medicine. Having received his DiplAC at Ruseto College in Boulder, Colorado, he later went on to pursue graduate studies in Daoist history in the East Asian languages and cultures at Indiana, University Bloomington, and received his PhD in medical history from UCL in 2013. He is a twenty-year practitioner of yoga, taiji, and martial arts. His research is concerned with the broader therapeutic culture of medieval China, especially that which is recorded in the Daoist Canon.

Marius Turda is Director of the Centre for Medical Humanities and Reader in Central and Eastern European Biomedicine at Oxford Brookes University. He is the author of *Modernism and Eugenics* and *Eugenics and Nation in Early 20th Century Hungary* (2010), and the editor of *The History of Eugenics in East-Central Europe, 1900–1945* (2017). His main areas of interest include the history of eugenics, racism, anthropology, and medicine in East-Central Europe, with a particular focus on Hungary and Romania. He has just completed a book on the history of race to be published in 2018.

1

One World, One Health?

Towards a Global History of Medicine

Mark Jackson

In October 2010, Haiti experienced the first outbreak of cholera in the country's history. Over the next four years, approximately 700,000 Haitians contracted the disease, over 8,000 people died, and cholera spread across the Caribbean region, with cases reported in the Dominican Republic, Cuba, and Mexico. The causes of the epidemic can be traced to a number of interlocking social, economic, and environmental factors. A devastating earthquake in January 2010 had killed over 300,000 people, displaced communities, exacerbated poverty, and disrupted sanitation, providing the conditions for the rapid diffusion of disease through vulnerable populations. At the same time, evidence that the strain of cholera in Haiti resembled strains prevalent in Africa and South Asia was used to suggest that cholera had been introduced to the Caribbean by Nepalese troops serving as part of a United Nations peace-keeping force. It would appear that the organism had hitchhiked across the world to infect a nation already rendered susceptible by ecological disaster and socio-economic conditions.[1]

It is tempting to interpret the trajectory of the recent Haitian cholera epidemic, as well as the outbreak and spread of other diseases such as Middle East Respiratory Syndrome, as a contemporary phenomenon, as a product of the ways in which modern globalization has accelerated the circulation of people, commodities, and organisms around an integrated and interconnected world. There is some merit to this argument. Whether we regard globalization in terms of the global economy, the transfer of information, or cultural exchange, there is no doubt that recent and rapid global change has transformed the ways in which we interact with each other and with our environments across what had previously seemed to be natural boundaries of space and time. Increasingly connected networks of trade, travel, and technology have served to realize Marshall McLuhan's vision of a 'global village', a world in which local cultures and practices always interact with global economic, political, and cultural forces, reshaping not only processes of production and consumption, but also patterns of health and disease and approaches to health governance.[2]

However, it is also clear that globalization is not a new phenomenon. Places and populations, as well as economies and cultures, have always been connected to some degree. Diseases have travelled and been transmitted through the movement of people and produce, leading to the fear of migrants and traders and to the creation of public health policies designed to separate or quarantine infected animals and humans. Medical knowledge and practice have been communicated and exchanged across spatial and temporal borders, helping to produce new understandings of the body and new forms of healing. Historical examples of the impact of global transactions on patterns and experiences of health and disease are not difficult to identify. The opening in 1914 of the Panama Canal, the construction of which had resulted in many thousands of deaths from malaria and yellow fever, raised the spectre of fresh epidemics, including cholera and plague, as trade routes became shorter.[3] The cholera pandemic of 1865–66 originated in an outbreak of the disease in Mecca apparently imported by pilgrims from India.[4] Even earlier outbreaks of cholera and other infectious diseases in Japan and China were similarly patterned not merely by local topographical and socio-economic conditions, but also by the movements of boatmen and dock labourers along canals, the opening of trade routes for tea and opium, and interactions between humans and non-human animals.[5]

These specific examples of global connections and continuities reveal another dimension of the history and geography of medicine, namely the parallel importance of understanding the local determinants of health and disease. Although we can discern global patterns linked to the interconnectedness of regions and nations, personal experiences, professional discourses, and state interventions have always been dependent on local social, political, cultural, environmental, and biological contexts. For example, while the rising life expectancy and declining mortality rates associated with the modern epidemiological and demographic transition are evident in many parts of the world, developments have not been evenly distributed across populations and places. Historical evidence suggests that the Western model of mortality decline cannot be readily transposed to other countries and continents. In 1901, male life expectancy at birth in Britain was in the region of forty-five years; amongst Indian populations life expectancy only reached that level in the 1960s.[6] As historians, epidemiologists, and medical geographers have pointed out, neither can we assume that mortality rates amongst particular communities or groups were reflected in the experiences of others: in the twentieth century, maternal mortality rates varied widely across England and Wales; and in the United States, maternal deaths followed different trajectories amongst urban and rural, white and black, and rich and poor populations.[7] By accentuating economic disparities, measured in terms of Gross Domestic Product (GDP), more rapid globalization may have amplified, rather than mitigated, health inequalities: in 2015, a World Health Organization (WHO) survey revealed that average life expectancy continued to vary widely across the world, ranging from 83.7 years in Japan to 50.1 years in Sierre Leone.[8]

Understanding the history of medicine therefore requires attention to both global and local dimensions of health and disease or, as the anthropologists Akhil Gupta and James Ferguson pointed out many years ago, remaining sensitive to 'locally lived lives in a globally connected world'.[9] Of course this commitment to exploring fully the complex relations between place, space, and time, as well as tracing the pathways along which people, animals, germs, food, ideas, norms, standards, practices, and diseases have travelled, raises methodological, conceptual, political, and ethical difficulties. The aim of this volume is to equip scholars with some of the knowledge and tools to confront those challenges. In the first instance, the following chapters introduce the history of health and illness, of medical knowledge and practice, across different periods and locations. Although structured largely around continents and regions, these overviews do not reinforce simplistic notions of distinct and static medical traditions or cultures associated with particular places. Instead they reveal the plurality and porosity of practices, experiences, and knowledge, as well as the dynamic social structures and political processes that have shaped the manifestation and distribution of disease, and the manner in which individual, professional, state, and international resources have been mobilized in order to maintain or restore health.

Secondly, contributors reflect on how to research and write histories of medicine that are sensitive to promiscuous linkages between global, regional, and local dimensions of health and disease. What sources, skills, and methods are required to connect histories convincingly across time and space? How can we challenge tenacious preoccupations with the 'rise' of Western bioscience as the dominant model for narrating the history of medicine? How can we reveal and resist the asymmetries of power that are concealed within the binary analytical frameworks that often structure and constrain our histories, lives, and practices: local/global; centre/periphery; state/voluntary; population/individual; East/West? Can we edge towards a global history of medicine that does not superficially reduce space, place, and culture to countries and continents, but instead considers the ways in which migration, commerce, war, and travel, amongst other human and non-human factors, have enabled healing practices to be constructed and reconstructed across borders, communities, and identities that are both real and imagined? How can we impartially navigate the always tangled roots and contours of medicine in the past and acknowledge their enduring pulse into the present?

Entangled Histories

Emerging at the intersection of global history and postcolonial studies, 'entangled history' constitutes an approach that challenges the ways in which historians have uncritically embraced nations, empires, and civilizations as 'the exclusive and exhaustive units and categories of historiography'.[10] According to Sönke Bauck and Thomas Maier, the notion of entanglement enables historians to adopt a trans-cultural perspective that foregrounds 'historic power structures and their constitution in space' and more carefully examines 'the multidirectional character of transfers'.[11] This form of historiographical renewal not only prioritizes local, regional, and trans-national connections and exchanges between populations, institutions, and practices, but also questions the 'hegemony of Eurocentric teleologies' of global development and modernization.[12]

Historians of medicine have sometimes mobilized the concept of entanglement to capture the complexity of interdependencies and exchanges between disciplines and cultures in the past and present, or to explore interactions between humans, animals, and their environments.[13] Through their work on colonial and postcolonial medicine, in particular, historians such as Warwick Anderson, Mark Harrison, and Alison Bashford have also contributed directly to the historiographical and political aspirations of entangled history, helping to decentre the global West and the North Atlantic from historical narratives and tracing the networks of power that sustain health inequalities.[14] However, attempts to write entangled histories of medicine also reveal the difficulties of pursuing historical analysis of this nature. At a pragmatic level, as Marius Turda points out in his chapter in this volume on the history of medicine in Eastern Europe, they demonstrate how convincingly disentangling scrambled histories of health and disease requires multi-lingual and multi-disciplinary expertise.[15] They also illustrate how even empirical studies of medical knowledge and practice that juxtapose different national contexts in order to develop comparative analyses tend to reproduce familiar temporal and geographical divisions, simplify the direction of flow between Western and Eastern forms of health care, and consolidate overly rigid distinctions between global and local sites of innovation and intervention.[16] Comparative studies have certainly opened up new questions about the circulation of information, experience, and practice and often move well beyond habitual preoccupations with Western biomedicine, but many of them have continued to narrate national experiences as parallel, rather than entangled, occurrences and, in doing so, to strengthen rather than trouble the binary analytical categories that have sustained both medical and historical professional hegemony.

Going global in these ways also raises uncomfortable questions about the potential for collusion between history and the politics of globalization. As Sarah Hodges has pointed out in a discussion of what she terms the 'global menace', there is a tension between 'the global as descriptor and an analytics of the global'. At best, she argues, the term global has simply replaced 'international', 'world', or 'colonial' as a description of the geographical range of a particular historical study. At worst, however, framing the history of medicine in global terms threatens to reinforce the notion of universality and commonality (or context-neutral objectivity) that characterizes both Western medical science and economic globalization. In this way, global histories of medicine can compress and obscure the unevenness and heterogeneity of places and periods and reproduce rather than critique 'globalisation as a set of institutions, discourses and practices'.[17]

Hodges' caution about the perils of globalizing the history of medicine, and her advice to historians of medicine to engage more effectively with postcolonial studies and environmental history, has not been ignored by other scholars seeking to colonize new historical and historiographical territories. In his recent reflections on global health history, Warwick Anderson has highlighted how postcolonial analysis can enable historians to generate 'critical and realistic histories of scale making in biomedicine, of the configuring of the local and global in global health' in ways that resist the hydraulic metaphors of circulation and flow that tend still to privilege the global North.[18] As Anderson's own work on biomedicine and biotechnology demonstrates, a postcolonial perspective allows historians to hold different contexts and trajectories 'within the same frame'; to 'interrupt a globalisation that lacks history or politics'; to 'recognise the entanglements of multiple agents'; to reveal 'the mutual reorganisation of the global and the local'; and to track the 'increasing transnational traffic of people, practices, [and] technologies'.[19]

It is important to recognize that, in these contexts, the term postcolonial does not refer merely to a chronological framework of analysis. It also captures a historiographical approach that, as Kavita Sivaramakrishnan has argued, 'traces the persistence of colonial power structures' and their impact on contemporary 'ideas and practices in global health'.[20] A similar lens has been used by environmental historians, such as Gregg Mitman, Michelle Murphy, and Chris Sellers, to scrutinize the links between health and disease, on the one hand, and structural and ecological change, on the other. New scholarship in these areas, they argued in their introduction to a special issue of *Osiris* some years ago, demands interdisciplinary research partnerships that enable us 'to explore the nexus of place, health and political economy in diverse sites and times around the world'.[21] By weaving together the methods and insights of history, geography, anthropology, and sociology, it becomes possible to develop multi-sited analyses that identify the relational aspects of health, unravel and confront the historical 'tangles of economy and flesh', and expose the manner in which 'privilege and violence' are built into exposure to diseases, poisons, and pollutants.[22] Here the conceptual and empirical work of scholars such as Doreen Massey on the intimate connections between space and time, Margaret Lock on how pathology and place interact to produce 'local biologies', and Arjun Appadurai's articulation of five dimensions of global cultural flows offers historians of medicine the resources to avoid 'grand narratives' at the same time as they acknowledge the global scale and complexity of many threats to health and well-being.[23]

The scholar who has arguably done most to bring these issues to the attention of historians of medicine in the last few years is Mark Harrison, whose own research not only charts the reciprocal relationships between commerce, labour migration, and war, on the one hand, and health and disease, on the other, but also invites historians to focus on networks rather than nations, to adopt longer-term perspectives on structural and ecological change, and to include chronic non-infectious diseases of prosperity in our evaluation of how local and global factors intersect.[24] Particularly valuable is Harrison's emphasis on recognizing the role of modern trade and warfare in establishing new world orders, marked by decolonization, the rise of multinational corporations, the global impact of neoliberal ideologies, and the emergence of foreign aid and global health governance especially after the Second World War. In addition, his examination of the construction of, and responses to, pandemics reminds us to situate historical studies of medicine and disease within wider, and contested, discourses of security, uncertainty, and risk.[25] As Harrison points out, the aspirations of international or global health policies to provide a common framework for disease prevention and health promotion are often obstructed or fragmented by the need to protect national security and trade.[26]

Harrison's provocation is persuasive and has elicited warmly critical responses from other scholars, who have drawn on his work to reinforce arguments for adopting historical perspectives that link global and local, as well as human and non-human, dimensions of disease and health care. As J. R. McNeill has pointed out, any global historiographical turn should incorporate attention to the movement of animals and animal pathogens, as well as products and people, around the world.[27] Alison Bashford has encouraged historians of medicine to broaden Harrison's vision by focusing on the manner in which neoliberal formulations of production and reproduction are gendered. A new mode of analysis, she argues, would be to identify issues, such as childbirth, that can serve as what some scholars have referred to as 'glocal' objects of enquiry, that is those that constitute 'matters simultaneously intimate and international, private and public, individual and aggregate'.[28] In proposing that historians of medicine adopt a 'zig-zag' perspective, Kavita Sivaramakrishnan reminds us that we need to explore alternative scales and sequences in order to combat the universalizing and teleological narratives of global history. New narratives, he argues, are necessary to expose the 'regional circuits of knowledge and exchange that often circumvented geopolitical dichotomies' and to decentre the West–rest dialectic that shapes our histories of medicine.[29] Sivaramakrishnan's call to complement history with ethnographies, oral histories, and the study of artefacts, manuals, and memories highlights the importance of assembling multi-disciplinary teams of scholars in order to develop relational approaches that connect largely synchronous and entangled histories of health, disease, and medicine.

Patchworks of Practice

In her wonderfully lucid reflections on space, place, and time, the geographer Doreen Massey argued that we should understand places not as static, bounded units that equate in any straightforward way to communities, which can exist 'without being in the same place', but as unique points of intersection between social relations, movements, and communications:

> Instead then, of thinking of places as areas with boundaries around, they can be imagined as articulated moments in networks of social relations and understandings, but where a large proportion of those relations, experiences and understandings are constructed on a far

larger scale than what we happen to define for that moment as the place itself, whether that be a street, or a region or even a continent. And this in turn allows a sense of place which is extroverted, which includes a consciousness of its links with the wider world, which integrates in a positive way the global and the local.[30]

Massey's insistence that globalization refers to more than spatial reach, but that it also signifies and realizes 'the stretching out of different kinds of social relationships over space', constitutes a fruitful reminder that historians of medicine need to continue to puncture national narratives in favour of accounts that unveil the pluralism, permeability, and power that saturate medical practice. At the same time, it suggests that we need to avoid what Barbara Weinstein has called the 'assimilationist discourse of the postcolonial era', which takes for granted Western superiority, and dispense with the notion of a single 'point of origin' to explain the emergence of diseases, medical knowledge, and health-care systems. Rather, Weinstein has argued, we should think in terms of 'multiple "contact zones"', where ideas, practices, and disease become entangled in complex ways.[31] Here then is a mandate for a more vibrant global history of medicine that focuses not on static traditions or grand narratives, but instead on how the 'patchworks of practice' that constitute medicine have been variably constructed, maintained, transmitted, and transformed across space and time.[32]

By challenging superficial notions of tradition, a concept that tends to close down any awareness of either changing historical contexts or the politics of practice, this volume explores not only how medicine has been plural and permeable in the past, but also how it has routinely reflected and reinforced power. As the chapters by Vivienne Lo and Michael Stanley-Baker, Hal Cook, Anne-Emanuelle Birn, and Mark Harrison in particular demonstrate, there have always been 'plural healing environments', in which responses to disease vary according to the human and non-human actors and agents involved. Although these chapters explore the history of medicine across large countries and continents, they also argue for a greater awareness and analysis of regional diversity, for recognizing what Ed Ramsden refers to in his chapter on North America as the presence of 'nations within nations'. As a number of historians have pointed out, experiences of health and the practice of medicine in the American South were different from those elsewhere across the continent partly because of climatic differences but also because of its distinctive regional history of slavery and plantations.[33]

While acknowledging that multiple medical approaches existed at any one moment in time, it is important not to draw simplistic boundaries between different modes of practice. Medical practitioners and their patients certainly adopted particular approaches to health and disease, dictated for example by religion and culture, but they did not always oppose or resist alternative diagnostic or therapeutic positions. However they were defined, orthodox and heterodox practitioners existed alongside each other, sharing as well as rejecting aspects of their alternate world views, integrating complementary dimensions of theory and practice as and when they saw fit. This introduces a further feature of the historical accounts of health and medicine presented in this volume, namely the extent to which healing practices have routinely been porous or permeable, marked by dynamic processes of exchange through time and between places. The chapters by Hormoz Ebrahimnejad, Linda Bryder, and Sanjoy Bhattacharya illustrate how the history of medicine has been shaped by the movements of people, organisms, lifestyles, ideas, and practices as a result of trade, travel, pilgrimage, and war. From this perspective, the notion of 'tradition' becomes especially problematic since it regards 'civilizations' or 'cultures' as static, bounded entities rather than as the result of active processes of transmission between and across generations: what we regard as Islamic medicine was the product of bilateral exchange between prophetic and Galenic forms of knowledge; so-called 'traditional Chinese medicine' was never a uniform or isolated system, but one that bestowed and borrowed diverse forms of knowledge and practice;[34] and medicine in Western Europe has always been open to, in fact invited or exploited, the importation of alternative medicinal compounds, new theories of disease transmission and different healing practices from other regions of the world.

Experiences and understandings of illness have also been mediated by politics and privilege. Gregg Mitman's fine historical study of asthma in North America and Richard Keller's provocative analysis of morbidity and mortality during the Paris heatwave of 2003 demonstrate how differential distributions of disease, as well as variations in the availability of, or access to, health-care resources, are neither natural nor inevitable. Rather they are dependent on the social, cultural, and ecological conditions in which different populations live, conditions themselves generated by different forms of biopolitics inspired by human concerns about race, gender, class, and commerce.[35] In this way, political systems can be bolstered by investment in certain forms of medicine. As many of the chapters in this volume indicate, medicine should not be seen as forever progressive, but needs to be understood as part of the wider historical context in which diseases are always, but uniquely, regarded as social and political commodities.

It is important to acknowledge that academic histories of medicine are similarly determined by socio-economic and political contexts. Historical accounts of medical 'traditions', for example, have been powerfully shaped by hegemonic Western preconceptions that non-Western forms of knowledge are in some ways naïve or derivative. As Lyn Schumaker makes clear in her chapter on medicine in sub-Saharan Africa, these historiographical perspectives are, like the patterns of disease and health care that they investigate, products of power. The relative paucity of studies of indigenous healing practices in Africa, she argues, can be traced to institutional resistance to interdisciplinary creativity, such as the effective integration of historical and anthropological methods, as well as to the absence of suitable mechanisms for funding such research. Global asymmetries in our histories need to be challenged as vigorously as the asymmetries in health and disease that have been generated by the economic forces of globalization. Attentive to the interplay of biological, social, cultural, political, economic, and environmental factors, historians of medicine must make visible and audible the lives and voices of people who have often been marginalized and silenced, but not always oppressed, by the medical and the historical record.

Conclusion

It is not possible to disentangle these global complexities and historiographical conundrums in a single volume. It is possible, however, to point to the key themes and challenges that historians of medicine need to address if we are to understand how lives have been lived locally 'in a globally connected world'. The contributors take different approaches to researching and writing history, but they share a commitment to reflecting critically on what a global history of medicine might begin to look like, even if written from a regional perspective. Collectively, they argue for more comparative work that is sensitive to cultural particularity as well as processes of alignment and exchange; for the need to assemble teams of scholars with the linguistic and analytical skills to pursue synchronous histories of health, disease, and medicine; for approaches that challenge the Western-dominated 'master narrative' of progress; for the use of new sources, methods, and ways of working to render visible the invisible and to reveal the diversity of everyday experiences of health and illness; for appreciation that health and medicine are always emergent and more than human, that is that we need to understand dynamic interactions between animals, humans, and environments;[36] and for recognition that we should always think globally, even if we act locally.[37]

A number of contributions to this volume also indicate that understanding the history of medicine in global terms is not only about the past, but that it carries resonance for contemporary populations. In her chapter on Latin America in this volume, Anne-Emanuelle Birn points out that the 'extensive borrowing back and forth among healing traditions has left footprints into the present', shaping patterns of disease and health policies into the twenty-first century. Such footprints are everywhere evident: health and medicine across the world are still structured by racial and class-based prejudices and by lingering colonial configurations of power; the treatment and prevention of chronic 'diseases of affluence', such as diabetes, cancer, and heart disease, continue to be predicated on an amalgam of ancient and medieval, Eastern and Western, formulations of balance and regimen; and recent calls for policies that embrace the notion of 'one world, one health, one medicine', as well as arguments for protecting and promoting planetary health, are often directly descended from Hippocratic and Aristotelian notions of the literal and metaphorical correspondences, interrelations and exchanges between animals, environments, and the cosmos.

The potential for the history of medicine and other disciplines within the humanities and social sciences to contribute to contemporary debates about health care has been acknowledged by a variety of national, regional, and global organizations. In particular, the forms of qualitative evidence that are made available by humanities scholars have become increasingly important within the aspirations of the WHO to develop a common health-policy framework that recognizes cultural specificity, values subjective experience, adopts participatory approaches to policy formation, and works across governments, societies, and sectors to enhance health and well-being.[38] For some years, the seminar series coordinated by the WHO Collaborating Centre for Global Health Histories at the University of York has been promoting dialogue between historians, medical practitioners, and policy-makers across the world.[39] And understanding the cultural contexts of health in order to improve the design and delivery of health-care policies has emerged as an important focus for the WHO Collaborating Centre on Culture and Health at the University of Exeter, where historians, anthropologists, ethnographers, geographers, health economists, and philosophers work together to provide tools and resources for health-care workers and policy-makers across the European region.[40]

Recent developments in global or entangled history, like those in global health and environmental policy, signal our intention to take seriously the interconnectedness of lives. At the same time, however, commitments to a global historical gaze, or to 'one world-ism' in health research and policy, can obscure the ways in which local conditions interact with global contexts to shape the health of populations, communities, families, and individuals at specific moments in space and time.[41] Writing histories of medicine that manage to hold global, regional, and local experiences and perceptions within the same frame therefore becomes pivotal not only to understanding the complexity of the past, but also to analysing and critiquing persistent inequalities in health and confronting the power and privilege that still inflect our health and medicine. Whether focusing on the outbreak of cholera in Haiti in the early twenty-first century, the rise of chronic non-infectious diseases across the twentieth century, disputes about traditional practices of midwifery in colonial Mexico, or the forms of state intervention implemented during the late eighteenth-century epidemics of plague in Moscow, histories can help us to reimagine and redirect future global health initiatives that are judiciously informed by an awareness of the entangled and uneven cultural, social, political, economic, and environmental factors that have shaped the patchwork of medical practices of today.[42]

Notes

1 For more detailed discussion of the role of travellers in spreading infectious diseases in Haiti and elsewhere, see: Stephen M. Ostroff, 'Perspectives: The Role of the Traveler in Translocation of Disease', on the Centers for Disease Control and Prevention website, https://wwwnc.cdc.gov/travel/yellowbook/2016/introduction/perspectives-the-role-of-the-traveler-in-translocation-of-disease, accessed 9 May 2017.

2 For discussion of the impacts of globalization on disease and health governance, see: Christine McMurray and Roy Smith, *Diseases of Globalisation: Socioeconomic Transitions and Health*, (London, Earthscan, 2001); Kelley Lee (ed.), *Health Impacts of Globalization: Towards Global Governance*, (Basingstoke, Palgrave Macmillan, 2003). McLuhan articulated his notion of a 'global village' or 'global theater' in a number of works, most notably: Marshall McLuhan, *The Gutenberg Galaxy: The Making of Typographic Man*, (Toronto, University of Toronto Press, 1962); Marshall McLuhan, *Understanding Media: The Extensions of Man*, (New York, McGraw-Hill, 1964); and Marshall McLuhan and Wilfred Watson, *From Cliché to Archetype*, (New York, Viking, 1970).

3 See Anne-Emanuelle Birn's chapter in this volume.

4 See Mark Harrison's chapter in this volume.

5 Robert Peckham, 'Symptoms of Empire: Cholera in Southeast Asia, 1820–1850', in Mark Jackson (ed.), *The Routledge History of Disease*, (Abingdon, Routledge, 2017), pp. 183–201; Akihito Suzuki, 'Disease, Geography and the Market: Epidemics of Cholera in Tokyo in the Late Nineteenth Century', in Jackson (ed.), *The Routledge History of Disease*, pp. 202–20.

6 For provocative discussions of international and regional patterns of mortality and life expectancy, see: James C. Riley, *Rising Life Expectancy: A Global History*, (Cambridge, Cambridge University Press, 2001); J. M. Winter, 'The Decline of Mortality in Britain 1870–1950', in T. Barker and M. Drake (eds.), *Population and Society in Britain, 1850–1950*, (London, Batsford Academic, 1982), pp. 100–20.

7 Irvine Loudon, 'Maternal Mortality: 1880–1950. Some Regional and International Comparisons', *Social History of Medicine*, 1 (1988), 183–228.

8 See the World Health Statistics Data Visualisations Dashboard, at http://apps.who.int/gho/data/node.sdg.le-1-map, accessed 12 May 2017.

9 Akhil Gupta and James Ferguson, 'Beyond "Culture": Space, Identity, and the Politics of Difference', *Cultural Anthropology*, 7 (1992), 6–23.

10 Sönke Bauck and Thomas Maier, '"Entangled History", InterAmerican Wiki: Terms—Concepts—Critical Perspectives', (2015), http://www.uni-bielefeld.de/cias/wiki/e_Entangled_History.html, accessed 28 April 2017.

11 Ibid.

12 Ibid.

13 See, for example, Tatsuya Mitsuda, 'Entangled Histories: German Veterinary Medicine, c. 1770–1900', *Medical History*, 61 (2017), 25–47.

For a discussion of entanglement as a way of framing or strengthening interdisciplinary modes of enquiry, see: Des Fitzgerald and Felicity Callard, 'Entangling the Medical Humanities', in Anne Whitehead, Angela Woods, Sarah Atkinson, Jane Macnaughton, and Jennifer Richards (eds), *The Edinburgh Companion to the Critical Medical Humanities*, (Edinburgh, Edinburgh University Press, 2016), pp. 35–49; Des Fitzgerald and Felicity Callard, 'Social Science and Neuroscience Beyond Interdisciplinarity: Experimental Entanglements', *Theory, Culture & Society*, 32 (2015), 3–32.

14 Warwick Anderson, 'Making Global Health History: The Postcolonial Worldliness of Biomedicine', *Social History of Medicine*, 27 (2014), 372–84; Mark Harrison, 'A Global Perspective: Reframing History of Health, Medicine, and Disease', *Bulletin of the History of Medicine*, 89 (2015), 639–89; Alison Bashford, *Medicine at the Border: Disease, Globalization and Security, 1850 to the Present*, (Basingstoke, Palgrave Macmillan, 2006); Alison Bashford, 'Bioscapes: Gendering the Global History of Medicine', *Bulletin of the History of Medicine*, 89 (2015), 690–5.

15 For comments on the need for multidisciplinary teams, see the chapters by Hormoz Ebrahimnejad and Marius Turda in this volume.

16 For examples of constructive edited volumes of this nature, see: John Woodward and Robert Jütte (eds), *Coping with Sickness: Historical Aspects of Health Care in a European Perspective*, (Sheffield, European Association for the History of Medicine and Health Publications, 1995); Mark Harrison, Margaret Jones, and Helen Sweet (eds), *From Western Medicine to Global Medicine: The Hospital Beyond the West*, (Hyderabad, Orient Blackswan, 2009); and Laurence Monnais and Harold J. Cook (eds), *Global Movements, Local Concerns: Medicine and Health in Southeast Asia*, (Singapore, NUS Press, 2012).

17 Sarah Hodges, 'The Global Menace', *Social History of Medicine*, 25 (2011), 719–28.

18 Anderson, 'Making Global Health History'.

19 Warwick Anderson, 'Postcolonial Technoscience', *Social Studies of Science*, 32 (2002), 643–58.

20 Kavita Sivaramakrishnan, 'Global Histories of Health, Disease, and Medicine from a "Zig-zag" Perspective', *Bulletin of the History of Medicine*, 89 (2015), 700–4, at 701, n.3.

21 Gregg Mitman, Michelle Murphy, and Christopher Sellers, 'Introduction: A Cloud Over History', *Osiris*, 19 (2004), 1–20, at 4.

22 Ibid., pp. 10, 13. On the relational dimensions of the history of health and the environment, see: Gregg Mitman, 'In Search of Health: Landscapes and Disease in American Environmental History', *Environmental History*, 10 (2005), 184–210.

23 Doreen Massey, *Space, Place and Gender*, (Minneapolis, University of Minnesota Press, 1994); Margaret Lock, *Encounters with Aging: Menopause in Japan and North America*, (Berkeley, University of California Press, 1995); Margaret Lock and Patricia Kaufert, 'Menopause, Local Biologies and

Cultures of Ageing', *American Journal of Human Biology*, 13 (2001), 494–504; Arjun Appadurai, *Modernity at Large: Cultural Dimensions of Globalization*, (Minneapolis, University of Minnesota Press, 1996).

24 For an overall discussion of these factors, see Harrison, 'A Global Perspective'. Harrison's expansive contributions to the field include: Mark Harrison, *Disease and the Modern World: 1500 to the Present Day*, (Cambridge, Polity Press, 2004); Mark Harrison, *Medicine in an Age of Commerce and Empire*, (Oxford, Oxford University Press, 2010); Mark Harrison, *Contagion: How Commerce has Spread Disease*, (New Haven, Yale University Press, 2013).

25 Mark Harrison, 'Pandemics', in Jackson (ed.), *The Routledge History of Disease*, pp. 129–46. Similar issues relating to the links between global health, globalization, geopolitics, and risk have also exercised geographers in recent years, but as yet there are only limited conversations between the two disciplines. For a discussion of some of the ways in which geographers are now engaging with global health as an object of enquiry, see Clare Herrick (ed.), *Global Health and Geographical Imaginaries*, (London, Routledge, 2017).

26 Harrison, 'A Global Perspective', p. 678.

27 J. R. McNeill, 'Harrison, Globalization, and the History of Health, Medicine, and Disease', *Bulletin of the History of Medicine*, 89 (2015), 696–9.

28 Bashford, 'Bioscapes', 693.

29 Sivaramakrishnan, 'Global Histories of Health', 701. For a discussion of the place of narratives in constructing regional histories, albeit in a British context, see: Keir Waddington, 'Thinking Regionally: Narrative, the Medical Humanities and Region', *Medical Humanities*, 41 (2015), 51–6.

30 Massey, *Space, Place and Gender*, pp. 153–5.

31 Barbara Weinstein, 'History Without a Cause? Grand Narratives, World History, and the Postcolonial Dilemma', *International Review of History*, 50 (2005), 71–93.

32 The original term, 'patchwork of practices', is taken from a recent critique of the 'One world one health' movement, which, it is argued, tends to 'under-value the local, contingent and practical engagements that make health possible': Steve Hinchliffe, 'More than One World, More than One Health: Re-configuring Interspecies Health', *Social Science and Medicine*, 129 (2015), 28–35.

33 Todd Savitt and James Harvey Young (eds), *Disease and Distinctiveness in the American South*, (Knoxville, University of Tennessee Press, 1988).

34 See the chapter by Vivienne Lo and Michael Stanley-Baker in this volume. See also Kim Taylor, 'Divergent Interests and Cultivated Misunderstandings: The Influence of the West on Modern Chinese Medicine', *Social History of Medicine*, 17 (2004), 93–111.

35 Gregg Mitman, *Breathing Space: How Allergies Shape our Lives and Landscapes*, (New Haven, Yale University Press, 2007); Richard Keller, 'Social Geographies of Sickness and Health in Contemporary Paris: Toward a Human

Ecology of Mortality in the 2003 Heat Wave Disaster', in Jackson (ed.), *The Routledge History of Disease*, pp. 279–97.

36 For overviews of how we need to include animals in our histories of medicine and recognize the historical linkages between human and veterinary medicine, see: Robert G. W. Kirk and Michael Worboys, 'Medicine and Species: One Medicine, One History?', in Mark Jackson (ed.), *The Oxford Handbook of the History of Medicine*, (Oxford, Oxford University Press, 2011), pp. 561–77; Abigail Woods and Michael Bresalier, 'One Health, Many Histories', *Veterinary Record*, 174 (2014), 650–4.

37 The phrase 'think globally, act locally' has been variably attributed to the Scottish biologist Patrick Geddes, the American microbiologist René Dubos, and the Canadian self-styled 'business futurist' Frank Feather. The term has become a defining feature of many environmentalist arguments to consider the impact of local actions on planetary health.

38 For WHO publications in this area, see: WHO Europe, *Health 2020: A European Policy Framework Supporting Action Across Government and Society for Health and Well-being*, Copenhagen, WHO Regional Office for Europe, 2012, http://www.euro.who.int/__data/assets/pdf_file/0009/169803/RC62wd09-Eng.pdf, accessed 30 September 2015; WHO Europe, *Taking a Participatory Approach to Development and Better Health*, (2015), http://www.euro.who.int/en/health-topics/health-policy/health-2020-the-european-policy-for-health-and-well-being/publications/2015/taking-a-par ticipatory-approach-to-development-and-better-health.-examples-from-the-regions-for-health-network-2015, Copenhagen, WHO Regional Office for Europe, 2015, accessed 11 June 2017; WHO, *The European Health Report 2012: Charting the Way to Well-being*, Copenhagen, WHO Regional Office for Europe, 2013, http://www.euro.who.int/en/data-and-evidence/european-health-report/european-health-report-2012, accessed 30 September 2015; WHO, *The European Health Report 2015: Targets and Beyond—Reaching New Frontiers in Evidence*, Copenhagen, WHO Regional Office for Europe, 2015, http://www.euro.who.int/en/data-and-evidence/european-health-report/european-health-report-2015/european-health-report-2015-the-targets-and-beyond-reaching-new-frontiers-in-evidence, accessed 4 November 2015; WHO, *Cultural Contexts of Health and Well-being, No 1: Beyond Bias: Exploring the Cultural Contexts of Health and Well-being Measurement*, Copenhagen, WHO Regional Office for Europe, 2015, http://www.euro.who.int/en/data-and-evidence/cultural-contexts-of-health/beyond-bias-exploring-the-cultural-contexts-of-health-and-well-being-measurement-2015, accessed 9 October 2015.

39 For details of the Centre, which is directed by Sanjoy Bhattacharya, see https://www.york.ac.uk/history/global-health-histories/, accessed 11 June 2017.

40 See http://cultureandhealth.exeter.ac.uk/, accessed 11 June 2017.

41 For critical discussion of 'one world, one health', see the contributions to a special issue of *Social Science and Medicine* published in 2015, in particular:

18 *Mark Jackson*

Susan Craddock and Steve Hinchliffe, 'Introduction: One World, One Health? Social Science Engagements with the One Health Agenda', *Social Science and Medicine*, 129 (2015), 1–4; Meike Wolf, 'Is there Really Such a Thing as "One Health"? Thinking about a More than Human World from the Perspective of Cultural Anthropology', *Social Science and Medicine*, 129 (2015), 5–11; Hinchliffe, 'More than One World, More than One Health'.

42 An important set of reflections on global health that are sensitive to historical and geographical specificities and set agendas and challenges for future health policies can be found in Paul Farmer, Jim Yong Kim, Arthur Kleinman, and Matthew Basilico, *Reimagining Global Health: An Introduction*, (Berkeley, University of California Press, 2013).

Select Bibliography

Anderson, Warwick, 'Making Global Health History: The Postcolonial Worldliness of Biomedicine', *Social History of Medicine*, 27 (2014), 372–84.

Bashford, Alison, *Medicine at the Border: Disease, Globalization and Security, 1850 to the Present*, (Basingstoke, Palgrave Macmillan, 2006).

Curtin, Philip D., *Death by Migration: Europe's Encounter with the Tropical World in the Nineteenth Century*, (Cambridge, Cambridge University Press, [1989] 2010).

Harrison, Mark, *Medicine in an Age of Commerce and Empire*, (Oxford, Oxford University Press, 2010).

Harrison, Mark, *Contagion: How Commerce has Spread Disease*, (New Haven, Yale University Press, 2013).

Harrison, Mark, 'A Global Perspective: Reframing History of Health, Medicine, and Disease', *Bulletin of the History of Medicine*, 89 (2015), 639–89.

Jackson, Mark (ed.), *The Routledge History of Disease*, (Abingdon, Routledge, 2017).

Jackson, Mark (ed.), *The Oxford Handbook of the History of Medicine*, (Oxford, Oxford University Press, 2011).

Jackson, Mark, *The History of Medicine: A Beginner's Guide*, (London, Oneworld, 2014).

McMurray, Christine and Roy Smith, *Diseases of Globalisation: Socioeconomic Transitions and Health*, (London, Earthscan, 2001).

Lee, Kelley (ed.), *Health Impacts of Globalization: Towards Global Governance*, (Basingstoke, Palgrave Macmillan, 2003).

Riley, James C., *Rising Life Expectancy: A Global History*, (Cambridge, Cambridge University Press, 2001).

Watts, Sheldon, *Epidemics and History: Disease, Power, and Imperialism*, (New Haven, Yale University Press, 1999).

2

Chinese Medicine

Vivienne Lo and Michael Stanley-Baker

Those active in living traditions of medicine, either as practitioners or patients, have often imagined a long empirical tradition stretching back to a golden age in pre-history. Historians and anthropologists have too easily identified the essential characteristics of the medicine of a specific place, even when that place, particularly in the case of China, has been geographically and culturally diverse. In contrast, new research is concerned in teasing out more complex dynamics between continuity and change as traditions constantly reinvent themselves in order to remain relevant, appropriate, and effective.

Excavated records recovered from Shang dynasty (traditional dates: 1766–1122 BCE) archaeological sites do indeed testify to very early divinatory techniques for identifying the cause and progress of illness, which is attributed to the malevolence of spirit ancestors.[1] Yet while modern forms of 'traditional Chinese medicine' (TCM) bear the marked vestiges of astro-calendrical divinatory traditions, concerted attempts have been made in the twentieth century to eradicate its most obviously religious aspects.

In the half-century since Joseph Needham began his project to write a history of science, technology, and medicine in China in its fullest social and intellectual context, the approaches of social and cultural historians have provided new tools to unlock the many dimensions of more popular (that is, pervasive) or religious healing practices. New evidence from texts written on bamboo and silk recently excavated from late Warring States (fourth to second centuries BCE) and Han dynasty (202 BCE–220 CE) tombs has also upset the traditional narratives that sourced the origins of medicine in the word of the legendary

Yellow Emperor, 5,000 years ago.[2] With these first medical treatises, set down in the late Warring States, we have a direct window onto the circumstances within which classical medical knowledge and practice initially emerged. These new sources add depth and richness to the 10,000 extant pre-Communist (to 1949) medical works listed in the 1991 National Chinese Medicine Union Catalogue.

This chapter does not attempt to describe the 'evolution' of a single entity that some imagine Chinese medicine to be. From a discussion of its mythic origins, through the coalescence of many theories about astro-physiology in early China to the medieval heyday of religious healing pluralism, it charts the changing emphases in what was always a plural healing environment. Indeed the ethnic and cultural boundaries of China itself are contested. Nevertheless there are clearly elements that pervade the scholarly and religious medicine of the Chinese empire. Most vividly, the extension of imperial bureaucracy reached into the body, whether controlling the body's fluids as if they were the imperial waterways, imagining the organs as officials, or submitting petitions for cure to deity-officials in the afterlife. The rupture of imperial authority at the hands of foreign aggression, contemporaneous with the large-scale arrival of European and American doctors and scientists, promised to ring the death-knell for Chinese healing traditions. Yet they have continued to prove tenacious at reinventing themselves according to the ever-changing social and political priorities of the twentieth and twenty-first centuries. We conclude with some observations about how the sensory modalities of Chinese medical thought speak powerfully to a modern global audience who frequently feel their own individual experience of health and sickness devalued in the processes of modern standardized medicine.

Mythic origins and classical texts

The beginning of imperial China is dated to 221 BCE, when the military machine of Qinshi Huangdi 秦始皇帝 (259–210 BCE), first emperor of the state of Qin, put an end to centuries of disunity during the Warring States period of the Zhou dynasty (1045–256 BCE), and established the short-lived Qin dynasty (221–206 BCE). With brutal efficiency, the Qin regime moulded a collection of small feudal kingdoms into a highly centralized imperial authority, broadly corresponding in geographic terms to what we know as China today. The Han dynasty (202 BCE–220 CE), which came to power shortly after Qinshi Huangdi's death, embraced the Qin's realpolitik and forms of governance, but at the same time sought to distance itself from its influential but hated predecessor by drawing authority from the sage rulers of a golden age at the dawn of Chinese civilization, after whom the new administration was supposedly modelled. To this end, the myth-makers and history-writers of the Han retold the stories of the lost golden age for their own times. In traditional Chinese accounts, the origins of medicine and the authoritative wisdom of the medical classics are ascribed to the revelations of sages and cultural heroes. The medical aspects of Chinese mythic history attest to the range of healing traditions that existed in early imperial China.

The task of civilizing and domesticating a savage world fell to the five Sage Emperors, each of whom corresponded to one of the five directions: north, south, east, west, and centre.[3] Two of them, the Yellow Emperor (Huangdi 黃帝), and the Red Emperor (Yandi 炎帝), also known as The Divine Farmer (Shennong 神農), are intimately associated with medicine and healing. Other mythic patrons of medicine include the 'Medicine King' Bian Que 扁鵲, sometimes represented as a human-headed bird, and the enigmatic Mr. White (Bai Shi 白氏). The names of these legendary figures occur repeatedly in the titles of medical texts, or as their putative authors.

Cultural heroes are thus credited with formulating various ideas that are central to Chinese views of the world, the body, and human society. The legend of the Divine Farmer, in whose name the *Shennong bencao jing* 神農本草經 (Divine Farmer's materia medica, *c.*first century CE) is written, enshrines the empirical spirit of Chinese medicine, and the concomitant belief that knowledge of the virtues of drugs and food had to be obtained through trial and error. The Divine Farmer's main role was to rescue human beings from a state of savagery, where they fed on the raw flesh of the animals they hunted, drank their blood, and dressed in their skins, and to lead them towards an agrarian utopia. Famously, he tasted all living plants to ascertain their properties and, according to later accounts, struck all the plants with a magical whip to make them yield up their essential flavours and smells. He subsequently classified the plants and distinguished those that were safe and suitable for consumption and medicinal use. Testifying to the importance of this tradition of empirical testing, his name occurs in the titles of many famous materia medica texts.

The best-known patron of medicine, the Yellow Emperor, is particularly associated with knowledge of how cosmic patterns were inherent in all things (laws, punishments, and the calendar) and he played a role in divination. These attributes link him with the specialized medical arts of understanding the body's relationship with the cycles and phases of Heaven and Earth, and of accurately predicting the progress and outcome of disease. Prognostications regarding sickness and health were framed within numerological sequences first found in calendrical systems; thus the 'Daybook' (*rishu* 日書) divinatory calculations, which served to determine propitious times and places for human activities, became part of everyday health and hygiene practices.[4]

In China, medical practitioners were often literate, and their knowledge and practice can be reconstructed both from their own writings and from the written records of scholarly and religious traditions allied to medicine. Through 2,000 years of empire, the authority and competence of the Chinese state were constantly embodied in a multitude of texts generated by the organs of government at every level and medical practice was enmeshed in this bureaucratic process. Access to the upper echelons of the civil service was obtained via a succession of competitive examinations essentially testing mastery of the Confucian canons. A similar hierarchy existed in scholarly medicine: increasingly, social status depended on the possession, knowledge, and authorship of written texts.

In the course of the Han period, a vast corpus of medical knowledge came to be ascribed to the Yellow Emperor. Compilations known as *jing* 經 (translated as 'classic' or 'canon') set out many of the cardinal principles of Chinese medical theory.[5] Today the Yellow Emperor corpus is known only through three recensions based on a printed edition published in the twelfth century. The three texts differ in subject-matter, but together describe medical theory: the human body as a microcosm, the origins of disease, and some therapies, principally acupuncture and moxibustion (a form of cautery or heat treatment generally using *artemisia vulgaris* or mugwort) and a few drug prescriptions.[6]

Important treatises in the 'Numinous Pivot' *Lingshu* 靈樞 are the earliest evidence for *qi* (the essential stuff of life that fuels and animates everything in the universe) moving round the body in a regular rhythm through channels called *mo* or *mai* (脈), a term variously translated as 'channels', 'vessels', 'meridians', or 'pulse'. In the theory and practice of healing, those channels, concepts of *qi*, blood, and yin and yang current during the Warring States period were woven together and brought to bear on the human body. The *mai* were structural elements in a linear configuration of the inner body, foreshadowing the familiar tracts and channels of acupuncture. According to context, *mai* could refer to tracts underneath the skin (recognizable by the valleys between the raised ridges of the muscles), blood vessels, or the pathways of pain and other internal bodily sensations experienced as travelling or responding to palpation along a given plane. At certain locations on the surface of the body, the channels emerged in the form of pulses, which could be read for clues to the state of the body's *qi* and the condition of the internal organs through which *qi* passed. Pulse diagnosis became the supreme diagnostic tool for elite medicine throughout the Chinese empire, and it retains primary importance for practitioners of TCM today.

As Han physicians and thinkers came to grips with the puzzling behaviour of sickness, they were guided by a vision of a microcosmic body, united in its essence with the cosmos and the state, and inhabited by the same spirits, which lent it their potency. Just as *qi* connects every phenomenon in nature with the movements of the heavenly bodies and thus with the deities and the spirits of the ancestors, the imperial rulers aspired to extend their sway everywhere under heaven—and even to the body's innermost depths where organs functioned as ministers of the empire, the heart as the ruler, the liver as the general. In an increasingly centralized state, the emperor played the crucial role of mediator between heaven and earth, which required him to carry out a cycle of complex rituals. Pursuing virtue, venerating one's ancestors, and performing the rituals correctly were ways of securing the gods' approval and ensuring order on earth. Disorder, in the form of civil unrest, natural disasters, famine, or disease, was a sign and consequence of the gods' displeasure.[7]

The flow of *qi* around the body was like the flow of essential traffic through the network of roads and waterways that provided for the well-being of the Chinese empire. If the flow was blocked or disrupted, analogous consequences would ensue, and the same kinds of remedies were called for. By the Former Han period, in the last two centuries BCE, this analogy was generally applied to a newly constructed acupuncture body with fourteen channels. For example, in part of the *Yellow Emperor's Inner Canon* the acupuncture channels are correlated with natural water courses.[8]

In the literature of this formative era, we find a variety of theories about the number of channels, their paths, and their physical nature, in relation to ideas about circulation. Often, these theories reflect alternative views of celestial movements and the structure of Heaven and Earth. For instance, there are traces of an archaic number system based on the number eleven, in which the number six belongs to heaven and five to the earth.

The treatises from the Yellow Emperor canon are mainly in the form of dialogues, which take place between the Yellow Emperor and a cast of learned ministers, including Lord Thunder (Leigong 雷公) and most notably the legendary minister Qibo 歧伯, who specialized in acupuncture and esoteric matters. In one dialogue, the Yellow Emperor asks Qibo about perceived contradictions in the ways in which the channels of the body reflect patterns in the heavens. In his reply, Qibo 歧伯 correlates particular days in the calendar with each channel.[9] It is clear that the *mai* channels carried no fixed or pervasive numerical associations in early Han times, as inconsistencies are apparent in the assignation of time markers to organ systems and even to yin and yang. Dialogue form is frequently utilized in expository writing of the Han era as a device for exploring conflicting viewpoints and reconciling diverse ideas. By depicting the perfect architecture and rhythms of the human body with the same broad brush-strokes as the larger model of the cosmos, medical theorists were able to find intelligible structure in an inchoate mass of information, without which it would have been impossible to make predictions or to chart anomalies and sickness, but a single system was slow to emerge.

The precursors of what is known today as 'acupuncture'—the practice of adjusting bodily essences by the use of fine needles—emerged in the Han period out of a diverse range of healing arts: *qi* and yin and yang practices, numerology, divination, petty surgery, bloodletting, and aspects of spirit healing. The material origins of acupuncture are found in 'medicinal stones' or *bian* 砭,[10] which by the beginning of the second century BCE were clearly being used with the specific aim of influencing the flow of *qi* along the *mai* channels so as to remove blockages believed to cause illness. An initial focus was fixed especially on locations where the channels crossed and the vicinity of the joints, where pain and discomfort were most frequently felt. Evidence for this therapy reveals an awareness of danger about the radical nature of this intervention. The '*Jiu zhen*' 九鍼 ('Nine Needles') chapter of *Lingshu* records the Yellow Emperor criticizing the clumsy use of stone needles in *qi* therapy.[11]

Needles intended for moving *qi* were as slender as a fine hair and of very high quality, but most references in this text do indicate petty surgery or bloodletting rather than *qi* therapy as such. Chinese smiths certainly possessed the technology to produce very fine needles at this period, but no actual examples have survived. It is not until the first century CE that we find archaeological records of fine needles that can be linked with *qi* therapy at named acupuncture points. At all events, the use of needles still evoked a lingering disquiet even much later on.[12]

At the gentle end of the therapeutic spectrum, heat treatment or massage could be carried out at the blockage sites. Heat treatment tended to be regarded as a cheaper and more user-friendly alternative to needling, and the most widespread and most popular form of this was *jiu* 灸, translated as moxibustion. Moxibustion embraces a range of heat and cauterization techniques using various materials. It is sometimes spoken of as cauterization or cautery in the broad sense of the application of extreme heat, but it was used only occasionally to sear wounds.

It has often been noted that anatomical research and dissection are conspicuous by their absence from the medical scene in early China. Yet from the first millennium BCE there are moral exempla of tyrants dissecting the bodies of officials and pregnant women, of the careful weighing and measurement of the viscera of an executed rebel leader (Wang Mang 王莽 r. 9–23), and records of the results of such cadaver dissections in the canonical medical works.[13] In the second century, Hua Tuo 華佗 famously performed abdominal surgery with the aid of an anaesthetic called *mafeisan* 麻沸散, which apparently rendered his patients insensible as though drunk.[14] Chinese theorists were not indifferent to the physical body. However, they viewed it first and foremost as a dynamic system of functions and relationships, governed by the same regularities observable in the external world. The body was not a discrete object to be considered in isolation but a piece of a correlative universe that echoed with sympathetic resonances and significant similarities. It was this that made the body susceptible to medical diagnosis and treatment.

Interlocking theories of cosmogenesis and statecraft, structured around the polarity of yin 陰 and yang 陽 and the *wuxing* 五行 'Five Agents', provided the framework for sets of correspondences that, by the third century BCE, had started to dominate ritual and technical thinking. For instance, *Lüshi chunqiu* argues that the emperor's conduct, diet, vestments, and place of residence must be aligned with a ritual schedule based on astronomically calculated calendrical divisions.[15] Around the dawn of empire they also organized classical Chinese medical thought, sometimes known as the Medicine of Systematic Correspondence.[16] Yin and yang are not substances or fixed properties, and are most satisfactorily described as relational categories that organize the *wanwu* 'myriad things' in 'complementary opposition'. Expressed most fundamentally in spatial alternation, such as back/front and inner/outer or in temporal contrasts such as day/night or the alternation between warm and cold seasons in the yearly cycle, yin and yang were to become key criteria for classifying physical substances and describing physiological and pathological processes and, thus, all the vicissitudes of health and sickness as well as stages in the development of diseases. The Five Agents schema extended the correlative basis for understanding the body by means of interrelated series of five: five seasons (spring, summer, late summer, autumn, and winter), five sapors or flavours, five viscera, and so on. It offered an overarching template for relations between the world and the human body, rooted in a fivefold division of the year.

The sets of correspondences summarized here model the natural (that is proper and salutary) relationship of the body with its surroundings, and the structure and form of what Joseph Needham called the 'organismic' universe.[17] The image of the microcosmic body was further strengthened by social and political analogy. This is particularly obvious in the yin and yang correlations of the *Yellow Emperor's Four Canons*, that is noble/lowly and controlling/being controlled.

Whereas the treatises compiled into the Yellow Emperor's inner corpus do not bear witness to their authors, the late Han period saw the publication of a number of medical texts that speak to us in a more individual voice. In particular, the work of the scholar-physician Zhang Zhongjing 張仲景 (*c*.mid-second to third century) had a decisive influence on the later course of Chinese medical theory. A foreword to the received text, attributed to Zhang himself, relates that he published two monographs on febrile disease in response to an epidemic that devastated his town. These two treatises were subsequently combined to form the much-cited *Shang Han Lun* 傷寒論 (*Treatise on Cold Damage*), which describes the course of febrile disease and includes a compendious materia medica with medicines for each stage. The 'cold damage' of the title is a systematic aetiological theory of febrile disease due to external attack in light of the progress of yin and yang. Eight centuries later, during the Song Dynasty (960–1279), Zhang's magnum opus gained a fresh lease of life when it was identified by government officials desperately searching for sources of ancient wisdom to combat a deadly series of epidemics.[18] They prepared a new edition, which is still published and consulted today, and enjoys particular popularity in Japan.

Religion and Medicine

Society in early China was peopled by religious figures who mediated spirit presences, including gods, nature spirits, and deceased ancestors. The *wu* 巫—diviners, mediums, shamans, or specialists in ritual, both male and female—were employed at court to avert demonic influences, resolve inauspicious events, and perform the work of communicating with the invisible realm. As an integral part of exorcisms and sacrifices to the spirits of nature at the correct times in the annual and seasonal cycle and summoning up the spirits of the departed at funeral ceremonies, they issued proclamations to expel illness and its causes, and used effigies and talismans to intervene in the course of disease. Female *wu* performed ritual songs, dances, and prayers, and participated in healing ceremonies alongside priests and medical practitioners of various kinds.[19]

The religious arena provided crucial continuity in face of dynastic rupture and political transformation. In medieval times, certain medical ideas were able to thrive and evolve in the context of religious movements.[20] At the beginning of the first century CE, millennial cults sprang up across China, some of them posing a threat to the power of the state, like the Yellow Turbans sect of Zhang Jue or Zhang Jiao (張角, d.184), which led an uprising against the Han ruling house. Though the uprising was crushed, it signified the beginning of the end for the Han empire, which collapsed in 220 amid local wars, famine, epidemics, and waves of refugees. One of the ways in which the Yellow Turbans won converts for their cause was by offering to heal the sick, often by such ancient practices as incantation, and burning talismans and administering the ashes in water. Their main sacred text was the *Taiping Jing* 太平經 (*Canon or Scripture of Heavenly Peace*), a text grounded, on the one hand, in the theory of the Unity of Heaven and Humanity (天人合一), wherein individual virtue was thought to invite corresponding response from Heaven. On the other hand, it also contained theoretical descriptions of the body comparable to those found in *Huangdi neijing*, as well as numerous longevity prescriptions encompassing meditation, breath and *qi* techniques, self-cultivation, diet, plant and animal drugs, and the use of charms and talismans. It was later assimilated into the Daoist canon.[21]

The Way of the Celestial Masters (*Tianshi Dao* 天師道), which also originated in this period, marked the beginning of Daoism as an organized religion. Religious Daoism found many adherents among the medieval ruling classes. The Celestial Masters held that illness was a punishment for evil deeds and could be cured by confession, submitting petitions in due form to the Celestial Bureaucracy, and atonement through acts of benevolence and public charity such as building roads and donating food to the poor.[22]

The *Shangqing* 上清 (Highest Clarity) school of Daoism, which grew out of the same tradition, was in part a reaction to the southward migration of the Celestial Masters, interfering with local religious structures. The *Shangqing* school rose to prominence in the fifth century under the guidance of Tao Hongjing 陶弘景 (456–536). A key figure in the history of alchemy and medicine as well as religious Daoism, he not only compiled the Shangqing corpus, but also wrote treatises on alchemy and published the first known critical edition of the Shennong pharmaceutical canon. He enjoyed imperial favour and patronage, especially for his work in the field of alchemy.[23]

The conjunction of medicine, alchemy, and high office is a recurrent theme in the lives of prominent medieval authors.[24] A distinguished example is the scholar-physician Sun Simiao 孫思邈 (581–681/2 CE), who held government posts at the beginning of the Tang period. Sun Simiao was noted for his eclectic intellectual and religious views, which are exemplified in two massive and wide-ranging medical works where Buddhist chants and demonic medicine stand on an equal footing with classical scholarly medicine.[25] Like Tao Hongjing, Sun Simiao was a seminal figure in the development of alchemy.

Classic Chinese alchemy set out to understand and master the workings of the cosmos by studying its physical nature. By scrutinizing a substance in all its stages of transformation from its primordial state, an alchemist could learn to apply powerful analogies with cosmic time cycles—from the dawn of time to its end, wherein lies its beginning. Through a carefully calibrated process of successive heating and cooling, the alchemists attempted to speed up the sequences of time so as to transmute imperfect base metal into perfected 'gold'. These practices were known as *waidan* 外丹 (external alchemy).

The alchemists' desire to master the physical world led them on a quest for elixirs of longevity and immortality. Highly toxic minerals like cinnabar, mercury, lead, and arsenic were used to preserve the material body in life as well as death. Arsenic, a commonly used 'mineral drug', is a nerve poison: when consumed over an extended period, even in small quantities, it results in lapses of consciousness, weakness, cardiac abnormalities, peripheral neuropathy, diarrhoea, and delusions. However, it may also induce hallucinations and ecstatic visions; and it seems that this, together with the gradual character of the pathology, allowed users to embrace the symptoms of poisoning as acceptable side-effects. Countless Chinese literati and even some of the emperors of the Tang dynasty are said to have perished from the effects of immortality elixirs over the centuries and this tragic irony brought about the demise of external alchemy.[26]

As commercial and cultural interchange between China and the outside world intensified in the first century CE, Buddhism began to spread into China along the Silk Roads. Early Buddhism was at times misinterpreted (sometimes deliberately) in China as a Daoist sect and Buddhist terminology, thought, and symbols were adopted by Daoist sects.[27] Buddhism offered a radical new view of the afterlife centred on the idea of progressive incarnations of an immortal personal soul, and it proposed meditation and prayer as the main path to salvation and healing. The Buddhist devotion to deities struck a particular chord with indigenous popular religion and the Buddha was readily assimilated into the local pantheon, often in the role of Medicine King, as were the boddhisatvas of healing, undergoing thorough sinicization in the process.

Both Buddhism and Daoism prospered greatly in the Sui (581–618) and Tang (618–907) period, when China was unified once more after centuries of division. The Sui emperors especially were active patrons of Buddhist institutions. At its apogee in the early Tang, Buddhism was the main form of religious observance across the entire social spectrum. Under the auspices of the Tang ruling house (the Li family), debates among exponents of the major religious traditions were staged at Court, creating a lively, competitive intellectual environment conducive to the fusion of religious ideas and the exchange of healing practices.[28]

With increasing prosperity, Buddhist monasteries became important cultural and social centres, some of them providing cheap hostel accommodation, epidemic relief, or free in-patient care in infirmaries called *Beitian fang* 悲田坊 (fields of compassion).[29] As ever, healing proved to be an effective mode of evangelism. However, the increasing material wealth and influence of monastic institutions brought them into collision with the state. Literary depictions of monk and nun healers play upon stereotypes of debauchery and immorality, much as in medieval Europe and India. Monks specializing in the treatment of women's illnesses bore the brunt of these prejudices. In the great suppression of Buddhism under the Tang emperor Wuzong from 842 to 845, thousands of monasteries were closed down or destroyed, their accumulated wealth was seized, and their infirmaries were taken over by the imperial authority.[30] But despite this persecution, monastic centres continued to play a vital role in the preservation and scribal transmission of medical literature. Our current knowledge of Chinese medicine in the Middle Ages is derived in great part from manuscripts copied by Buddhist monks living in far-flung communities along the Silk Roads.[31]

The Song Period and Politics

Medicine received strong state support in the Northern Song dynasty (960–1127), owing to the personal involvement and interest of successive emperors, coupled with pressure on the Song government to tackle a series of major epidemics. The Song government sponsored the publication of medical texts, founded the first Imperial Medical School, and established a formal system of medical education. It launched an empire-wide initiative to collect and record local herbs and remedies, which greatly expanded the repertoire of materia medica. This in turn stimulated the production of new illustrated herbals and prompted a reappraisal of drug classifications. Seeking ways to combat the epidemics, theorists and practitioners revisited ancient medical learning and reintegrated it into current practice. In this climate, a new elite of scholarly physicians, the *ru yi* 儒醫 (literally 'Confucian physicians'), emerged.[32]

Towards the end of the first millennium, in the period spanning the close of the Tang dynasty and the beginning of the Song, the empire entered a period of rapid and continuous economic change. With population growth and greater prosperity came a general expansion of the educated classes. As a consequence, competition for posts in the imperial bureaucracy—the traditional career destination for the educated elite—grew ever more fierce. A career in medicine came to be seen as an increasingly attractive alternative.

From the outset, the Northern (early) Song Dynasty (960–1125) was marked by intense political debate focusing on the role of government and the appropriate extent of state intervention. This reached a crescendo in the late eleventh century, when the reforming statesman Wang Anshi 王安石 (1021–86) introduced a radical package of 'new policies' designed to modernize finance, agriculture, and administration. In this interventionist climate, the Bureau for the Editing of Medical Texts was established in 1057 to identify and publish an official canon of medical literature. This yielded thirty editions of canonical medical and pharmaceutical treatises and remedy collections and essentially shaped the corpus of early medical literature as we know it today. The rediscovery and promotion of the *Treatise on Cold Damage* of Zhang Zhongjing (second century) belongs to this period.

A combination of factors at work from the twelfth to the fourteenth centuries (during the Song and Jin (1127–1235) and Yuan (1279–1368) dynasties) had far-reaching repercussions for the production of knowledge, especially in the area of medicine. Advances in printing technology enabled the official canons to be widely disseminated and also meant that medical knowledge could be accessed and transmitted outside closed medical lineages. The scale of the medical bureaucracy and of state involvement in medical training during these two centuries was unparalleled before or since, until the twentieth century at least. Some officials had medical texts inscribed or displayed in public places as a public information service and as a way of enhancing the government's image. One official took it upon himself to demonstrate the efficacy of medicines by having them forcibly administered to the people of the district.[33]

The Southern Song (1125–1275) government made real efforts to address public health issues, commissioning elite doctors to dispense drugs as epidemic relief, but uptake in the southern regions was poor. Officials reported that the populace shunned and isolated the sick, or entrusted them to the care of *wu*, traditional practitioners specializing in religious healing.[34] Some officials responded by punishing spirit healers, smashing their altars, giving them official medical texts to study, and requiring them to renounce their old occupation and become farmers or medical practitioners.

Urbanization and the growing market economy favoured the development of knowledge networks, and provided the rising elite of scholarly physicians with unique opportunities to engage in the production of texts and innovative forms of medical activity. After the abolition of civil service examinations under the Yuan (Mongol) dynasty (1279–1368), publishing medical texts became a key way for a scholar and gentleman to exhibit his intellectual and social status while also 'accumulating virtue'—a meritorious activity with both private and public aspects, and both moral and practical advantages.

Intersections

From the late Han period onward, and probably far earlier (although the scarcity of evidence makes this more problematic), the history of medicine and healing in China needs to be viewed in a larger geographical context that extends eastward into what is now Korea and, in the Middle Ages, beyond that to Japan, and westward and southward to Mongolia, Tibet, India, and all the nations and cultures that lie along the overland routes linking the ancient capitals with Persia and the lands further west. The medieval manuscripts recovered in the library cave at the Dunhuang shrines in today's Gansu province, north-west China, offer a rich mine of source material to investigate the connections and tensions between periphery and centre, or rather between multiple peripheries and centres. Recent research into these sources, most of which are held at the British Library and the Bibliothèque Nationale de France, shows the remarkable degree of penetration of the official medical texts generated in the capital, but it also reveals an enthralling range of local medical material and international influences that have left little trace in the official canons and other transmitted literature.[35]

Far away from the Chinese borders, at the end of one of the Silk Routes in Mongolian Ilkhanid Persia, scholars and translators from China, Tibet, Kashmir, India, Europe, and Arabia congregated, around the turn of the thirteenth and fourteenth centuries, at the court of the Judeo-Muslim scholar and Vizier Rashid al-Din (1274–1318)—one of the great intellectual melting pots of its time. Himself a court physician, Rashid al-Din sponsored medical translations and produced a monumental collection of medical knowledge edited and collated from a vast range of sources including Chinese sources. This literature is only now being studied in light of its significance for cross-cultural transmission.[36]

In the end, however, one is left questioning how much influence scholarly translations like these can have had on actual medical practice. A more accessible point of entry into the practical business of transmitting knowledge may be provided by translating and analysing books of remedies and recipes. In translating concrete details and practices, the present-day translator is brought up against some of the same problems of identifying and interpreting substances and techniques that must have challenged earlier translators, merchants, and ordinary end-users. The *Yinshan zhengyao* 飲膳正要 evokes a vision of Mongolian expansion that is very different from the popular clichés of rape and pillage.[37] Viewing the Mongolian imperial presence through the sensual, subtle medium of ingredients and spices, and the technology and philosophy of cookery and diet, we see how it functioned as a vehicle for cultural dissemination and assimilation throughout thirteenth- and fourteenth-century Asia. *Yinshan zhengyao* incorporates and interprets dietary and technical knowledge from Muslim and Arabic areas, often sinicizing it in the process. Paul Buell's ongoing work is an English translation of *Huihui yaofang* (Muslim pharmaceutical prescriptions), a Chinese text dating to the Mongolian Yuan dynasty that includes many Arabic prescriptions, with Arabic and Persian drug names noted after the Chinese equivalents. It provides a fascinating window on the network of commercial, religious, and ethnic interchange that formed Chinese medical culture in and after the period of the Mongol emperors.[38]

The reception of new medical technologies from abroad was played out against the background of an empire in crisis, under attack from the imperialist powers of Europe, Japan, and America. As the increasingly fragile Qing dynasty lost its grip on central power, new medical techniques were entering the country, mainly through Christian missions. The first Treaty of Tianjin (1858), which granted foreigners immunity from Chinese laws and the freedom to travel, enabled foreign missionaries, for the first time, to acquire property and to live outside the treaty ports. By the 1890s, missionary clinics had been set up in large towns and cities in many parts of the country, and it was commonly acknowledged that free medical care could win converts where preaching failed. Missionary medicine appealed directly to the poor; wealthier people, who had the alternative of paying for expert medical care, were apt to despise missionary medicine and to be suspicious of its religious and political agenda.[39]

From the early eighteenth century, European anatomical texts had been available in China in Jesuit translations but, as long as they were not backed up by verifiable methods of treatment, they were regarded as little more than an exotic intellectual curiosity.[40] This changed in the middle of the nineteenth century, with the advent of impressive new foreign techniques, mostly surgical and anaesthetic.[41] However, spectacular though some of these were (including cataract surgery and the removal of tumours, cysts, and stones), they tended by their nature to align Western surgeons not with learned scholar-physicians, but with humbler medical artisans. Since antiquity, many kinds of petty and skin-deep surgery had been routinely carried out in China, including bloodletting, lancing abscesses, suturing wounds, removing projectiles, repairing hernias, surgical treatments of haemorrhoids, castration, and acupuncture.[42] A small number of foreign miracle drugs, notably chloroform and quinine, were added to the repertoire of materia medica.

Smallpox prevention provided an arena for the negotiation of indigenous and foreign technologies. Since the end of the first millennium, symptoms identifiable retrospectively as smallpox are known to have been endemic among young children. These symptoms were classified under the rubric of 'cold damage', the syndrome pattern used since the Han period to explain feverish diseases and other, frequently infectious, conditions deemed to be caused by external pathogens. However, in the 1500s, medical practitioners in southern China had begun to carry out variolation (introducing infected matter from a patient with smallpox into the body of a healthy child so as to achieve immunity). There were five types of variolation, with accompanying rituals, intended to remove 'foetal poisoning'—according to Chinese medical theory, a hereditary disease arising partly from a disorderly lifestyle, and sexual, emotional, or dietary excess, and thus an oblique moral indictment of the sufferer's mother.[43]

Variolation did indeed prove effective. Thus when Edward Jenner vaccine was first introduced into China in 1805 by Dr. Alexander Pearson, it was cast as the competitor of variolation, creating tension and conflict particularly in rural areas. While variolation was carried out privately, Jennerian vaccination was offered free of charge by some Chinese charitable organizations; however, the vaccine was difficult to obtain, preserve, and distribute. Compared with variolation, vaccination had a firmer methodological basis and better safety record, was easier to deliver, and did not carry the risk of spreading smallpox, making it suitable for institutional mass provision. Nonetheless, each side claimed that their own technique involved less human suffering and left fewer disfiguring pockmarks, and variolation continued to be practised into the twentieth century.[44]

Within the Qing (Manchu) administration, the cause of technological Westernization was espoused by a hard core of ethnic Chinese officials who especially favoured the adoption of foreign military technology. These fundamentally conservative reformers established the Self-Strengthening Movement (1860–95) under the slogan 'Chinese

learning for our foundation, Western learning for practical application'.[45] There followed a limited programme of industrialization,
which gave rise to the Fuzhou dockyard and Jiangnan arsenal in
Shanghai. In a similar spirit, the Tianjin Medical School was founded
in 1881 as the first state institute for training in 'Western medicine'.[46]

The urgency of reform was underlined by China's defeat in the
Sino-Japanese war of 1894–5 and the debacle of the Boxer Uprising,
which further strengthened the hold of the imperialist powers over the
ailing Qing state.[47] Opinion in China was polarized: while conservative Qing officials repudiated any form of institutional modernization,
many of their reformist opponents saw wholesale Westernization as
the only way forward. Numerous Chinese intellectuals went abroad to
pursue studies in medicine or natural science, particularly in Japan,
which had instituted a thorough-going top-down programme of
reform after the 1868 Meiji Restoration. Medical training abroad is
a common theme in the lives of the major Chinese revolutionary
writers and reforming politicians of the early twentieth century.[48]

Reading the Body Culturally: Sense and Sensuality

China's most notable contribution to the mapping of the human body
may lie not so much in the visual representation of its functionality as
in descriptions of the sensory apprehension of the inner body. In his
work on the cultural and social history of perception, Shigehisa
Kuriyama explores the contrasting perceptual modalities whereby
European and Chinese images of the body were constituted, and
describes how different ways of understanding the body privilege
distinct ways of seeing. For example, Chinese complexion diagnosis,
which identifies bodily imbalances in the aura or colours of the face, is
grounded in botanical metaphors deeply embedded in early Chinese
language and culture. Like the flower of a plant, the complexion is a
visible outward manifestation of the underlying health and strength of
the human organism. Beyond the modern hegemony of the outward
eye, Kuriyama finds differences between knowledge derived from
touch (haptic knowledge) in the Chinese and European traditions.
He contrasts the knowledge of the pulse derived from ancient Greek
tradition with the Chinese palpation of the *mai* 脈—a term in which
ideas about bodily channels merge with the sensory awareness of the

rhythmic pulsation of the vessels—illustrating how direct experience of the body is inseparable from culture-bound preconceptions and theoretical constructs.[49]

The social historian's desire to encompass human experience in its broadest sense has led a growing body of scholars to a new methodological turn, known as 'sensory history', that challenges the presumption that 'the past is best seen rather than, say, heard or smelled'.[50] By exploring culturally specific styles of perception, this approach holds out the possibility of making histories that are situated within the sensibilities of their subjects. It has produced intriguing and richly evocative histories alive with sounds, tastes, and smells. China has a great deal to offer this methodological turn in terms of both sources and perspectives.[51]

In documenting the felt, internal experience of being well, fit, and strong, and the sensations of pain, pleasure, and passion, the Chinese healing arts also medicalized the world of the senses.[52] Out of this culture of attending to the life of the inner body, and the language and theories that it generated, emerged the single most crucial innovation in early Chinese medicine—the concept of *qi*. The semantic circuits summoned up by *qi* confound any simple distinction between mind, body, and emotions, uniting them as changing states of the experienced self.[53] The persistence of the concept of *qi* evokes the aesthetics of a time when the boundaries between these ways of experiencing the self and the world were not clear-cut.[54]

Inner body *qi* cultivation has always had political resonances. Scholars studying contemporary manifestations of self-cultivation often point to the use of the body as a locus of resistance to authority or the state. Undoubtedly, some forms of *qi* cultivation, and allied religious and medical rituals, have functioned as expressions of political and personal autonomy. This can be seen in the bodily cultivation practices of hermits and political recusants from pre-imperial times onwards and of the early revolutionary armies, as well as the purportedly passive protests of the Falun Gong 法輪工, which have recently aroused such concern in the Chinese authorities.[55] Equally, working with inner body *qi* can be a deeply conservative and conformist practice. 'Studies of culture need to pay at least as much attention to sites of concentrated cultural practice as to the dispersed sites of resistance.'[56] Traditionally, self-cultivation forms part of the culture of artistic expression and refined leisure expected of retired government officials, living out their remaining years in tranquil rural seclusion. Today's bands of post-menopausal, sword-wielding women practising their *taijiquan* in Chinese municipal parks are no more likely to endanger the status quo.

Conclusion

Most of the researchers cited in this chapter have, in one way or another, challenged the premise that we can valuably look back at historical events from the perspectives of our current concerns. Certainly those histories that seek to understand sources as they were understood in their own time are more likely to provide rich sociocultural contexts and so capture the historical moment. For the ancient worlds this has meant that recent histories are more intent upon the ritual and religious worlds within which classical medical ideas formed and flourished. For China, what earlier historians left out was, for example, the pervasive power of calculating auspicious times and places, the plurality of beliefs attendant on any medical encounter, and accounts of healing in religious organizations. Yet, it is a folly to think that we can entirely extract the concerns that shape us as readers and writers in our own time from our historical narratives. Nor should we. Both authors of this chapter are as much practitioners of modern *qi gong*, martial arts, and Chinese medicine as we are historians. Our readings of primary text and interpretation of sources consciously lean towards practice-orientated accounts, as textured through our own experience. Such historical enterprise dignifies itself with the idea that it is possible to share something of the sensory and perceptive style of the originators of early Chinese healing practices, and that doing so is germane, indeed essential, to deepening our appreciation of their textual legacies. Added to textual filiation and institutional histories, body-centred readings enable one to observe more readily the fluid interplay between exercise, diet, pharmacology, cuisine, ritual, and cosmography, in the constitution of Chinese healing practice. With these methodological tools at our disposal, the door also opens into a rich inter-regional cultural and material history, into a narrative not only concerned with internal 'Chinese' genealogical developments but also ready to tackle the transitions, transformations, and transmissions that happen to medical knowledge as it is exchanged between different peoples across physical domains as well as down through generations of healers.

Notes

1 David N. Keightley, 'Shamanism, Death, and the Ancestors: Religious Mediation in Neolithic and Shang China (ca. 5000–1000 B.C.)', *Asiatische Studien/Études Asiatiques* 52 (1998), 763–828.

2 Donald Harper, *Early Chinese Medical Literature: The Mawangdui Medical Manuscripts* (London/New York: Kegan Paul, 1998).

3 Anthony Christie, *Chinese Mythology* (London: Hamlyn, 1968), 84–91.

4 Martin Palmer, *T'ung shu, the Ancient Chinese Almanac*, 1st edn (Boston: Shambhala, 1986); Roel Stercx, 'Religious Practices in the Han Dynasty', in Michael Loewe and Michael Nylan (eds), *China's Early Empires, a Re-Appraisal* (Cambridge: Cambridge University Press, 2010); Michael Nylan, 'Yin-yang, Five Phases and Qi', ibid. 398–414; Vivienne Lo, '*Huangdi Hama jing* (Yellow Emperor's Toad Canon)', *Asia Major* 14 (2001), 61–99.

5 Nathan Sivin, 'Huang ti nei ching 黃帝內經', in Michael Loewe (ed.), *Early Chinese Texts: A Bibliographical Guide* (Berkeley: Society for the Study of Early China, 1993), 196–215.

6 Paul U. Unschuld, *Medicine in China: A History of Ideas: Comparative Studies of Health Systems and Medical Care* (Berkeley: University of California Press, 1985), 263–95.

7 *Suwen* 3.8. The *Suwen* is part of the *Inner Canon of the Yellow Emperor*. For a study of the *Suwen* see Paul U. Unschuld, *Huang di nei jing su wen: Nature, Knowledge, Imagery in an Ancient Chinese Medical Text* (Berkeley/Los Angeles: University of California Press, 2003).

8 *Lingshu* 12. See Wu Jing-Nuan, *Ling shu or The Spiritual Pivot* (Honolulu: University of Hawaii Press, 1993), 69.

9 *Huangdi neijing taisu* 黃帝內太经素 5; *Lingshu* 4.15 'Wushi ying' 五十營, in Wu Jing-Nuan, *Spiritual Pivot*, 83.

10 Vivienne Lo, 'Spirit of Stone: Technical Considerations in the Treatment of the Jade Body', *Bulletin of the School of Oriental and African Studies* 65 (2002), 99–128.

11 Wu Jing-Nuan, *Spiritual Pivot*, 258–63.

12 Bridie Jane Andrews, 'The Making of Modern Chinese Medicine, 1895–1937', doctoral thesis, University of Cambridge, 1996, 20–48.

13 John Knoblock and Jeffrey Riegel, *The Annals of Lü Buwei* (Stanford: Stanford University Press, 2000), 596; Louis Fu, 'A Forgotten Reformer of Anatomy in China: Wang Ch'ing-Jen', *ANZ Journal of Surgery* 78 (2008), 1052–8; *Lingshu* 12, 'Channels and Rivers' 經水. See Wu Jing-Nuan, *Spiritual Pivot*, 69, or Fu, 'A Forgotten Reformer of Anatomy', 1052.

40   *Vivienne Lo and Michael Stanley-Baker*

14 Zheng Bocheng, 'The Miracle-Working Doctor', *Journal of Traditional Chinese Medicine* 5 (1985), 311–12.

15 *Lingshu* 11.77. See Wu Jing-Nuan, *Spiritual Pivot*, 254–67; Shigehisa Kuriyama, *The Expressiveness of the Body and the Divergence of Greek and Chinese Medicine* (New York: Zone Books, 1999), 244–5; Sun Xiaochun and Jacob Kistemaker, *The Chinese Sky during the Han: Constellating Stars and Society* (Leiden/New York: Brill, 1997), 96–7.

16 Unschuld, *Medicine in China*, 51–92.

17 Joseph Needham and Ling Wang, *Science and Civilisation in China*, Vol. 2: *History of Scientific Thought* (Cambridge: Cambridge University Press, 1956), 291–2.

18 Asaf Moshe Goldschmidt, *The Evolution of Chinese Medicine: Song Dynasty, 960–1200* (London: Routledge, 2009), 69–102.

19 Lothar von Falkenhausen, 'Reflections on the Political Role of Spirit Mediums in Early China: The Wu Officials in the Zhouli', *Early China* 20 (1995), 279–300; Michael J. Puett, *To Become a God: Cosmology, Sacrifice, and Self-divinization in Early China* (Cambridge, MA: Harvard University Press, 2002); Harper, *Early Chinese Medical Literature*, 148–83; and Unschuld, *Medicine in China*, 17–50.

20 Unschuld, *Medicine in China*, 117–53; Sakade Yoshinobu 坂出祥伸, *Taoism, Medicine and Qi in China and Japan* (Osaka: Kansai University Press, 2007); Ute Engelhardt, 'Qi for Life: Longevity in the Tang', in Livia Kohn and Yoshinobu Sakade (eds), *Taoist Meditation and Longevity Techniques* (Ann Arbor: Center for Chinese Studies University of Michigan, 1989), 263–96.

21 Barbara Hendrischke, *The Scripture on Great Peace: The Taiping jing and the Beginnings of Daoism* (Berkeley: University of California Press, 2006).

22 Peter S. Nickerson, 'The Great Petition for Sepulchral Plaints', in Stephen R. Bokenkamp (ed.), *Early Daoist Scriptures* (Berkeley: University of California Press, 1997), 230–60; Terry F. Kleeman, 'Licentious Cults and Bloody Victuals: Sacrifice, Reciprocity, and Violence in Traditional China', *Asia Major*, 3rd series, 7 (1994), 185–211.

23 Michel Strickmann, 'The Alchemy of T'ao Hung-ching', in Holmes Welch and Anna K. Seidel (eds), *Facets of Taoism: Essays in Chinese Religion* (New Haven, CT: Yale University Press, 1979), 123–92; Michel Strickmann and Bernard Faure, *Chinese Magical Medicine* (Stanford: Stanford University Press, 2002).

24 Strickmann, 'Alchemy'; Strickmann and Faure, *Chinese Magical Medicine*; Nathan Sivin, *Chinese Alchemy: Preliminary Studies* (Cambridge, MA: Harvard University Press, 1968).

25 Sivin, *Chinese Alchemy*; Sabine Wilms, 'The Female Body in Medieval China: A Translation and Interpretation of the "Women's Recipes" in Sun Simiao's *Beiji qianjin yaofang*', doctoral dissertation, University of Arizona, 2002; Elena Valussi, 'The Chapter on "Nourishing Inner Nature" in Sun Simiao's *Qianjin yaofang*', MA thesis, School of Oriental and African Studies, 1996; Fang Ling, 'La tradition sacrée de la Médecine Chinoise ancienne. Étude sur le Livre des exorcismes de Sun Simiao (581–682)', doctoral dissertation, Ecole Pratique des Hautes Etudes, 2001, x.

26 Joseph Needham, 'Elixir Poisoning', in *Clerks and Craftsmen in China and the West: Lectures and Addresses on the History of Science and Technology* (London: Cambridge University Press, 1970), 316–39.

27 Erik Zürcher, *The Buddhist Conquest of China; The Spread and Adaptation of Buddhism in Early Medieval China* (Leiden: Brill, 1959); Stephen R. Bokenkamp, 'Daoism: An Overview', in Lindsay Jones (ed.), *Encyclopedia of Religion* (Detroit: Macmillan Reference USA, 2005), 2176–92.

28 Christine Mollier, *Buddhism and Taoism Face to Face: Scripture, Ritual, and Iconographic Exchange in Medieval China* (Honolulu: University of Hawai'i Press, 2008).

29 Charles D. Benn, *Daily Life in Traditional China: The Tang Dynasty*, 'Daily Life through History' series (Westport, CT: Greenwood Press, 2002), 227.

30 Stanley Weinstein, *Buddhism under the T'ang* (Cambridge/New York: Cambridge University Press, 1987); Needham, *Clerks and Craftsmen in China and the West*, 277–8.

31 Vivienne Lo and Christopher Cullen (eds), *Medieval Chinese Medicine*, trans. Penelope Barrett (London/New York: Routledge Curzon, 2005).

32 Goldschmidt, *The Evolution of Chinese Medicine*, 103–46; Unschuld, *Medicine in China*, 154–88.

33 T. J. Hinrichs, 'The Medical Transforming of Governance and Southern Customs in Song Dynasty China (960–1279 C.E.)', PhD dissertation, Harvard University, 2003, 33–4.

34 Ibid. 31.

35 Lo and Cullen (eds), *Medieval Chinese Medicine*; Vivienne Lo, 'Acuponcture et Moxibustion', in C. Despeux (ed.), *Médecine, religion et société dans la Chine mediévale: Etude de manuscrits chinois de Dunhuang et de Turfan (Paris: L'Institut* des Hautes Etudes Chinoises, College de France, 2010).

36 V. Lo and Wang Yidan, 'Blood or Qi Circulation? On the Nature of Authority in Rashīd al-Dīn's *Tānksūqnāma* [*The Treasure Book of Ilqān on Chinese Science and Techniques*]', in Anna Akasoy, Charles Burnett, and Ronit Yoeli-Tlalim (eds), *Rashid al-Din as an Agent and Mediator of Cultural Exchanges in Ilkhanid Iran* (London: Warburg Institute, 2011).

37 Paul D. Buell and Eugene N. Anderson, *Soup for the Qan: Chinese Dietary Medicine of the Mongol Era* (Leiden: Brill, 2nd edition, 2010).

38 Ibid.

39 Paul Cohen, 'Christian Missions and Their Impact to 1900', in Denis Twitchett and John King Fairbank (eds), *The Cambridge History of China*, Vol.10: *Late Ch'ing, 1800–1911, Part 1* (Cambridge: Cambridge University Press, 1978), 543–90; W. G. Lennox, 'A Self-Survey by Mission Hospitals in China', *Chinese Medical Journal* 46 (1932), 484–534.

40 Daniel Asen, 'Manchu Anatomy: Anatomical Knowledge and the Jesuits in Seventeenth- and Eighteenth-Century China', *Social History of Medicine* 22 (2009), 23–44; Marta Hansen, *Speaking of Epidemics in Chinese Medicine: Disease and the Geographic Imagination in Late Imperial China* (London: Routledge, forthcoming).

41 Andrews, 'The Making of Modern Chinese Medicine', 55–9.

42 Adrian Le Tellier, *La Chine: essai ethnographique, médical et hygiènique* (Paris: Baillière et fils, 1899), 45–52.

43 'Inoculation', in Joseph Needham, with Lu Gwei-Djen, *Science and Civilisation in China*, Vol. 6: *Biology and Biological Technology*, Part 6: *Medicine*, ed. Nathan Sivin (Cambridge: Cambridge University Press, 2000), 114–74.

44 'Introduction of Jennerian Vaccination', in Chi-Min Wang and Lien-teh Wu, *History of Chinese Medicine: Being a Chronicle of Medical Happenings in China from Ancient Times to the Present Period* (Tientsin: Tientsin Press, 1932), 271–301.

45 Liu Kwang-Ching, 'Self-strengthening: The Pursuit of Western Technology', in Twitchett and Fairbank (eds), *The Cambridge History of China*, Vol. 10, 491–542; and Edward L. Shaughnessy, *China: The Land of the Heavenly Dragon* (London: Duncan Baird, 2000), 85–6.

46 Wang and Wu, *History of Chinese Medicine*, 437–62.

47 Philip A. Kuhn, 'The Taiping Rebellion', in Twitchett and Fairbank (eds), *The Cambridge History of China*, Vol. 10, 264–317.

48 Andrews, 'The Making Of Modern Chinese Medicine', 149–76.

49 Kuriyama, *Expressiveness of the Body*.

50 Mark M. Smith. 'Making Sense of Social History', *Journal of Social History*, 37 (2003), 165–86.

51 Alain Corbin, *The Foul and the Fragrant: Odor and the French Social Imagination* (Cambridge, MA: Harvard University Press, 1986); Judith Farquhar, *Appetites: Food and Sex in Postsocialist China. Body, Commodity, Text* (Durham, NC: Duke University Press, 2002).

52 *Mawangdui Hanmu boshu*, ed. by Organising workgroup, Vol. 4 (Beijing: Wenwu chubanshe, 1985); *Shi wen* 十問 30–32; *Suwen* 16; Unschuld, *Huang di nei jing su wen*; Vivienne Lo, 'Tracking the Pain', *Sudhoffs Archiv* 83 (1999), 191–211.

53 Vivienne Lo, 'Pleasure, Prohibition and Pain: Food and Medicine in China', in Roel Sterckx (ed.), *Of Tripod and Palate: Food, Politics, and Religion in Traditional China* (New York/Basingstoke: Palgrave Macmillan, 2005), 163–65; Thomas Ots, 'The Silenced Body—The Expressive Leib: On the Dialectic of Mind and Life in Chinese Cathartic Healing', in Thomas J. Csordas (ed.), *Embodiment and Experience: The Existential Ground of Culture and Self* (New York: Cambridge University Press, 1994), 116–36.

54 Robert Jütte, *A History of the Senses: From Antiquity to Cyberspace*, trans. James Lynn (Cambridge: Polity Press, 2005), 25–31.

55 Nancy N. Chen, *Breathing Spaces: Qigong, Psychiatry, and Healing in China*, (New York/Chichester: Columbia University Press, 2005), 369–74.

56 W. H Sewell, 'The Concept(s) of Culture', in Victoria E. Bonnell, Lynn Hunt, and Richard Biernacki (eds), *Beyond the Cultural Turn : New Directions in the Study of Society and Culture* (Berkeley/London: University of California Press, 1999), 35–61, at 56.

Select Bibliography

Buell, Paul D. and Eugene N. Anderson, *Soup for the Qan: Chinese Dietary Medicine of the Mongol Era* (Leiden: Brill, 2010).

Harper, Donald, *Early Chinese Medical Literature: The Mawangdui Medical Manuscripts* (London/New York: Kegan Paul, 1998).

Hinrichs, T. J., 'New Geographies of Chinese Medicine', *Osiris* 13 (1998), 287–325.

Kuriyama, Shigehisa, *The Expressiveness of the Body and the Divergence of Greek and Chinese Medicine* (New York: Zone Books, 1999).

Lo, Vivienne, and Christopher Cullen (eds), *Medieval Chinese Medicine: The Dunhuang Medical Manuscripts* (London: Routledge Curzon, 2005).

Pregadio, Fabrizio, *Great Clarity: Daoism and Alchemy in Early Medieval China* (Stanford, CA: Stanford University Press, 2006).

Unschuld, Paul U., *Huang Di nei jing su wen: Nature, Knowledge, Imagery in an Ancient Chinese Medical Text, with an Appendix: The Doctrine of the Five Periods and Six Qi in the Huang Di nei jing su wen* (Berkeley: University of California Press, 2003).

Zhan, Mei, *Other-Worldly: Making Chinese Medicine Through Trans-national Frames* (Durham, NC: Duke University Press, 2009).

3

Medicine in Western Europe

Harold J. Cook

Attempting a short introduction to medicine in Western Europe can be daunting. It is quite a different project from summarizing what is sometimes called the Western medical tradition.[1] The phrase 'medicine in Western Europe' encourages discussion of the multiplicity of sometimes rapidly changing practices that have always surrounded the maintenance of health and treatment of illness, whereas the 'Western medical tradition' suggests a coherent body of ideas and practices persisting for many centuries that made Western Europe special. Of course, from the beginning of written records in Europe, authors showed an awareness of texts and traditions from previous generations, often commenting explicitly on their predecessors, a literary legacy conveyed to many other regions via settlement, colonialism, imperialism, and adaptation. In recent centuries, the literary legacy of Greece and Rome, and Christianity, helped to create an idea of a common 'European' heritage, in medicine as in other aspects of life. Since the late nineteenth century, great medical libraries have been founded in Europe, Britain, and the Americas in order to associate modern medicine with this learned tradition. During the Cold War, 'the West' came to stand for an expansive form of civilization that united western parts of Europe, Canada, the USA, and Japan in a system of progressive 'development' based on technology and science underpinned by democratic institutions.[2] The Western medical tradition was therefore meant to indicate the best parts of the medicine of Western civilization as it first took root in antiquity, blossomed in the Renaissance and Enlightenment, and found fruition in progressive modernism. Indeed, 'modern medicine' itself held out a large part of the West's promise for humankind's material and moral betterment.

Since civilizations were considered to be very large groupings based on canonical textual traditions,[3] the Western medical tradition was organized according to certain key ideas. These were said to originate in the 'rational' medicine of the Hippocratic tradition and its heirs in classical antiquity, picked up and reformulated in the first few hundred years of the Islamic world, then passed back to Europe by translation and commentary in the Middle Ages, analysed and purified in the Renaissance, and then built into scientific medicine from the seventeenth century onwards, through the Paris clinics and German laboratories, English sanitary innovations, and American research institutions, to yield the powerful biomedicine of today. To this core intellectual history, scholars have added historical accounts of professionalization, disease, and, most recently, class, gender, race, and the patient's point of view. Most historians of medicine, and a very large group of medical professionals, have developed skills of textual criticism and archival research in order to teach and write about the Western medical tradition, which has framed almost all accounts of medicine's histories, even when they have set out to counter it or to add experiences of other 'traditions' to this narrative.[4]

However, if the Western medical tradition can be regarded as a construct, finding other ways to retell a coherent account of the history of medicine in Western Europe is no easy task. 'Medicine' is itself a problematic category, being an abstraction built upon a rich variety of activities that differed considerably across both time and space. Moreover, the region itself is hard to define: what we now call Europe has no clear geographical boundary to distinguish it from Asia, nor is there a line between Eastern and Western Europe. The closest to a natural division is linguistic, with Western Europe being the shifting and permeable territory in which Germanic, Romance, and Celtic languages are predominant. Then, too, Western Europe has always been connected to the rest of the world. The proportion of territory lying within a few days' travel of the sea is great, while the many navigable rivers means that very few parts of the subcontinent can be considered landlocked: it was relatively easy to move people and goods from place to place, and to reach across the surrounding seas and Eastern steppes to other regions and peoples, so that even in the modern period of 'scientific' medicine, the commercial, colonial, and imperial relations of Europeans with other regions helped to shape European medicine.[5]

No master narrative of medicine in Western Europe is possible, then. What is attempted below is rather to locate one main theme in order to gain an impression of change in a general region. It points to one of the ways in which some medical activities in Western Europe were channelled in ways unlike most other regions of the world: the legal form of a 'corporation' grew rapidly in the past millennium, making many informal social institutions into self-conscious and stable bodies. It was such formal institutions, from guilds, universities, and colleges of physicians to hospitals, laboratories, and collective but 'private' businesses, to which much of what is taken as special about medicine in Western Europe can be attributed: the embodying and empowering of a collective 'tradition' handed down the generations in each body that was also capable of adapting to critical challenges without losing its identity because it was more than a set of ideas, practices, and individuals.

Custom and Use

Western Europeans have always been connected to other places. Indeed, the first agriculturalists had moved into Eastern and Central Europe from the Near East around 5500 BCE, while the major Indo-European languages of Western Europe (Celtic, Germanic, and Italic) had been introduced by the late second and first millennia BCE from parts far to the East. Early Bronze Age metallurgy, also invented elsewhere, could be found in the Iberian Peninsula by around 2400 BCE, and throughout Western Europe over the course of the next 1,000 years. Presumably, such people sought help when the need arose where they could—mainly in consultation with family, friends, neighbours, and people in the community who had a reputation for medical knowledge or practice—and often obtaining it. The case of the recently discovered Neolithic 'iceman' given the name Ötzi, who lived about 5,000 years ago, is instructive: he had on him a birch fungus that may have been useful as an antibacterial and perhaps as an anthelminthic (anti-worming agent). More surprisingly, perhaps, Ötzi's body also had tattoos over his lower spine, behind his left knee, and on his right ankle, which have been suggested as spots marking points for something to be inserted to relieve pain. If this is, as some have argued, an early form of acupuncture, it indicates that some medical practices were common across Eurasia.[6] The hint of practices widespread throughout large regions should not surprise us, since people had not only come to Europe from far distances but engaged in certain kinds of commerce that moved precious objects across lengthy human chains of contact.

Later immigrants established cities and composed written records, some of which are extant. Romans, for instance, mainly encouraged a domestic medicine that combined empirical methods with religious practices, documented in parts of some handbooks written for male heads of households. Indeed, in the case of one of the greatest such compilations, by Celsus (fl. *c.*25–*c.*50 CE), only the medical parts remain, commonly going by the title *De medicina* (*On Medicine*). While it contains much information about what people like Celsus himself knew and thought about medicine elsewhere, as among the Greeks, on the whole his work mainly offers practical advice of a mixed religio-empirical kind about treatments—quite in line with the approach of his fellow encyclopaedist, Pliny the Elder, who also wrote of the medicinal virtues of various substances. However, Greek-speaking immigrants, who were known for their philosophical agility, also came to Rome from the East: Archagathus is said to have arrived about 219 BCE and to have been given citizenship because of his medical abilities, while about a century later, Asclepiades of Bythnia made his reputation as an outstanding 'dietetic' physician, that is, the kind of doctor who argued that he understood the underlying causes of natural events, and so could advise on how to live in accordance with one's true constitution in order to maintain or restore health. However, philosophy also grew more respectable among Romans, and in the year 46 CE citizenship was offered to Greek doctors and teachers in Rome, while other major cities within the empire came to appoint municipal physicians conversant in philosophical medicine to help the poor and advise the magistrates. Indeed, Greek philosophy grew well enough for a Greek-speaking philosopher-physician, Galen of Pergamon, to travel to Rome around 161 CE, where he became famous. Over the next fifty years or so he wrote many books, which were so encyclopaedic in character, so astute in formulating questions and answers in clear and precise philosophical language, and so venomous against his rivals, that few of the works of his medico-philosophical predecessors or contemporaries survive.[7]

There were also many new remedies introduced from abroad to Western Europe during the Roman period, flowing in over long-distance trade routes. For instance, cloves and pepper—both from South East Asia—seem to have first appeared in Roman receipts for cooking and medicine around the first century AD. Pliny knew of cane sugar starting to be grown in Egypt after arriving from South Asia, but it was too expensive to be used except as a medicine. It was never easy to match what was known about the medical uses of plants, animals, and minerals with general philosophical principles about the functioning of the body, however. Like encyclopaedic works, then, written pharmaceutical information—even that of the famous compiler Dioscorides (*c.*65 CE), who listed approximately 600 simples—remained empirical, with sources and underlying meanings that are still difficult to decode.[8]

The 'decline of Rome' (evidenced in the sacking of the city in 410) also meant a decline in written medical sources. An in-depth knowledge of ancient philosophical learning, including Greek medicine, remained alive in the Eastern parts of the Roman Empire, but only elements of it remained in the Latin West. One of the places where some basic written traditions about philosophy and learned medicine was retained was the Christian Church. A founder of a monastic group in Italy, Cassiodorus (480–575), wrote down a set of rules that included the requirement to copy texts, ensuring that some literature would survive; such monasteries also set up schools and had infirmaries for the care of inmates and pilgrims. However, the main focus of Christian efforts remained the further development of their religious ideas and practices; indeed, there was a growing reaction against 'pagan' philosophy. When around 600, Isidore, Archbishop of Seville, attempted a summary of all knowledge, including learned medicine, in his *Etymologies*, he was able to squeeze everything into a length amounting to perhaps 300 modern printed pages. By the end of the next century, Western European trade with other places reached a nadir. Since most people relied on local medicines and customary practices, these changes probably indicate little alteration in their resources, although the increased levels of local violence and population decline north of the

Alps from perhaps 12 million in 200 to about 10 million in 600 must have made for some grim moments in many lives.

By around 800, imported spices were again being noticed in Northern Europe, used more for medicine than cooking, and the first drugs related to Arabic pharmacology also began to appear, suggesting that with the revival of urban commerce the pharmacopoeia was expanding. When Anglo-Saxon handbooks began to be written, they were like their Roman predecessors in many ways, including containing a great deal of information about medicines, as well as charms, amulets, and other curative practices.[9] The following centuries brought relative prosperity and a doubling of population between 1000 and 1348. By the later tenth century, a person like Gerbert could acquire a good foundation in Latin classics at his monastic school, put his talents for learning and administration at the service of various powerful political masters, help the Archbishop of Rheims revise and expand the monastic curriculum in the seven liberal arts, and rise to become Pope (as Sylvester II). Some of his followers in southern Italy—a region mixing Latin, Byzantine, Islamic, and Jewish cultures—helped to lay the foundation for an intellectual renaissance in the second half of the eleventh century around the ancient Benedictine Abbey of Montecassino and the nearby archbishopric of Salerno, where Graeco-Latin sources were arranged and epitomized for teaching. One of the translators there, Constantinus Africanus—a merchant born at Carthage in North Africa who had travelled for many years in the East—developed what became a legendary reputation for medical translations from Arabic to Latin produced between about 1077 and 1087. In the next century, Gerard of Cremona became the most famous of the translators, working with Arabic- and Hebrew-speaking colleagues in the religious borderlands of Iberia to make available Latin texts of both ancient and Islamic works, including medical works of Galen, Ibn Sinā's *Al-Qānun*, and al-Rāzi's *al-Hāwi*.

The early history of medicine in Western Europe therefore saw people mainly reliant on local skills and resources, and oral traditions, supplemented from time to time by the availability of texts and practitioners who devoted themselves to medical learning and practice. Medical knowledge might be passed down in families or through apprenticeships. Anyone with a personal interest in finding out more about what could be known through the study of various texts and traditions could set off on the road, inquiring after teachers of reputation and moving on again when they thought the time was right, perhaps eventually settling somewhere and taking on pupils themselves. While there might be 'schools' of thought, there were no formal medical schools, degrees, or licences, only a range of medical practitioners, from the blacksmith who might set broken bones to the local wise woman who knew herbs and spells, to merchants who sold drugs and self-proclaimed philosophers who could read (and sometimes write) medical books, many based on the wisdom of previous generations who lived in far-off lands. Given the widespread movement of people, medicines, and even ideas, few places were cut off from the rest of Europe or the rest of the world: indeed, from what can be discerned about long-distance medical trade and efforts to translate Arabic texts into Latin, medicine was a part of life that showed how willing people were to borrow and adapt if the opportunity occurred.

Corporations and Formulations

One of the consequences of the revival of learning that would change the nature of organizations in Western Europe was the development of something that formalized medical groups in ways unknown elsewhere: the corporation. While the word is used loosely today mainly to indicate large business concerns, it is best understood more generally as a legal fiction derived from Roman law allowing a group of people to stand before the law as one person or body (*corps*). For the particular purposes that brought them together they could sue or be sued, hold property, owe certain defined obligations, and exercise certain defined rights just like a person, but to go on doing so beyond any one person's lifetime. Inside the virtual body, members also had specified rights and duties. Corporations did not depend on or represent the view of one person, but acted as a group according to their governing rules, usually after formal discussion. While medical innovations were produced by individuals, it was very often the acceptance of such innovations by collective and formal organizations, their amalgamation and adaptation to previous work, and their passing on to new generations as good practice that gave them authority. In other words, a new kind of agent or organization now took part in medical interactions, one of long memory and many powers.

By the eleventh and twelfth centuries, it was common for cities to have secured their rights as corporations and, within the cities, groups of merchants and craftspeople to have secured theirs through establishing subordinate corporations, in English usually called guilds: in many places, such as London, the right of citizenship (which granted a person the right to come before a city court and to have a voice in electing certain officials) was itself conferred mainly through membership in one of these corporations. The guild in turn acted to protect the privileges of its members against individual interlopers or corporate rivals.[10] People in medical occupations could be found in some of the early guilds, who over the next centuries split off and founded their own corporations, particularly those of barber-surgeons, surgeons, and apothecaries (the merchants who imported exotic medicines and spices).

Similarly, the founding of the early universities was also the result of teachers or students obtaining corporate rights. At places where large numbers of people gathered to learn from masters—such as at Bologna, a gathering point for teachers of law and their pupils— students banded together to form corporations (around 1150 in this case, using the Latin term *universitas*). By the thirteenth century, by threatening to withdraw from Bologna as a group, the university gained the right to fix the prices of books and lodgings, to set rules for their education, and so forth; the professors in turn formed their own corporation, or *collegium*, which set strict requirements for admission to their group, most importantly the ability to teach a subject as judged by their peers. They therefore established what was in effect a hierarchy of licences to teach, which became the degrees of Master of Arts, and Doctor of Laws, Medicine, and Theology. Given the student-run nature of universities at places such as Bologna, Pavia, and Montpellier, teaching tended to emphasize practical studies, particularly law and medicine. Another kind of university came into being further north that gave more emphasis to philosophy and theology, being governed by the masters rather than students. It is best illustrated by the example of Paris, where the Chancellor of the Cathedral of Notre Dame had the right to license teaching in the diocese. As its reputation as a centre of learning grew, however, not all the students flocking to it could be accommodated by licensed instructors, causing many teachers to establish themselves outside the

Cathedral's legal remit, on the Left Bank of the Seine (or Latin Quarter). When in 1200, conflicts between town and gown grew so heated that some students were killed, the King of France issued a legal declaration granting students and their servants special protections and recognizing an independent body of teaching masters. Further conflicts a couple of decades later led the Pope to grant special privileges to students and masters, introducing a formal certificate of learning (the baccalaureate degree), which became an entry ticket into the rapidly expanding bureaucracies of church and state. The division of faculties came to be fourfold: arts, medicine, law, and theology. In the three higher faculties, teaching rights were granted and degrees conferred based upon the ability to comment upon and debate the content of ancient philosophical texts from the most up-to-date commentaries, which in medicine were based mainly on works translated from Arabic. The university's corporation of professed physicians—the medical faculty—not only came to control teaching, but also attempted to regulate practice as well, sometimes fining or even exiling from Paris those practitioners who refused to obey them. Similar conflicts arose in other university towns.

The significance of the new corporations can be seen during the deadly pandemic known as the Black Death, which first struck Western Europe in 1348–9 and then returned many times over the next three centuries in epidemic waves. It was first introduced into Genoa by merchants returning from the Black Sea, and then spread outward to most of the rest of Europe. A few locales escaped while others experienced up to 90 per cent mortality, with the total loss of life in Western Europe generally estimated to have been well over 30 per cent. Western Europe's population would take two centuries to return to pre-plague numbers. By the time of the Black Death, however, university-educated physicians and apprenticed surgeons and apothecaries could be found in most large cities and in the households of many great men. More importantly to modern eyes, many European cities came to enact quarantine measures overseen by the corporately certified medics in order to prevent anyone suffering from the plague to interact with the healthy. Such steps seem to have been important for gradually limiting the recurrent effects of the disease, until it disappeared from Western Europe. The last major outbreak was confined to Marseilles in 1720.

Despite the high mortality rates from epidemic disease in the late fourteenth and fifteenth centuries, commerce and corporations allowed the cities of Europe to continue to flourish, while efforts were also launched to find sea-borne trade routes south and east around Africa to the wealthy spice-producing lands of South and East Asia. Within Western Europe, as military means of domination shifted from feudal levies to the use of engineers and artillery officers, paid from state revenues, taxable commercial activities were encouraged. Some of the profits of commerce were also reinvested in efforts to rediscover the secrets of antiquity, while others supported innovations in machinery, architecture, and the fine arts. By the end of the fifteenth century, as European commercial ventures expanded into the Indian Ocean and beyond, and into the New World, a flood of entirely new information about the world accumulated rapidly, while grave doubts about accepted opinion also gained ground. The confluence of such developments led to what is called the Renaissance, while the spread of materialist values meant that the struggle for the future of Latin Christendom took on renewed vigour, breaking the Church into multiple and competing institutions during the Reformation.

For medical learning, the critical textual methods of the Renaissance brought to light many classical alternatives to widely received views, while commercial interests also emphasized the importance of accurate information. At the same time, from Asia and the New World came new substances that their proponents claimed were as good or better for treating diseases than anything found earlier. Examining all these claims required physicians to be not only competent in the study of texts and philosophy but also as knowledgeable about natural details as apothecaries, or even more so, causing the first professorship of materia medica to be established at the papal university in Rome in 1514; by the later sixteenth century, almost every university medical faculty with aspirations to conveying up-to-date botanical knowledge sought to have a garden. Municipally employed physicians also asserted their authority over apothecaries by writing pharmacopoeias, which established lists of officially approved simples.[11] However, challenges to accepted methods of treatment emerged from similar sources, such as the introduction of guaiac wood from the Caribbean, which became a very well-regarded treatment for syphilis, although china root and then sarsaparilla (also from the Americas) replaced it. Individuals who offered their own medical innovations flourished and often took advantage of the new medium of print to distribute their views. As an example of what to our eyes was a successful innovation, an incorporated French surgeon, Ambroise Paré (1510–90), famously wrote about his experience in treating gunshot wounds in a military campaign, where he ran out of the hot oil with which it was customary to cauterize them, substituting a mild ointment (the receipt, or recipe, for which he had earlier obtained from an empiric), thereby discovering that those treated by cautery did much worse than the others. While not all empirical remedies had a similar success, a great many lent strength to the voices of practitioners who argued that improvements to human health would come from personal experience rather than study in books. For their part, incorporated practitioners took on board some of the innovations, sometimes adapted new practices and ideas, and other times pushed back or even tried to suppress those they considered to be dangerous.[12]

The most serious challenges to the incorporated medical establishment came from the medical chemists (iatrochemists), whose many successful innovations were often based upon ideas and practices that had no place in the universities or guilds. Partly this was because they fitted badly into the classical tradition. Processes such as glass-making had been known to the Romans, but chemical methods of distillation and other processes of separating substances into their essences (or active substances) and inert matter (or dross) came to Europe in the early medieval period from Asia—probably originally from China—and often bore Arabic names, such as alcohol, alkali, and alchemy. By the thirteenth century, distilling apparatus had become powerful enough to extract the 'quintessence' of wine in the form of *aqua vita* (the water of life), while by the later fifteenth century, all kinds of alcoholic essences (liqueurs) could be extracted from plants, making for powerful cordials (originally, as the name implies, meant to warm and strengthen the heart). Other methods worked with heavy metals such as gold and mercury in order to make them potable, again to strengthen the corporeal powers of the recipient. Many alchemists also struggled to produce a substance called the 'philosophers' stone', or the prime substance from which both gold and the elixir of life could be derived. In the middle of the sixteenth century, the publication of works by a Swiss iatrochemical practitioner and religious reformer best known by his pen name, Paracelsus (1493–1542), became a particular focus for controversy. Thus, while iatrochemistry had the support of many monarchs such as Emperor Rudolph II, Queen Elizabeth I, and King Philip II, its un-classical methods and ideas, and its association with heterodox figures like Paracelsus, also caused many religious and political authorities, as well as the medical establishment, to be suspicious about the implications of this branch of medicine.[13]

Over time, however, corporately affiliated physicians and apothecaries adopted iatrochemical procedures while taming its radicalism with materialism. While one of the best-known chemical authors of the early seventeenth century, the physician and nobleman Joan Baptista van Helmont (1579–1644), further developed Paracelsian ideas about the source of vital powers in the *archeus*, a professor of medicine at Leiden, Franz de le Boë Sylvius (1614–72), discarded previous speculation about immaterial powers. Based on further experimental investigations—by the mid-seventeenth century chemical teaching was a common supplement to the regular medical curriculum—he wrote about fermentation and effervescence (being the first to clearly distinguish them), and divided material substances into fixed salts, acids, and 'volatile salts' (alkalis), which reacted to one another without the intervention of occult powers. The influential textbook published in 1675 by the French royal apothecary Nicholas Lémery (1645–1715) further attacked the 'superstitions' of the alchemists and accounted for chemical reactions according to the sizes and shapes of the particles of which material bodies were made.

Materialism can also be noticed making in-roads in two other famous areas of medical learning, anatomy and physiology. Dissection to inspect the remains of the deceased had begun both among late medieval nuns and other religious groups who were trying to establish the presence of unusual marks in the bodies of those who might be considered to have been particularly saintly, and among surgeons called on to confirm cause of death in cases of possible violence; by the fourteenth century, at the university of Bologna, there also developed occasional public lecturing on anatomy to point out the organs described in the texts. By the early sixteenth century, however,

medical professors and their students were investigating bodies more
closely in order to confirm or deny details found in the freshly edited
classical texts, often coming to criticize sharply the ignorance of the
past. Most famous for this was Andreas Vesalius (1514–64), who
lectured on anatomy at the university of Padua and produced a richly
and carefully illustrated compendium of human anatomy entitled *De
humani corporus fabrica* (*On the Fabric of the Human Body*), first printed in
Basel in 1543.[14] Within a century, the careful materialism of the new
anatomy had led to a radical revision of physiological theory, too, with
the experimental finding that the blood moved in a circuit throughout
the body without the need for spirit to drive it. The Englishman who
published on this in 1628 in *De motu cordis et sanguinis* (*On the Motion of the
Heart and Blood*), William Harvey (1578–1657), fundamentally challenged the view of interdependent relationships among the organs
that had been accepted since Galen's time, throwing open questions
about the purposes of all the bodily parts, and launching a host of new
investigations that were carried out at many places. It also raised
questions about the causes of the motions, which Harvey refused to
speculate about; indeed, he had argued against using older terms such
as *spiritus*. For many thinkers, his account was one of the key ideas that
opened up possibilities for offering complete descriptions of the living
body as a set of material structures operating more or less self-
sufficiently, without the need to invoke a soul. René Descartes
(1594–1650), for example, took a deep interest in chemistry and
anatomy and, based upon the latest research as well as his own
investigations, developed a mechanical account of the body.[15]

At some university medical faculties, then, a subterranean strand of
materialism grew up and persisted, becoming a resource for radical
new views of humankind. At Leiden, for example, Herman Boerhaave
(1668–1738), the most famous medical professor of the early eighteenth century, may have held to a strong personal religious faith, but
he taught that true medical knowledge came from attention to the
material facts, so that understanding the first causes of things was no
business of the physician. Julien Offray de la Mettrie, who had
travelled to Leiden to study with Boerhaave, developed ideas about
how organic processes in the brain and nervous system could account
for all necessary features of life; his book, *L'Homme machine* (1748),
came to be almost universally condemned as a source for radical

sensualism and atheism. In opposition, professors like Georg Ernst Stahl (1659–1734) of Halle, and a variety of teachers at Montpellier, continued to be explicit that vital processes could not be explained without invoking animal spirits of some kind, but they, too, considered chemical and physical investigations to be critical in the discovery of new knowledge.[16]

The sense that true knowledge was tangible also helped to support the rise of surgeons to medical prominence. Much of the growing authority of surgeons came from their usefulness to the state in caring for soldiers and sailors who fought in the numerous wars. However, some came from the surgical techniques developed in the burgeoning hospitals. In France, for instance, after Charles-François Félix (1650–1703) operated successfully on Louis XIV for an anal fistula in 1686 (after practising on numerous hospital inmates), the surgeons gained new legal powers, while under Louis XV and Louis XVI, the Paris surgeons almost became the equals of the university physicians. In their constant encounters with bodies, surgeons also furthered the materialistic point of view.[17]

New treatments also signified the domestication of 'folk' remedies inside corporate medicine. The use of foxglove to stimulate the circulation of the blood, for instance, was introduced to learned physicians by William Withering (1741–99) in a book of 1785, although it started with a complex recipe for dropsy from a traditional healer who worked with charms as well as herbs. Considering that the remedy must derive from a material property of one of the simples in the recipe, Withering finally identified the effects with foxglove (*Digitalis purpurea*). Two other famous methods derived from folk traditions helped to prevent the spread of smallpox. The first was the practice of inoculation, imported to Britain from the Near East and Africa in the second decade of the eighteenth century by Lady Mary Wortley Montague (1689–1762). In 1798, Edward Jenner (1749–1823) published a much better variation on the theme. Instead of inoculating with a mild form of smallpox, he gave his subjects cowpox, following the example of dairymaids in Gloucestershire, who believed that those of them who had contracted this milder disease would not get smallpox. Jenner's method, which came to be called vaccination (after the Latin word for cow, *vaccus*), was quickly taken up and spread throughout the world.

By the eighteenth century, in other words, the waning power of religious institutions and the growing authority of medical commerce and corporate medical bodies that served the state enabled even the professors to agree that the foundations of medical knowledge had been renewed by empirical and experimental studies and, in some cases at least, that the functions of animal bodies and their treatment could be accounted for without recourse to a disembodied soul. While innovations in practice and pronouncement arose from personal initiative, collective debate within the universities and the growing number of other medical institutions of the period, whose governing structures often gave their members security and confidence, enabled such views to be assimilated and to flourish as a new orthodoxy.

The Nation-State and Medicalization

From the end of the eighteenth to the end of the nineteenth century, Western Europe was transformed by urbanization, industrialization, and colonialism, and from the later nineteenth onwards by nation-states that offered material benefits to large segments of the citizenry, including medical services. Medical materialism provided an evidential and theoretical framework for 'improvement' in the conditions of life for Europeans and their fellows, while medical relationships themselves came to depend increasingly on the provision and regulation of public services, from hospitals to health insurance. Informal medical relationships persisted of course, but the redistribution of wealth through taxation, and the control of medical licensing and reimbursement through bureaucratic mechanisms, gave national governments large powers and responsibilities. Their ministers came to see laboratory science and other fields of materialist knowledge as fit devices for making choices about what kinds of changes would most benefit citizens. The state therefore attempted to resolve many problems by placing them under the rubric of medicine, even measuring the success of domestic government itself by counting population figures and disease rates. The 'medicalization' of life in the past century and more has therefore come to be seen as an indication of the power of collective expertise in the service of the state. However, in Western Europe, at least, medicalization was possible due to the expansion and proliferation of corporate bodies and professional organizations, which continued to protect the interests of their members and, in their view, their members' patients.

The most powerful cause of change in the modern era has been the demographic revolution, initially spurred by higher fertility rates rather than falling mortality rates, which led to more than a doubling of the population of Western Europe from about 120 million in 1750 to about 265 million in 1850, despite emigration abroad, particularly to the Americas. Population pressures sped the pace of agricultural and industrial revolution, urbanization and emigration, wealth creation and impoverishment. A feared new epidemic disease, cholera, caused a feeling of occasional public crisis after it first appeared in Europe in 1830 (with subsequent outbreaks in 1847, 1853, and afterward). Many governments stepped in to promote better poor relief, including medical assistance. As always, Europe's connections to the rest of the world had major effects: large portions of the taxable wealth of many European countries that made public improvements possible came from overseas trade and colonies.

Many state policies depended on the collection of numerical information about the population; regular censuses became mandatory in many countries from the late eighteenth century. Statistical studies blossomed. For example, early in the nineteenth century Louis Villermé (1782–1863) studied public hygiene based on numerical data first gathered from the army, then from prison populations, and finally from Parisian neighbourhoods, trying to understand differentials in mortality rates. He assigned the chief reason for disease (and so mortality) to filth, which he in turn associated with poverty. In 1839, England appointed a Registrar General, William Farr (1807–83), who undertook remarkable studies of the causes of mortality; about the same time, the new chief of the Poor Law Commissioners in London, Edwin Chadwick (1800–90), commissioned an initial report and follow-up study to look into the connections between disease and poverty. His *Report on the Sanitary Condition of the Labouring Population of Great Britain* (1842) demonstrated the connections between disease and poverty, making a utilitarian argument for public investment in the means to control disease as a method for holding down the poor rates (and so paying for itself). Friedrich Engels (1820–95), a businessman who was radicalized by what he saw and read, drew heavily on Chadwick's *Report* in his own manifesto of 1845, *The Condition of the*

Working Class in England, which concluded that since society knew that the conditions under which it made people live brought them to premature and unnatural deaths, their deaths should be considered premeditated murder. By the mid-1850s, municipally appointed Medical Officers of Health appeared in London and soon elsewhere, being the eyes and ears on the ground for government officials. While the details of similar arrangements varied in other countries, everywhere the combination of rising urban populations and the linked burdens of poverty and disease made the gathering of medical intelligence critical to government.[18]

By the 1850s, the emphasis in arguments about the causes of disease focused on the ubiquitous organic dirt. In Vienna, in 1847, Ignaz Semmelweis (1818–65) demonstrated that washing of hands in a solution of chlorinated lime prevented the spread of organic morbific particles from the mortuary to the birthing clinic. The outbreak of cholera in London in 1854 pointed to something similar when John Snow (1813–58) traced many deaths from the disease to the Broad Street pump and had its handle removed, after which the disease declined dramatically in that neighbourhood. Florence Nightingale (1820–1920) also waged war against dirt and disease in a successful attempt to lower mortality rates in British hospitals during the Crimean War of 1853–6, and made fresh air and cleanliness the first principles of her subsequent campaigns. The great stinks emanating from urban rivers like the Seine and Thames began to be tackled in massive public works projects that channelled organic filth away and piped in clean water. Although it is difficult to estimate precisely how much sewerage and water projects ameliorated the weight of urban disease and death, the example of the city of Hamburg in 1892 was a lesson to many, when it was devastated by an epidemic of cholera because it had not sufficiently invested in clean water.[19]

The shift in thinking from organic dirt to 'germs', which began in the 1860s, further aided governments in allowing for a more precise determination of the cause of many communicable diseases. It was in turn the product of a new form of corporate organization: the laboratory team, supported by state, university, and philanthropic funding. The idea also had roots in a series of scientific developments in physiology and chemistry that emerged from universities, hospitals, and agricultural research institutes. Publications in 1838 and 1839 by

Matthias Schleiden (1804–81) and Theodore Schwann (1810–82) announced that all parts of living bodies—even teeth—arose from cells; Rudolf Virchow (1821–1902) took this further in the mid-1850s by developing the concept of cellular pathology (thus in his view finally ending humoral pathology), in which the seat of disease was always to be sought in the cell. However, the idea that the causes of disease might themselves be cellular organisms came from a chemist, Louis Pasteur (1822–96), a professor who believed in placing his knowledge at the service of the State. Ingenious experiments concerning the ancient problem of spontaneous generation allowed him to show that micro-organisms did not arise simply from the presence of life-giving air mixed with nutriment, but only from other micro-organisms floating in the air. Even more convincingly, in the later 1870s a German state-sponsored physician, Robert Koch (1843–1910), demonstrated the life cycle of a micro-organism and how it caused the disease of anthrax. During the 1880s and 1890s, increasing numbers of laboratory investigators found a vast range of diseases to be caused by germs.[20] The best field for such studies was often found to be in the European colonies.[21]

Germ theory had large implications for public health. Using government-paid field investigators supported by laboratories, sources of infection could be identified convincingly and cleaned up; waste products could be treated chemically to avoid the circulation of bacteria; the sources of the provision of meat, milk, and other foods could be inspected and withdrawn from commerce if found to harbour dangerous germs; public campaigns could be launched to fight germs in home and kitchen; disease carriers could be identified and treated even if (as in some famous cases of typhoid) they showed no signs of illness themselves. Such measures could be controversial, while some writers, such as Max Joseph von Pettenkofer (1818–1901), a professor of hygiene in Munich, argued that the false optimism of narrowly contagionist arguments like the germ theory would undermine the beneficial effects on health of continuing to fight the causes of poverty and poor living conditions: to make his point, he publicly swallowed a vial of cholera vibrio without ill effects.

The new laboratory science nevertheless quickly gained the backing of governmental authorities, who believed that it would alleviate many social problems by preventing the rampant communicable diseases that so devastated the lives of rich and poor alike. The development of laboratory methods as an adjunct to clinical medicine also held out to governments the possibility to educate, sustain, and distribute through society a new kind of scientific doctor. A newly unified medical profession came into being through bureaucratically controlled medical regulation, the provision of health insurance, and the development of a hospital medicine used by all parts of the social spectrum. It sometimes pitted eminent clinicians, who wanted to retain their own professional autonomy, against ordinary doctors, who welcomed state finance. However, it also established a relatively expensive and effective scientifically oriented medicine as the standard against which any other alternatives would be judged.

Hospitals became one of the chief sites for scientific medicine in the nineteenth and twentieth centuries. In most of Europe, these medical establishments for the sick were part of governmental provision for the poor, but this changed by the end of the nineteenth century. The development of anaesthetic and antiseptic surgery, newly professionalized nursing, and access to the latest techniques of laboratory diagnosis and treatment increasingly caused ordinary people to think of entering hospitals—which had formerly been for the sick poor alone—and paying for treatment there. During the same period, medical staff came to have control over the criteria for admission. The development of a variety of technically difficult diagnostic and treatment regimes turned the attention of admitting doctors to patients who needed specialized services, and doctors in turn became more common members of hospital boards. In all countries of Western Europe, more complicated surgical operations that required special operating theatres, teams of well-trained staff, and special recovery procedures received much attention; but so too did the attached laboratories, which allowed definitive diagnosis in many diseases, radiological procedures following the introduction of X-ray and other electrical devices, blood-typing and blood-banking (after the First World War), and so on. As the 'best' medical care became increasingly associated with the 'most scientifically advanced', hospitals benefited, and medical practitioners had increasing incentives to gain access to hospitals, or at least to gain admitting rights for their patients.[22]

Such spaces helped to shape a new kind of medical profession. The details of how a single medical profession arose differed from country to country, but can be observed to be general throughout Western Europe. In Britain, for instance, while the old corporate bodies survived, the Medical Act of 1858 set up the General Medical Council to oversee the certification processes of the various groups and to establish an official 'list' of all those so qualified. In the German territories, both certification by universities and examination by the state were common, and by the end of the nineteenth century various laws strictly prohibited the practice of anyone not sanctioned by the state. So, too, governments increasingly regulated methods of reimbursement for their state-sanctioned professionals. Between 1883 and 1911, Germany, Austria, Belgium, France, Denmark, Norway, Sweden, and Britain all passed national health insurance legislation, providing reimbursements in cases of sickness, accident, old age, and death. Doctors who wished to participate in the insurance system could often count on a steady income in return for heavy case-loads, although the possibilities for conflict between doctors and bureaucrats over medical treatment also arose. From the early twentieth century, national governments also intervened in the medical market by establishing regulations for foods and drugs. Such measures, coupled with a great investment in sanitation and public health, had important consequences, shifting the burden of disease in the twentieth century from infectious to chronic illness.[23]

By the beginning of the twentieth century, then, Western Europe had been 'medicalized'. Government-sponsored scientific medicine had come to dominate not only measures for the prevention of communicable disease but the provision of health care, the regulation of foods and medicines, and even the possibilities of medical consultation for ordinary people. Stimulated by the crisis of the Second World War and the subsequent 'welfare state', medicine in Western Europe continued to become ever more scientized and bureaucratically controlled, although from the later 1960s onward, alternative strategies were at work to encourage a more patient-centred approach within the overall framework of government-provided health care. On the other hand, as governments have come to regulate, pay for, and even control institutions managing the delivery of health care, the corporate groups that have overseen medical education and training, professional ethics and standards, and the approbation of new methods and ideas have come to feel more and more disempowered:

fear of the loss of professional autonomy remained powerful in the twentieth century.

Conclusion

Simple models of the contemporary world often pit the private sphere against the public sphere, with government provision of medical care contrasted to privately paid care. Obviously, this is far too simple a view. When in need, people still often rely on themselves, family, friends, neighbours, and nearby medical practitioners, whom they may compensate by returning favours or other personal credits, or by payment. But they also turn to 'regular' medical practitioners, that is, those regulated by a corporation or government body. Corporations of various kinds have, since the eleventh century, taken on the responsibility of certification and licensing, and inspection and regulation, of their members and other practitioners. Governments—at first municipal, and later national—found it in their interest to enable corporations, and to referee disputes among them, as a means of allying these 'private' bodies with a view of the public interest. In more recent decades, patients may seek out only those practitioners allowed compensation through insurance or public payment—which are in turn regulated by national governments or backed by public revenues—or they may simply appear at clinics or hospitals overseen and funded by government. In that sense, the layers of medical assistance continue to range from the personal to the public, and payment to range from the informal to the monetary to a form of public investment. Practitioners and educators themselves, however, remain aware of the importance of professional corporations, which can still mobilize voluntary work on behalf of their members. Western Europeans have always been connected to other places and practices as well, and owe much of their knowledge and wealth to them. But it may be in the legal form of corporate groups, whose members engage in activities that continue to form a kind of citizenship in their institutions, with associated duties and privileges, that one of the most important and enduring legacies of the medicine of Western Europe can be seen, however much they may now be considered under threat from new forms of the nation-state. National governments in turn feel as never before an intense public scrutiny on the question of provision of medical services and a public health infrastructure. Medicine is certainly no longer a private affair, although it is not simply a public one, either.

It might be possible, then, to say this about medicine in Western Europe: when people inhabiting the region have attempted to prevent, ameliorate, or relieve the ills of body and mind, they have always done so in a variety of ways. However, the development of certain kinds of legal forms as constitutive of public life allowed both for long-lived corporations to come into being and for them to grow into formations that framed the collection of people, activities, and ideas that we call medicine. Medical activities organized around corporate bodies have shaped the recruitment and expenditure of effort and resources so as give rise to a kind of official medicine that has framed discussion of other ideas and practices and has furthered the development of political economies and populations that consider health to be one of the key measures of the good. Perhaps it is possible to begin to imagine a history of medicine in Western Europe that sees 'ideas' and 'practices' not as distinct subsets of a 'medical tradition', but as abstractions flowing from the organization of effort and attention on problems relating to preventing illness and prolonging life.

Notes

1 Lawrence I. Conrad et al., *The Western Medical Tradition, 800 bc to ad 1800* (Cambridge: Cambridge University Press, 1995); William F. Bynum et al., *The Western Medical Tradition 1800 to 2000* (Cambridge: Cambridge University Press, 2006).

2 For one clear formulation of the ideology, see the later edition of a book first published in 1960, W. W. Rostow, *The Stages of Economic Growth: A Non-Communist Manifesto*, 3rd edn (Cambridge: Cambridge University Press, 1990).

3 See, for instance, the definition of 'civilization' in Marshall G. S. Hodgson, *Rethinking World History: Essays on Europe, Islam, and World History*, ed. Edmund Burke, III (Cambridge: Cambridge University Press, 1993), 81–5.

4 For some recent examples, see Conrad et al., *The Western Medical Tradition*; Bynum et al., *The Western Medical Tradition 1800 to 2000*; Roy Porter, *The Greatest Benefit to Mankind: A Medical History of Humanity* (New York: Norton, 1998); Jacalyn Duffin, *History of Medicine: A Scandalously Short Introduction* (Toronto: University of Toronto Press, 1999). For further accounts of the historiography, see Frank Huisman and John Harley Warner (eds), *Locating Medical History: The Stories and Their Meanings* (Baltimore: Johns Hopkins University Press, 2004).

5 Paolo Palladino and Michael Worboys, 'Science and Imperialism', *Isis* 84 (1993), 91–102; Shula Marks, 'What is Colonial about Colonial Medicine? And What Has Happened to Imperialism and Health?', *Social History of Medicine* 10 (1997), 205–19; Warwick Anderson, 'Postcolonial Histories of Medicine', in Huisman and Harley Warner (eds), *Locating Medical History*, 285–306.

6 L. Capasso, 'A Preliminary Report on the Tattoos of the Val Senales mummy', *Journal of Paleopathology* 5 (1993), 173–82.

7 Owsei Temkin, *Galenism: Rise and Decline of a Medical Philosophy* (Ithaca: Cornell University Press, 1973).

8 For a fresh approach, see Laurence M. V. Totelin, *Hippocratic Recipes: Oral and Written Transmission of Pharmacological Knowledge in Fifth- and Fourth-Century Greece* (Leiden: Brill, 2009).

9 Michael McCormick, *Origins of the European Economy: Communications and Commerce, AD 300–900* (New York: Cambridge University Press, 2002), 791; Linda E. Voigts, 'Anglo Saxon Plant Remedies and the Anglo Saxons', *Isis* 70 (1979), 250–68.

10 Antony Black, *Guilds and Civil Society in European Political Thought from the Twelfth Century to the Present* (New York: Methuen, 1984).

11 Jerome J. Bylebyl, 'The School of Padua: Humanistic Medicine in the Sixteenth Century', in Charles Webster (ed.), *Health, Medicine and Mortality in the Sixteenth Century* (Cambridge: Cambridge University Press, 1979), 335–70.

12 Harold J. Cook, *The Decline of the Old Medical Regime in Stuart London* (Ithaca: Cornell University Press, 1986).

13 Bruce T. Moran, *Distilling Knowledge: Alchemy, Chemistry, and the Scientific Revolution* (Cambridge, MA: Harvard University Press, 2005); Charles Webster, *Paracelsus: Medicine, Magic and Mission at the End of Time* (New Haven, CT: Yale University Press, 2008).

14 Katherine Park, *Secrets of Women: Gender, Generation, and the Origins of Human Dissection* (New York: Zone, 2006); Andrea Carlino, *Books of the Body: Anatomical Ritual and Renaissance Learning*, trans. John Tedeschi and Anne C. Tedeschi (Chicago: University of Chicago Press, 1999).

15 Thomas Fuchs, *The Mechanisation of the Heart: Harvey and Descartes* (Rochester: University of Rochester Press, 2001).

16 Kathleen Wellman, *La Mettrie: Medicine, Philosophy and Enlightenment* (Durham, NC: Duke University Press, 1992).

17 Owsei Temkin, 'The Role of Surgery in the Rise of Modern Medical Thought', *Bulletin of the History of Medicine* 25 (1951), 248–59; Toby Gelfand, *Professionalizing Modern Medicine: Paris Surgeons and Medical Science and Institutions in the Eighteenth Century* (Westport, CT: Greenwood, 1980); Laurence Brockliss and Colin Jones, *The Medical World of Early Modern France* (Oxford: Clarendon Press, 1997).

18 Anne Hardy, *The Epidemic Streets: Infectious Disease and the Rise of Preventive Medicine, 1856–1900* (Oxford: Clarendon Press, 1993); François Delaporte, *Disease and Civilization: The Cholera in Paris, 1832*, trans. Arthur Goldhammer (Cambridge, MA: MIT Press, 1986).

19 Dorothy Porter (ed.), *The History of Public Health and the Modern State* (Amsterdam: Rodopi, 1995); Christopher Hamlin, *Public Health and Social Justice in the Age of Chadwick: Britain, 1800–1854* (Cambridge: Cambridge University Press, 1998); Richard Evans, *Death in Hamburg: Society and Politics in the Cholera Years 1830–1910* (Oxford: Oxford University Press, 1987).

20 Gerald L. Geison, *The Private Science of Louis Pasteur* (Princeton: Princeton University Press, 1995); Christoph Gradmann, *Laboratory Disease: Robert Koch's Medical Bacteriology*, trans. Elborg Forster (Baltimore: Johns Hopkins University Press, 2009).

21 Bruno Latour, *The Pasteurization of France*, trans. Alan Sheridan and John Law (Cambridge, MA: Harvard University Press, 1988); Mark Harrison and Biswamoy Pati (eds), *Health, Medicine and Empire: Perspectives on Colonial India* (New Delhi: Orient Longman, 2001); Warwick Anderson, *The Collectors of Lost Souls: Turning Kuru Scientists into Whitemen* (Baltimore: Johns Hopkins University Press, 2008).

22 Mary E. Fissell, *Patients, Power, and the Poor in Eighteenth-Century Bristol* (Cambridge: Cambridge University Press, 1991); Guenter B. Risse, *Mending Bodies, Saving Souls: A History of Hospitals* (New York/Oxford: Oxford University Press, 1999).

23 Dorothy Porter, *Health, Civilization, and the State: A History of Public Health From Ancient to Modern Times* (London: Routledge, 1999).

Select Bibliography

Brockliss, Laurence, and Colin Jones, *The Medical World of Early Modern France* (Oxford: Clarendon Press, 1997).

Bynum, W. F., *Science and the Practice of Medicine in the Nineteenth Century* (Cambridge: Cambridge University Press, 1994).

Carlino, Andrea, *Books of the Body: Anatomical Ritual and Renaissance Learning*, trans. John Tedeschi and Anne C. Tedeschi (Chicago: University of Chicago Press, 1999).

Delaporte, François, *Disease and Civilization: The Cholera in Paris, 1832*, trans. Arthur Goldhammer (Cambridge, MA: MIT Press, 1986).

Evans, Richard, *Death in Hamburg: Society and Politics in the Cholera Years 1830–1910* (Oxford: Oxford University Press, 1987).

Fissell, Mary E., *Patients, Power, and the Poor in Eighteenth-Century Bristol* (Cambridge: Cambridge University Press, 1991).

Geison, Gerald L., *The Private Science of Louis Pasteur* (Princeton: Princeton University Press, 1995).

Gradmann, Christoph, *Laboratory Disease: Robert Koch's Medical Bacteriology*, trans. Elborg Forster (Baltimore: Johns Hopkins University Press, 2009).

Hamlin, Christopher, *Public Health and Social Justice in the Age of Chadwick: Britain, 1800–1854* (Cambridge: Cambridge University Press, 1998).

Hardy, Anne, *The Epidemic Streets: Infectious Disease and the Rise of Preventive Medicine, 1856–1900* (Oxford: Clarendon Press, 1993).

Harrison, Mark, and Biswamoy Pati (eds), *Health, Medicine and Empire: Perspectives on Colonial India* (New Delhi: Orient Longman, 2001).

Nutton, Vivian, *Ancient Medicine* (New York: Routledge, 2004).

Park, Katherine, *Secrets of Women: Gender, Generation, and the Origins of Human Dissection* (New York: Zone, 2006).

Porter, Dorothy, *Health, Civilization, and the State: A History of Public Health from Ancient to Modern Times* (London: Routledge, 1999).

Risse, Guenter B., *Mending Bodies, Saving Souls: A History of Hospitals* (New York/Oxford: Oxford University Press, 1999).

Webster, Charles, *Paracelsus: Medicine, Magic and Mission At the End of Time* (New Haven, CT: Yale University Press, 2008).

Worboys, Michael, *Spreading Germs: Disease Theories and Medical Practice in Britain, 1865–1900* (Cambridge: Cambridge University Press, 2000).

4

Medicine in Islam and Islamic Medicine

Hormoz Ebrahimnejad

The term 'Islamic medicine' has appeared to many historians loaded with religious overtones, which they often found necessary to dispel by long warnings that it was not exclusively Islamic or Arabic, but included also works of non-Arab and non-Moslem scholars, such as Persians, Jews, Indians, or even Europeans.[1] 'Islamic medicine' suggests a homogeneous system, regardless of the fact that such a term was never used either by laity or by physicians in Islamic countries before the nineteenth century, whereas 'medicine in Islam' contained a wide range of practices and theories from humoral to folk practice and faith and magic healing. For two reasons, however, we might call this medicine 'Islamic': firstly, because it was developed under the Islamic rulers' patronage; and secondly, because it was part of the intellectual process of the formation of Islam itself by associating religion and science, illustrated in the curriculum of the *madrasa*s (Islamic colleges).

Medical histories produced since the nineteenth century have not delved into the intellectual and socio-political factors behind the choice of the term 'Islamic'. The aim of this chapter is not to provide a history of 'Islamic medicine', but to examine the key developments that led to its formation, by addressing its theoretical, practical, and institutional features and the ways in which these features were formed and developed in relation to both pre-Islamic and Islamic resources. The dilemma created by a pre-Islamic and Islamic dichotomy was experienced and discussed by Islamic scholars down to the modern period.[2] Yet, the 'superiority' and distinction of Islam, as a new religion and rising political power, was to be asserted all the more because it borrowed from pagan cultures. It was this endeavour that eventually informed the development of medicine in Islam examined in this chapter.

Medicine in Early Islam

Contemporary sources that could inform us about the state of medical knowledge and practice at the time of the prophet Mohammad (570–632) are extremely scant. The major reliable source would be the Koran itself but the Koran contains nothing about medicine other than advices such as 'how the faithful should wash for prayer when they are sick,' or 'honey has curing effect,' or 'eat and drink but not to excess.'[3] The sayings of the Prophet on the matter of health and medicine were transmitted orally through generations before being collected and published posthumously under the title of *Tibb al-nabi* (*Medicine of the Prophet*), and thus it may not represent the unaltered form of Bedouin medicine during Mohammad's time. Nevertheless, emphasis on invocation and the healing effect of prayers in Prophetic medicine is reminiscent of the supernatural healing methods in the Bedouin Arabia. Magic and supernatural healing were accompanied by physical treatments such as cupping, cautery, venesection, and bone-setting,[4] practices that may have had local origin and were not necessarily borrowed from Greek medicine.[5]

In the Koran, jinn, as a supernatural spirit, as well as man, are created to pray to Allah.[6] This concept of jinn is not unrelated to the jinn in contemporary popular culture, which can either cause illness or restore health.[7] The animistic conception of illness, according to which diseases were considered as spiritual beings inhabiting humans, might find its roots in the idolatry that was widespread among tribes of the Arabian Peninsula.[8] However, as in every other society, magic or faith healing was coupled or alternated with medical treatment, which in this case was predominantly based on everyday experience. Medicinal effects of herbs and foods were known and the same customs continued with Islam. In time, some of these items would carry religious connotations. The date, the staple food at the time of the Prophet, has become in some Islamic countries a sacred diet, and donating dates especially in religious festivals is said to be rewarded.

Affinities between Islam, Judaism, and Christianity, illustrated in the terms and concepts common to the Koran and the Old and New Testaments, had parallels in the field of medicine. Arab populations were either within the remit of the two empires of Persia and Byzantium or in relation with them, whence some similarities in medical knowledge and practice emerged.[9] The use of Greek terms in contemporary Arab poetry bears witness to the influence of Greek medicine there.[10] This influence grew in the century following Islam's conquering of regions belonging to the Byzantine and Persian empires. In the oral literature, one finds some anatomical knowledge of organs of the body, such as liver, heart, spleen, stomach, and bowels. The liver is the seat of hunger, thirst, and passion (including anger), the kidneys are the seat of greed, and the place of intellect is in the brain.[11] The Prophet, advising that in the treatment of headache by cupping the cup should not be placed in the nape of the neck, followed this popular physiology, according to which the cerebellum is the site of memory.[12]

Principles of Galenico-Islamic Medicine

Most Islamic medical tracts were meant to be comprehensive, dealing with pathology, aetiology, pharmacology, anatomy, psychology, rules for preservation or restoration of health, and so on. Al-Rāzi, or Rāzi (865–925), defines medicine as the 'art of preserving the health, combating disease and restoring health to the sick'.[13] Medicine, following the formulation of Ḥunayn ibn Isḥāq (809–73), is divided into theoretical and practical fields.[14] According to Ibn Sinā, or Avicenna (980–1038), theoretical medicine, *ṭibb nazari*, meant learning about the 'principles' of medicine; for instance, fevers are of three categories, and temperaments are of nine types. Practical medicine, *ṭibb 'amali*, consisted of methods of practice. 'To treat hot inflammation, for instance, the practitioner should apply a drug that stops the inflammation growing, followed by a cooling drug before adding to these an emollient drug.'[15] Sometimes practical medicine equates to 'manual' medicine or surgery. For Ibn Riḍwān (988–1061), practical medicine signified 'the study of restoration of fractured bones, luxation, incision, stitches, cautery, perforation, ophthalmology and all other surgical procedures'.[16] Usually, medical tracts begin with general and theoretical themes, such as humours, fevers, symptoms, and anatomy, and then explore pharmacology and the prescription of drugs to prevent or cure diseases.

The two main sources of Islamic pharmacology are Dioscorides' *On Medicinal Substance* and Galen's *On the Powers of Simple Drugs*. Dioscorides assigned to each substance (plant, mineral, and animal) attributes such as softening, warming, astringent, diuretic, and emetic. Galen fine-grained the quality of the drugs in four different degrees, from the weakest to the strongest, so that each drug was further qualified. Pepper is hotter than nard, because it is hot in the third degree while nard is hot in the second degree.[17] Physicians were not always unanimous on the quality of drugs. In India, *bannā'*, for instance, was considered to be cold but Hakim Mohammad Sharif believed that 'even the sour *bannā'* is not devoid of hot quality, while sweet *bannâ'*, a drug that increases potency and strengthens the stomach, is hot in the second degree and dry in the third.[18] In therapeutics, the appropriate degree of drugs' qualities was used according to the state of health or the intensity of the malady. To cure an illness, Rāzi recommended diet in the first place; but if the illness was too complicated to be healed by diet, he prescribed simple or compound drugs according to the strength of the disease.[19] According to Arzāni, *Qarābādin* is a Greek term that signifies a compound drug.[20] Ibn Sinā, who devotes the fifth volume of his *al-Qānun fi'l-Ṭibb* [*Canon of Medicine*] to this subject, attributes the necessity of compound drugs to the fact that usually diseases are complex and often develop from the combination of several pathological problems.[21]

The idea of humours circulating inside the body seems to be a projection of the image of observed liquids flowing out of the body (such as blood and pus). However, the theory of humour incorporating this universal concept belongs to Hippocrates, and in the form that is known today was elaborated by Galen (129–216).[22] According to this theory, the human body is made of three parts: organs (*aʿḍā*, plural of *ʿuḍv*), which are solid; humours (*akhlāt*, pl. of *khilṭ*), which are liquid; and spirits, or pneumata (*arvāḥ*, pl. of *ruḥ*).[23] There are four humours: blood (*dam*), black bile (*sawdā*), yellow bile (*ṣafrā*), and phlegm (*balgham*). Each humour (*khilṭ*) corresponds to two of the four primary qualities, which are also called *mizāj* (temperament)—*mizâj* literally meaning a mixture of different qualities: thus blood is hot and moist, black bile is cold and dry, yellow bile is hot and dry, and phlegm is cold and wet.[24] If the quality and quantity of these humours *(khilṭ* also means mixture) in the body are generally balanced, the person is healthy. An imbalance of humours causes illness, which can be cured when balance is restored.

Not only man but also everything in the universe, including seasons, planets, plants, animals, and drugs, was associated with humoral theory. An inflammation caused by excess or putrefaction of blood should be treated by applying drugs of cold temperament.[25] Each season, having specific temperament and quality (cold, humid, hot, or dry), can also cause illness or be useful for its treatment. The end of the autumn and the beginning of the winter is said to generate pestilences.[26] Prognosis of the course of a disease depended on the phases and motion of the moon and 'mineral, vegetal and animal products associated with the individual planets and zodiac signs were gathered at the astrologically favourable moments and were combined into drugs that were specific for diseases caused by the stars.'[27]

Greek Science and Islamic Medicine

In the middle of the eleventh century in the city of Neishābur, in the eastern part of the Abbasid Caliphate, a renowned physician, 'Abd al-Rahmān ibn Abi Sādeq-e Neishāburi (died after 1068), was surnamed Buqrāt-e Thāni (Hippocrates the Second). The use of such titles after the names of Greek physicians, frequent in Islamic history, demonstrates Greek intellectual influence in Islam. Although scholars differ in details, generally they support the idea that the assimilation of Greek science by Islam was the continuation of pre-Islamic Greek influence in the regions where Islam had expanded, a fact mainly due to the propagation of Hellenism in the aftermath of conquests by Alexander of Macedonia. Not only Eastern Christianity, represented by the Nestorians of Nisibis and Edessa, but also Zoroastrian religion was influenced by Hellenistic ideas, and particularly Aristotelianism.[28] The main channel of Greek influence was, according to Montgomery Watt, the living tradition in different schools in Alexandria (Egypt), Gondishāpur (southwest of Iran), and Harrān (southeast of Turkey). However, this influence gained particular momentum with the transfer of the Alexandrian school, dominated by Aristotelian philosophy, first to Antioch in about 718, and a century later to Harrân and then to Baghdad, in the form of immigration of teachers and partly their library.[29]

According to Manfred Ullmann, the key factor in the transmission of Greek sciences into Islam is to be found in the Christianization of the south and east of the Mediterranean. With Christianity the Greek language was no longer the lingua franca and Greek sciences were translated into local languages, such as Syriac, Coptic, and Pahlavi, and with the advent of Islam, they needed to be translated into Arabic. At the same time, Christianization also changed the syllabus by eliminating poetry, tragedy, and historiography and keeping philosophy, medicine, and exact sciences. This trend, Ullmann states, was inherited particularly by Islam because Islamic theology encouraged the adoption of these sciences due to the fact that logic and dialectic helped give Islamic religion dogmatic basis.[30] Dimitri Gutas, on the other hand, finds the origin of the integration of Greek sciences not in the continuation of the intellectual development under the aegis of the School of Edessa and the eastern Christian tradition, but in the transfer of a Sasanian imperial ideology to Islam, which encouraged the Abbasid caliphate to translate Greek sciences into Arabic.[31]

We should not, however, neglect religious opposition to the continuity of Greek culture. Conversion to Christianity in the Byzantine Empire led to the development of orthodoxy, which banned pagan Greek science. A similar phenomenon occurred in the Sasanian Empire. Consecutive with the centralization of power by Ardeshir-e Pâpakân and the reform of Zoroastrian religion by eliminating its pagan elements, the counsels of the Zoroastrian priesthood, who played an important role in the administration of the Empire, forbade all worship except the Zoroastrian faith and the 'sword of Aristotle (as the polytheism and philosophy of the Greeks was called) was broken'.[32] However, unlike the Byzantines, the Sasanids for political reasons accommodated the members of non-Magian religious groups. This strategy foreshadowed the way Moslems dealt with non-Moslem subjects.[33]

What gave Greek science special status in Islam, compared with the eclectic tendency of the Sasanian period, was the vital importance of Aristotelian theology for the elaboration of its dogma, via the Neo-Platonism borrowed from the Alexandrian School because its tenets were close to Koranic monotheism.[34] The intellectual debates and political conflicts between the Mu'tazilites and Ash'arites, and finally the triumph of the traditionalists, such as al-Ghazzāli (1058–1111), who were opposed to philosophy but made use of it, bear witness to the new dynamics created by the expansion and formation of Islam as religion and political power.

The inherent relationship between philosophy and medicine, embodied in the Arabic term *hakīm* (physician-philosopher) for physician, is based on Aristotelian natural philosophy (*hikmat tabī'ī*). The dilemma of 'essence' and 'matter', the order of their generations, their different qualities and temperaments, the composition of man from soul and body, the perennial character of the former and the decaying nature of the latter, and their link to the universe as conceived by Aristotle, gave a central place to medicine in the Islamic sciences. It is thus not surprising that medicine and astrology were, respectively, the first and second in importance in the translation movement.

Hunayn ibn Isḥāq (809–73) claimed to have translated no less than 129 works, most of them Hippocratic texts as summarized by Galen, including the Aphorisms of Hippocrates (*Foṣul Buqrât*). He also translated Aristotle's *Categories*, *Organon*, and *Physics*, Euclid's *Elements*, and Plato's *Republic*. In general, Hunayn translated ninety-five books of Galen into Syriac and thirty-nine into Arabic. Another seventy books were translated into Arabic and six into Syriac by his pupils.[35] Many other translations were made from Greek sciences into Arabic before Hunayn. Thanks to this culture of translation, many books authored by Greek scholars and later lost in their original survived in Arabic versions. For instance, Galen's *On the Examination of the Doctor* is not known in Greek, but there are two Arabic copies of this book in Alexandria and Bursa. Similarly, only four short passages of Galen's commentary on Hippocrates' *About the Atmosphere* have been preserved in Greek, quoted by Oribasius (320–400). However, in the ninth century, Ḥunayn translated this commentary into Syriac and his pupil Hubaysh translated the Syriac version into Arabic.[36] Fragments of lost Greek works have also survived in Arabic translation, such as the collection of twenty-one clinical reports from Rufus.[37] To these should be added other Arabic translations of Greek books no longer extant, but we know about them via their being quoted by later scholars. This is the case of Galen's *De demonstratione*, used by Rāzi and Ibn Rushd (d. 1198 CE).[38]

The integration of Greek medicine by Islam was part of the process
of the formation of Islam itself: 'The Abbasid caliphs could not allow
discord and differences between theologians and those interested in
legal questions and brought pressure to bear on them to overcome
their disagreement and form a common outlook.'[39] In this sense, the
development of science, including medicine, in Islam was tightly
linked to the establishment of their power and the elaboration of
Islam as a religion. This process influenced the way medicine in
Islam was conceived and practised. All aspects of knowledge and
techniques, which needed to be assimilated, received the blessing of
religion. In an important number of tracts, often after the tenth
century, an introductory passage refers to the sayings of the Prophet
or the Koran to bless medical knowledge and justify its education.
Al-ʿilm-ʿilmān: ʿilm al-abdān wa ʿilm al-adyān ('Sciences are twofold:
science of the body and science of religion') is the most often quoted.[40]
Some authors even go as far as claiming that the science of the body
(*ʿilm al-abdān*) is more important than the science of religion (*ʿilm al-
adyān*), because without a healthy body the faithful cannot accurately
perform their religion.

The Format of Islamic Medical Literature

The Greek literary format, adopted by Islamic scholars through
translation, framed the development of medical knowledge in Islam
and informed medical education. Most medical texts translated by
Hunayn and his pupils consisted of commentaries and summaries for
educational purposes. Hunayn perhaps followed the Alexandrian
medical literature that mainly comprised the canon of sixteen books
by Galen and the corresponding *Summaria alexandrinorum* (Alexandrian
epitomes). No less than thirteen commentaries were written on the
Canon of Ibn Sinā. Often the authors claim that the purpose of their
commentaries was to clarify obscure points or to correct erroneous
ideas or interpretations in medicine. Be that as it may, commentary in
the Islamic medical literature was a style and method of writing rather
than a method for providing critical work. For example, the *Shokuk ʿalā
Jālinus (Doubts on Galen)* of Rāzi, a criticism of Galen, was in turn
criticized by Ibn Abi Ṣādeq Neishaburi, known as Buqrāt thāni. An
illustrative example is the six commentaries written by Ibn Riḍwān on

Galen's books, despite the fact that Ibn Riḍwān criticized commentary literature as the cause of the decline of medicine: 'Summaries fail to encompass all Galen's ideas, while commentaries increase the length of the art, and distract [students] from studying, since, of necessity, these would have to be read for verification together with their [original] works.'[41]

The forms of question and answer or medical aphorisms in the style of poems represent other 'pre-Islamic' literary formats adopted by Islamic physicians. One of the ophthalmologic treatises of Hunayn, the *Masā'il fi l-'ayn* (*Book of Questions on the Eye*), on the physiology and pathology of the eye, was couched in the form of question and answer,[42] as was another major work by Hunayn, *Masā'il fi l-ṭibb* (*Questions on Medicine*). Commentaries on a master's work constitute perhaps the bulk of medical literature in Islam as they were popular in the medical circles of late Antique Alexandria.[43] Sometimes treatises were written by eminent physicians with exactly the same titles as those of their Greek predecessors. Rāzi wrote a tract called *Man lā yaḥḍuruhu Tabib* (*He Who Has No Physician to Attend Him*), following Rufus and Oribasius.[44] In the more recent period, too, physicians followed the model of their medieval predecessors. The abridged (*saghira*) and extended (*kabira*) formats of *vabā'iyye* (on cholera) of Shirāzi in the mid-nineteenth century[45] are reminiscent of the Small and Large Compendiums by Ibn Sarābiyun in the ninth century.[46]

Along with the external configuration of medical texts, different medical paradigms developed by the Greek, and particularly Alexandrian, schools of medicine, including clinical medicine, anatomy, and surgery, and the relationship between magic/religion and medicine, were introduced. The Alexandrian School was home to an intellectual movement much influenced by Aristotle and the dogmatics who laid emphasis on the importance of anatomy. Unlike Rufus, who focused more on clinical and bedside medicine, Galen reconciled philosophy, clinical medicine, and anatomy, producing a synthesis of various tendencies, such as dogmatism and empiricism, as well as various approaches found among the Hippocratics.[47] This synthesis is important because during the Hellenistic period these tendencies were irreconcilable to the extent of being considered as antagonistic sects. Even the Hippocratic authors were not unanimous on humoral theory.[48] Controversies divided also Islamic physicians. Mirzā Qāzi ibn Kāshef,

writing in the seventeenth century, in his Commentary on the work of
'Emād al-Din Mahmud on china root, contended that matters are not
made of one quality but of a combination of different humours and
qualities, and therefore treating diseases by prescribing a drug of
opposite quality (cold, hot, wet or dry) was not appropriate. For
instance, china root is hot according to the perceived opinion but it
is used to treat syphilis (*atashak*) that is also hot, which is a contradiction
in principle. The fact, however, is that china root, like many other
matters such as lentil, rose, or wine, is *morakkab-alqovā*, that is composed of different properties.[49]

Magic and Medicine

Magic and incantation were the dominant features of medical outlook
in pre-Islamic Arabia. The epidemic of plague in 541, for instance,
was attributed to jinn, commissioned by the enemies. A person
affected by fever was considered to have been penetrated by a supernatural spirit. These beliefs corresponded to the idolatry culture and
worship of objects and gods, which was opposed by the new mono-
theist religion preached by Mohammad. It comes thus as no surprise
to see that Islam opposed animism and incantation.[50] However, this
opposition was religiously or politically inspired and for this reason
magical outlook in diagnosis and healing was simply dressed in the
new Islamic garb: God replaced magical objects. Since He sent
disease, He was the only one who could remove it.[51] Just as in the
plague of the middle of the sixth century, magic played a significant
role in popular responses to the Black Death in the fourteenth
century.[52]

The outcome was the reconciliation of old customs with newly
introduced medicine based on humoral physiology, epitomized in
the medicine of the Prophet. This phenomenon set a theoretical
framework for blending or juxtaposing rational and irrational medicine in Islam. In the middle of the nineteenth century, Mirzā Musā
Sāvaji devotes the first part of his treatise on *vabā* (cholera) to the
standard medical methods of healing, based on humoral theories, and
the second part to prayers and cryptograms and 'letter magic' for both
prevention and treatment of cholera.[53] The systematic and sustained
juxtaposition of rational and magic medicine in Islamic medical

literature bears witness to the style borrowed from Greek literature while tapping into the above-said cultural and social heritage. Magic did exist in Galen's works, although in a reserved and moderate form in regard to medical treatment. However, Alexander of Tralles (late sixth century) allowed free rein to these irrational tendencies alongside exposing Galenic teaching.[54] Likewise, one finds close similarities between medical tracts, such as the *Mokhtaṣar-e mofid* and *Khavāṣṣ al-ashyā'*, in which the magic effects of objects and items are underlined in the treatment of diseases,[55] and the book of Xenocrates of Aphrodisias (*c*.70 CE), 'who recommended cures based on sympathetic magic using parts of organs, secretions and secreta from men and animals'.[56] Rāzi also occasionally recommended treatment by sympathetic magic.[57]

Anatomy and Surgery

Anatomy is the theoretical knowledge of the structure of the body, obtained through the practice of dissection, for the benefit of surgery, pathology, and medical treatment. All these branches of medicine were dealt with in the works of Hippocrates and Galen as translated into Arabic. The books on dissection translated into Arabic included *The Great Book on Dissection*,[58] *Dissection of the Dead Animals*, *Dissection of the Living Animals*, *On Hippocrates Knowledge of Dissection*, and *Aristotle's Knowledge of Dissection*.[59] But none of these texts appears in the *Summaria Alexandrinorum*, which comprised the textbooks of medical students in Islam.

Galenic discourse on the importance of anatomical knowledge, acquired through dissection, was always emphasized by Islamic physicians. However, such an emphasis was not to respond to the necessity of practical dissection. While commentaries or compendia, such as the Canon of Ibn Sinā and the Kāmel al-Ṣenāʻa of al-Majusi, include chapters on anatomy, Islamic physicians did not author even one book similar to Galen's books on dissection. The purpose of anatomy was to know the place and location of nerves, veins, and bones to avoid mistakes in bloodletting or bone-setting. The aim of acquiring knowledge of the body was also to be aware of the miracles of Creation and to be able to receive the knowledge of God.[60] Anatomical knowledge in Islamic literature was entirely based on Galen's findings, and anatomists did not seem concerned to state that 'since Galen had observed perfectly the body and described it, they did not need to undertake dissection of their own.'[61] It is highly significant that Rāzi, in his 'Examination of Physicians' (*Miḥnat al-aṭibbā wata'yeenihi*), specifies that in addition to theoretical and practical knowledge, students should also have knowledge of anatomy, vivisection, and astronomy.[62] However, as far as we know there is no record indicating that Rāzi himself undertook any vivisection or even dissection of humans or animals. It appears that Rāzi points to dissection or vivisection not because he found it necessary, but because Galen had indicated this necessity in his treatise on 'Examining Physicians'.[63]

The *Tashriḥ-e Manṣuri* of Ibn Elyâs is the only book that contains diagrams of veins, bones, and nerves not found in Galen's books. In some copies, illustrations of the fetus are added. However, it seems that Ibn Elyâs took these illustrations from the work of Paul of Aegina (*c.*625–90 CE), just as Abul-Qāsim al-Zahrāwi (936–1013) drew his surgical materials mainly from the sixth book of Paul's *Epitome*.[64] The only anatomical book based on dissection in Islamic medicine, but now lost, appears to be the *Kitāb al-Tashriḥ* by Yuhanna ibn Māsawayh.[65] According to Ibn abi Usaybi'a, referring to an event in the month of Ramaḍan 221 (August 836), Ibn Māsawayh was keeping monkeys for the purpose of 'dissecting them and composing a book on the same subject as Galen'. But he had abandoned his plan because 'in their bodies the arteries and veins and nerves are too fine'. However, 'upon receiving a large monkey as a gift from the caliph al-Mu'taṣim…he carried out his plan…and there was composed a work which even his enemies found fit to praise.'[66]

Even the discovery of the pulmonary circulation by Ebn Nafis was based not on anatomical observation but on inference. It occurred in a chapter of the commentary of Ibn Nafis on the Canon of Ibn Sinā, who, following Galen, believed that the passage of blood from the right ventricle to the left was mainly through invisible pores of the wall separating the two cavities although Galen had also observed that there were minute connections between the branches of pulmonary veins and arteries.[67] Ibn Nafis contended that:

> when the blood in the right cavity becomes thin, it must be transferred
> to the left cavity where the pneumata is generated. But there is no

passage between the two cavities, neither visible nor invisible, as Galen has thought…It must, therefore, be that when the blood has become thin, it is passed into the arterial vein (pulmonary artery) to the lung… in order to mix with the air. The finest parts of the blood are then strained passing into the venous artery (pulmonary vein) reaching the left of the two cavities of the heart, after mixing with the air and becoming fit for the generation of pneumata.[68]

It seems that this insight was accidental in Ibn Nafis' Commentary. In fact, Ibn Nafis, who was himself a jurisconsult, is explicit that 'the veto of the religious law and the sentiments of charity innate in ourselves alike prevent us from the practice of dissection. This is why we are willing to be limited to basing our knowledge of the internal organs on the sayings of those who had gone before us.'[69]

Lack of dissection in Islam has often been attributed to religious prohibition. However, such legal prohibition was not stated in the Koran or even among the sayings of the Prophet; it probably reflected technical or cultural impediments that made dissection impracticable. A parallel obstacle for experimental anatomy and dissection even on animals was epistemological. Knowledge, based on inquiry and research, a characteristic of Greek and Hellenistic medicine, was replaced in Islam by knowledge based on tradition, transmission, and the authority of the text. What prevented physicians investigating the inner body was the want of the 'freedom of scientific inquiry' that went against religious dogma,[70] whilst the pagan culture of the Hellenistic period left scientific investigations, such as those by Aristotle and Galen, unfettered.

Surgery consisted of a wide range of operations from phlebotomy and bone-setting to incision of abscesses and boils, and amputation of organs. Islamic physicians, men of bookish knowledge, never stained their mantle with the blood of surgery. This, however, did not stop them from inserting a chapter on surgery in their books.[71] Typical of medieval Islam, even surgery was more written about than actually practised, just as anatomy and dissection were primarily framed in books. Most cases of extreme surgery occurred during war or for the purpose of punishment. In *Zakhira ye Kāmela* (or *Jarrāḥiya*), composed some time before 1642, Ḥakim Mohammad includes thirty chapters relating to thirty kinds of injuries or diseases requiring surgical operation. Invasive surgery relates only to two kinds of injuries. Chapter 1 discusses injuries caused by sword, knife, arrow, and gun bullet, and Chapter 6, called *siyāsat-e pādeshāh* ('Punishment Ordered by the Shah'), enumerates injuries applied by surgeons to execute the royal order as a means of punishment, which included amputation of hands, legs, and penis, extraction of pupil, or deprivation of sight by approaching the red iron called mil (probe) to the cornea in order to damage the pupil.[72]

While clinical medicine was popular amongst learned physicians in Islam, surgery was left to surgeons (*jarrāḥ*) who often had no anatomical knowledge. Cyril Elgood quotes Amār b. 'Ali of Mosul as saying that he was accompanied only by two or three students when he operated. Elgood then compares this with the large number of students attending the clinical classes of Rāzi.[73] Al-Zahrāwi (Albucasis) celebrated for inventing various surgical instruments, emphasized that in his time a 'skilled practitioner of surgery is totally lacking', a statement in staggering contrast with the high status of medicine in Islam in the tenth century, when he was writing.[74]

The Medical Profession

State support was crucial in the formation of the medical profession in Islam. The early Islamic states, the Omayyad (661–750) and Abbasid (750–1258), recruited physicians from the existing medical profession in the regions they had conquered; hence most of them were Christians or Jews. State sponsorship also played an important role in the development of medical knowledge and literature. The state-sponsored translation movement set the model for the medical profession as closely linked to the state or the nobility. As Shelomo Goitein indicated, almost any doctor of distinction was also a member of the entourage of a king, a sultan, a vizier, or a governor.[75] Yahya b. Isā b. Jazlah (d. [473] 1080), for instance, could practise medicine thanks to the position and salary that the chief justice (the *qāḍi al-quḍāt*) of Baghdad offered him, probably because he converted to Islam. He apparently had such an income that he was able to treat patients and even provide them with medicine free of charge.[76] Major medical books commissioned by the court or a noble patient were later dispersed through individual copies, either for sale or for personal use. The impact of court medicine on the nature of medical literature is evident in its remarkable concern with dietetics, preservation of health, usefulness of sexual intercourse and the harm caused by its excess, and invention of new compound drugs to increase well-being. The treatise on hygiene by Maimonides, for example, was written for the son of Sultan Saladin, who for a short period occupied the throne of Egypt.

Nevertheless, the medical profession was not limited to the tiny number of learned or ranking physicians attending the court or the nobility. According to Franz Rosenthal, the existence of an elite group of physicians indicates that there must have been a broad supporting base offering medical services to a large portion of Moslem society.[77] This idea is corroborated by the important number of low-quality copies of famous books, or amateur compilations from other books. Many medical manuscripts are copied or scribed by poor hands and contain orthographic mistakes.[78] Most of those who believed that they could master medicine by self-learning used such manuals for medication or treatment of others' illnesses, a fact that could cause mishap in treatment or medication. Exceptionally one finds brilliant self-taught physicians such as Ibn Riḍwan or Maimonides.

The terms used to distinguish between learned physicians who were knowledgeable in both Islamic and pre-Islamic sciences, and those who held basic medical knowledge for practice were, respectively, *ṭabib* or *Ḥakim* (physician-philosopher) and *mutiṭabbib* (practitioner), although often learned physicians through modesty called themselves *mutiṭabbib*. According to Galen, 'only he is a perfect physician who is at the same time a philosopher.'[79] In practical terms, however, one can hardly attribute a definite level of knowledge or skill to each category, not least because there was no standard method for learning.[80]

The number of physicians able to master the books indicated above or even afford them for study was limited. On the other hand, a large number of people contented themselves with small tracts and a basic knowledge of medicine, without having to read and learn classical texts. There are, however, no figures for such practitioners, except anecdotal accounts. According to Ibn al Qifti, 'the number of those who were successful in the examination in 937 by Sinān b. Thābit b. Qurra, the court physician, amounted to about 860 in addition to those who were so prominent they did not need an exam and those who were serving at the court of the Caliph al-Muqtadar.'[81] Considering such educational and social contexts conditioning medical practice, it is hard to specify the boundaries of the Islamic medical profession.

Lay Medical Literature

Extant medical literature can be divided into learned and lay medical texts. A clear-cut distinction between folk and learned medicines is inaccurate because one finds elements of folk medicine in both learned and lay medical texts. The extent to which Galenic medicine penetrated both learned and folk medicine was due to the fact that it was integrated in the Islamic world-view. Although learned doctors mainly used rational methods to educate and to treat, at times they used magic or irrational methods to heal. In *Mokhtaṣar f'il Ṭibb*, which dealt with curing illnesses and the preservation of health by means of food and diet, 'Abd al Mālek b. Ḥabib referred to both the traditions of the Prophet and Greek humoral theories.[82] Mirzā Musā Savaji, writing in 1853, believed that there were:

> two causes of epidemics (*vabā*): a) the distant/heavenly causes (*asbāb-e ba'ida*), either the will of God or Destiny or the influence of the planets, in which cases one should seek healing in *ṣadaqa* (alms giving), penitence, invocation, and prayer; b) accessible/earthly causes (*asbāb-e qariba*), like the putrefaction of the air, the (prophylactic) solution to which was to flee the foul air...while they should also have recourse to prayer, *ṣadaqa*, and invocation for warding off affliction alongside other prophylactic measures like evacuation, retention and the use of appropriate diet.[83]

What, however, distinguished learned from lay medical literature was their quality, originality, and intellectual levels. Sometimes learned physicians wrote treatises destined for different types of readers. Rāzi's *al-Ḥāwi* (*Continent*) and the *Jodari va Ḥaṣba* (*Smallpox and Measles*) resulted from his clinical observations over a long period of time. Rāzi also wrote a book entitled *Man lā yuḥzar al-Ṭabib* (*What to Do in the Absence of Doctor?*), which was destined for the common people.[84] This book is also called the *Ṭibb al-fuqarā* (*Medicine for the Poor*), for those who could not afford a doctor. Allāh Ābādi, the author of the *Muḥibb al aṭibbā*, makes it clear in his introduction that he wrote this book in order for the reader to dispense with the need for a doctor.[85] Books like *Zād al-Mosāferin* (*Provision for Travellers*) were for use when travelling. Esmā'il Gorgāni, after his *Zakhira* (*A Medical Compendium*), abridged it under the title *Khuff-e 'Alā'i* (*The Boots of 'Alā'i* (*Exaltation*)), for the prince 'Alā-al-Dowla Khārazmshāh II (r. 1128–57), so that it might be placed in his boots when he went horse-riding.[86]

The assimilation of humoral theory into folk medicine and the adoption of folk or magic healing by learned physicians were based on existing cultural and religious beliefs that penetrated all layers of the population. In this situation learned physicians did not find it contradictory to pull together magical healing and rational medicine. Perhaps the social framework in which lay and learned medicine were combined should be assigned to the fact that the medical profession was institutionally loose. The lack of clear institutional and professional delimitation allowed the combination of various medical ideas and practices just as it favoured close contact and dialogue between learned and unlearned.

Prophetic Medicine

There are no less than nine works on the medicine of the Prophet and the Imams but only a few are extant or published. Ḥāji Khalifa, writing in 1658, mentions seven works known to him, including those by the Shiite Imām 'Ali b. Reza (*c.*765–818) and 'Abd ar-Raḥmān al-Suyūṭī (1445–1505). To these should be added works by Shams al-Din al Zahabi (1274–1348) and Ibn Qayyim al-Jawziyya (d. *c.*1350/1), to which al-Suyūṭī frequently refers.[87] It ought to be noted that Prophetic medicine was an apocryphal production of later date, narrated through a chain of several generations of scholars of different philosophical or ideological persuasions. Al-Suyūṭī, for instance, was one of the Shāfe'i scholars of the fifteenth century and well versed in Greek medicine. The opening chapter of al-Suyūṭī's *Ṭibb al-Nabbi* is on the principles of humoral medicine, the preservation of health, and aetiology based on the six non-naturals. As-Ṣanowbary (d. 1412), on the other hand, in his *Book of Mercy on Medicine and Wisdom*, makes a brief mention of humoral theory and one reference to Hippocrates and Galen, but devotes most of his book to quotation of *hadiths* and to magical and talismanic methods of healing.[88]

Al-Jawziyya and al-Suyūṭī under each entry provided a humoral description of the illness, a drug, or a food before relating *ḥadith*s of the Prophet about them. For headache, for instance, after giving its different kinds according to the anatomical location of the pain, al-Jawziyya enumerated their various causes, such as the predominance of one of the humours, stomach ulcer, and inflammation of the stomach veins. Amongst the remedies for headache as narrated from the Prophet, cupping and applying henna are cited. Henna counter-balanced the heat that ascended to the head and caused pain, because it was cold in the first degree and dry in the second.[89] The '*Ṭibb al-Nabbi* as composed by al-Jawziyya and al-Suyūṭī is concerned not only with transmitting the traditions of the Prophet, but also with justifying the tenets of humoral medicine by expounding on the sayings of the Prophet. In short, the literature known as Prophetic medicine follows the agenda of Galenico-Islamic medical tracts, with added references to the traditions of the Prophet.

Prophetic medicine was not thus a reaction against Greek medicine, but asserted that the tenets of Islam contained all knowledge necessary for the faithful. Prophetic medicine was a development within the general trend of assimilating Greek medicine into Islam. The assimilation was reciprocal. Physicians who were trained in, and adhered to, Galenico-Avicennian medicine also introduced religious concepts in their medicine. According to 'Aqili (eighteenth century), a physician should also learn other sciences, such as jurisprudence (*fiqh*) and tradition (*ḥadith*), moral philosophy, logic, natural science, geometry, astronomy, arithmetic, and the art of soothsaying and discernment (*kahānat va fārāsat*).[90]

Similar associations can also be found in folk medical literature. In the *Risāla-ye Dallākiyya*, a treatise on bathing, the author shares two divergent opinions: according to the first, bath was the invention of Solomon, and, following the second, it was the creation of the physicians. Infection is sometimes attributed to unclean tools (like towels), or stagnation of water in *Ḥammam* (public baths), factors that should be avoided. However, the treatise also states that water should be warmed by fire and not brought in from mineral sources because the warmth or heat of mineral sources originated in hell. While the removal of dirt by rubbing unblocks the pores of the skin allowing the transpiration of the body, it also depletes the means (dirt) through which Satan penetrates the body. The tract also warns against the use of the rubbing glove or towels of those infected by contagious diseases.[91] Hygiene as usual was braided with religious rituals.

Opposition to Greek medicine did not come from Prophetic medicine, but from a perception of medical knowledge and practice developed by 'traditionalist' scholars, who were themselves imbued with a 'rationalist' spirit. Ghazzāli, for instance, was a philosopher and theologian, who believed in natural sciences, including medicine, and made use of logic and dialectic in his arguments, but contended that natural philosophers (*Tbi'iyun*) could not see beyond the nature and the original cause that makes nature work.[92] He also argues that 'knowledge' is superior to belief and that knowledgeable men are closer to the Prophet than those who believe without knowing.[93] Ghazzāli did not reject medicine, but believed that medicine and doctors alone were not able to heal unless correct usage was revealed to the faithful via faith or by the angels. He stated that:

> People think that [for treating an illness] it suffices that they purchase drug prescribed by the doctor and apply it. This is wrong because prior to any action the best choice of doctor should be revealed to the patient first, and then the best and the most efficient drug, its dose and the time of its use must be revealed to the doctor via divine inspiration. Without faith and heavenly revelation, wrong treatment is mistaken for the right one. And the faith and inspiration cannot be found in any drugstore but in the treasury of the angels. There is no way to buy inspiration from the storehouse of the angles (*khazāneh-ye malaekeh*) other than by prayer.[94]

The Modern Period

All the factors that characterized 'Islamic medicine' and helped its development throughout the Middle Ages informed also the way it encountered modern Western medicine from the eighteenth century onwards. One crucial factor was state or princely support, without which medieval Islamic medicine could not have developed as it did. Likewise, in the modern period, without state sponsorship the introduction of modern medicine was inconceivable. Medical reform was not so much due to the impulse of social and political development as to the authoritative state planning for military modernization. It was the state agenda that brought about quick and mechanical, rather than gradual and conceptual, change.

The form, intensity, and extent of medical modernization depended on the structure or the nature of the state authority. In Tunisia, the growing influence of the colonial power by the end of the nineteenth century relegated local physicians to a tolerated status.[95] In Iran, the status of local medicine did not decrease but at the same time, modern medicine and Western doctors at the court became increasingly present and respected. In Egypt, which was not a colonial state, the French Dr Clot undertook modernization under the authority of Mohammad Ali, the ruler of Egypt, and sought to work in harmony with the local medical establishment, for instance by preparing textbooks for the study of modern medicine in Arabic.[96] At the end of the century, however, following the British occupation, medical education was deemed archaic and the remedy, according to a correspondent in 1894, was teaching medicine in a European language, rather than in Arabic, and the all-inclusive replacement of the teaching staff of the school.[97]

Although the conceptual in-road of modern sciences and biomedicine was crucial in sidelining traditional Galenic medicine, institutional factors were no less important. They played an even more important role in the demise of medieval Islamic medicine. Whenever traditional medicine found social, institutional, or cultural support, it survived even though some re-adaptation was necessary. One example is the medicine of the Prophet that is popular among Moslem communities even in the West.[98] The survival and wide practice of *Ayurveda* and *Unani* (Greek) medicine in the Indian subcontinent was closely linked to the anti-colonial movement. They were used as representative of the national identity and symbol of resistance to colonial sciences and medicine. In countries such as Iran and Turkey, on the other hand, where traditional humoral medicine lost state sponsorship, it was no longer dominant by the mid-twentieth century.

The major difference between the introduction of Greek medicine into Islam in the Middle Ages and the modernization of Galenico-Islamic medicine in the nineteenth and twentieth centuries seems to be that the former was introduced through the formation of Islam as a religion or worldview, while the latter was integrated through the introduction of modern science and the making of the modern nation-state. Galenico-Islamic medicine, accountable as it was to religion and faith, failed, in its later development, to meet modern conditions. Mohammad-Hosein 'Aqili, the outstanding physician of the late eighteenth century, when recommending the study of philosophy and dialectic and logic to medical students, insisted that this should not be used against religion or as a means of personal and independent inquiry according to one's own will and opinion, but for strengthening and understanding the *sharī'a*.[99]

Conclusion

Galenico-Islamic medicine followed Greek medicine in style and recycled its content. The strength of learned 'Islamic medicine' remains less in its innovations than in its pedagogical capacity. Authors such as Avicenna and al-Majusi were great organizers of the mass of information according to a coherent theory and classification that facilitated their assimilation. The question now is to see why 'Islamic medicine' turned medical theories into dogma and froze the spirit of inquiry and observation, which were the raison d'être of Hippocratic and Galenic writings, by sanctifying the latter. Any new development was delayed until the emergence in the eighteenth century of neo-Hippocratism that advocated a return to Greek sources.

This chapter has pointed to the adoption of Greek medicine within the framework of the formation of Islam as one factor in this outcome. It is from this vantage point that the term 'Islamic medicine' finds its historical grounds. No doubt, however, further explanations for such developments need to be found in the intellectual and social history of the Islamic East and the Latin West in the same vein that the emergence of Hippocratic medicine around 400 BCE needs to be understood in the context of the profound social transformation of ancient Greece.

Acknowledgements

This chapter was prepared as part of research funded by the Wellcome Trust. I am grateful to Lutz Richter-Bernburg for his thorough comments on an earlier version of this paper.

Notes

1 Lawrence I. Conrad, 'Arab-Islamic Medicine', in R. Porter and W. Bynum (eds), *Companion Encyclopedia of the History of Medicine* (London: Routledge, 1993), 1: 676–727; P. Pormann and E. Savage-Smith, *Medieval Islamic Medicine* (Edinburgh: Edinburgh University Press, 2007), 2; M. Ullmann, *Islamic Medicine* (Edinburgh: Edinburgh University Press, 1978), xi; D. Campbell, *Arabian Medicine and Its Influence on the Middle Ages*, Vol. 1 (Mansfield Centre: Martino, 2006), xi; De Lacy O'Leary, *How Greek Science Passed to the Arabs* (London: Routledge and Kegan Paul, 1979), 5. This edition is also available through Assyrian International News Agency, Books Online: http://www.aina.org

2 F. Rosenthal, 'Al-Biruni between Greece and India', in *Science and Medicine in Islam*, Variorum reprint (1990), 11–12.

3 Arthur John Auberry, *The Koran Interpreted* (Oxford: Oxford University Press, 1964), 79, 100, and 265–6.

4 Conrad, 'Arab-Islamic Medicine', 678–82.

5 G. E. R. Lloyd (ed.), *Hippocratic Writings* (London: Penguin Books, 1987), 166.

6 The Koran, sura 51/.ayah 56.

7 Conrad, 'Arab-Islamic Medicine', 679.

8 Ullmann, *Islamic Medicine*, 2.

9 Kamal S. Salibi, *A History of Arabia* (Delmar, NY: Caravan Books, 1980), 27 ff.

10 The use of mil, or 'probe' (from Mele, a Greek term), in surgery is underlined by Pormann and Savage-Smith, *Medieval Islamic Medicine*, 7–8.

11 Ullman, *Islamic Medicine*, 2–3, 6.

12 C. Elgood, *A Medical History of Persia and the Eastern Caliphate* (Cambridge: Cambridge University Press, 1951), 64.

13 Cited in S. Hamarneh, 'The Physicians and the Health Professions in Medieval Islam', *Bulletin of NY Academy of Medicine* 47(9) (1971), 1088–110, at 1090.

14 Ibid.

15 Ibn Sinā, *Qānun dar Ṭebb [Canon of Medicine]*, Persian translation, vol. 1: 3–4; Mohammad-Hossein 'Aqili, *Kholāsat al-ḥekmat [Digest of Medicine]*, lithograph edn (Bombay, [1261] 1845), 2.

16 A. Z. Iskandar, 'An Attempted Reconstruction of the Late Alexandrian Medical Curriculum', *Medical History* 20 (1976), 235–58, at 243.

17 Pormann and Savage-Smith, *Medieval Islamic Medicine*, 52–3; Y. Tzvi, 'Another Andalusian Revolt? Ibn Rushd's Critique of al-Kindi's *Pharmacological Computus*', in Jan P. Hogendijk and Abdelhamid I. Sabra (eds), *The Enterprise of Science in Islam: New Perspectives* (Cambridge, MA/London: MIT Press, 2003), 354.

18 Ḥakim Mohammad Sharif-Khan, *Ta'lif-e Sharif*, Persian manuscript ([1206] 1792), Wellcome Manuscripts (WMS.) Per. 582, fol. 12.

19 Ḥamarneh, 'The Physicians and the Health', 1091. For a debate amongst early Islamic scholars on the qualities of drugs and their classification according to their potency, see Tzvi, 'Another Andalusian Revolt?'.

20 Mohammad Arzāni, *Qarābādin-e qāderi*, WMS. Per. 544, fol. 2a. *Qarābādin*, or *aqrābādin*, is a corruption of the Greek term *graphidion* meaning 'prescription'—Pormann and Savage Smith, *Medieval Islamic Medicine*, 54.

21 *Qānun dar Ṭebb*, 5: 229–30.

22 Campbell, *Arabian Medicine*, 4.

23 Emād al-Din Mahmud Shirāzi, *Resāleh*, Persian MSS, WMS. Per. 293(A), fol. 2.

24 According to Ibn Sinā, mizâj is a quality that results from the combination of opposing matters. The interaction of these matters produces a unique state that is called mizâj (or temperament). See Ibn Sinā, *Canon*, p. 12.

25 *Qānun dar Ṭebb*, 1: 4.

26 Michael Dols, *Medieval Islamic Medicine: Ibn Riḍwān's Treatise on the Prevention of Bodily Ills in Egypt* (Berkeley: University of California Press, 1984), 100.

27 David Pingree, 'Astrology in Islamic Times', in E. Yarshater (ed.), *Encyclopaedia Iranica* (New York: Columbia University, 2008); see online version at http://www.iranica.com/articles/astrology-and-astronomy-in-iran-

28 Ullmann, *Islamic Medicine*, 15; F. E. Peters, *Aristotle and the Arabs: The Aristotelian Tradition in Islam* (New York: New York University Press, 1968), 35–47, 54.

29 W. Montgomery Watt, *Islamic Philosophy and Theology* (Edinburgh: Edinburgh University Press, 1962), 42–3.

30 Ullmann, *Islamic Medicine*, 7; Conrad, 'Arab-Islamic Medicine', 695–6.

31 D. Gutas, *Greek Thought, Arabic Culture* (London/New York: Routledge, 1998), Chapter 2.

32 Elgood, *A Medical History of Persia*, 37–8.

33 Michael G. Morony, *Iraq after the Muslim Conquest* (Princeton: Princeton University Press, 1984), 4.

34 Montgomery Watt, *Islamic Philosophy*, 46; Etienne Gilson, *La philosophie au Moyen Âge: des origines patristiques à la fin du XIVe siècle*, 2nd edn (Paris: Payot, 1952), 347–9, 352–7.

35 For a list of Hunayn's books, see: Dehkhodā, *Loghatnāmeh*, 6: 9226–7; Lucien Leclerc, *Histoire de la Médecine Arabe* (Paris, 1876), 1: 143–52.

36 Ullmann, *Islamic Medicine*, 31, 33–4.

37 Ibid. 36.

38 Peters, *Aristotle and the Arabs*, 19.

39 Montgomery Watt, *Islamic Philosophy*, 38–9.

40 'Aqili, *Kholāsat al-Ḥekmat*, 3.

41 Ibn Riḍwān, *Useful Book*, MS. Tibb 483, 31, ll. 2–18, cited in Iskandar, 'An Attempted Reconstruction of the Late Alexandrian Medical Curriculum', 242.

42 Elgood, *A Medical History of Persia*, 139.

43 Pormann and Savage-Smith, *Medieval Islamic Medicine*, 15.

44 Conrad, 'Arab-Islamic Medicine', 706, 725, quoting Fuad Sezgin, *Geschichte des arabischen Schrifttums*, vol. 3: *Medizin—Pharmacie—Zoologie—Tierheilkunde bis ca. 430 H.* (Leiden: Brill, 1970), 65, 154, 258.

45 Mohammad Taqi Shirāzi Malek al-Atebbā, *vabā'iyye-he Saqira* [*Lesser Treaty on Cholera*] ([1283] c.1867); *vabā'iyye-he kabira* [*Greater Treaty on Cholera*] ([1251] 1835), lithograph edn, Tehran, Library of Majles.

46 Pormann and Savage-Smith, *Medieval Islamic Medicine*, 35.

47 V. Nutton, *Ancient Medicine* (London/New York: Routledge, 2004), 140; Ullmann, *Islamic Medicine*, 21; H. Ebrahimnejad, 'Jālinus', in Yarshater (ed.), *Encyclopaedia Iranica*, 14: 420–7; also available online at http://www. iranica.com/articles/jalinus

48 Lloyd (ed.), *Hippocratic Writings*, 27.

49 *Montakhab az resālah—ye Mirzā Qāzi*, WMS. Per. 293 (B), 1–4. Similarly, Hakim Mohammad Hāshem Tehrāni, writing about china root, calls into question the principle of treating a disease by the drug of a temperament opposite to that of the disease by stating that *teriaq* is hot but is beneficial also for diseases of hot temperament (*Eyn al-hayāt dar sharāyet-e chub-e chini*, WMS. Per. 352, Fol. 6).

50 Conrad, 'Arab-Islamic Medicine', 683–4.

51 M. Dols, *The Black Death in the Middle East* (Princeton: Princeton University Press, 1977), 121–2. The saying attributed to the Prophet, فان الذي انزل الداء انزل الدواء ('The one who sent disease sent also its remedy') echoes this concept.

52 Dols, *The Black Death*, 122.

53 Mirzā Musā Sāvaji Fakhr al-Atebbā, *Dastur al-aṭebbâ fi 'alāj al-vabā* [*Prescription of Physicians for the Treatment of Cholera*] ([1269] 1852), lithograph edn, Tehran, Library of Majles.

54 Ullmann, *Islamic Medicine*, 22; Conrad, 'Arab-Islamic Medicine', 682, 688.

55 Anonymous Persian manuscript, Medical Library of UCLA, MS 80 ([1240] 1824), fols. 3–48; Hakim Mohammad Beg, *Khavāṣṣ al-ashyā'*, WMS. Per. 10, fols. 3–9.

56 Ullmann, *Islamic Medicine*, 19.

57 Ibid. 44. Supernatural healing could be seen in almost all human societies. The practice of seeking cure during sleep with the hope of visiting the spirit of the healer in a dream, or leaving the sick at the temple of the healing god in ancient Greece, can be seen amongst Jews as well as Moslems—Max Meyerhof, *Studies in Medieval Arabic Medicine*, ed. by P. Johnstone (London: Variorum, 1984), Chapter 8, 'L'oeuvre médicale de Maimonide', 136.

58 This book has been translated into English from the extant Arabic version: Galen, *On Anatomical Procedure*, trans. by W. L. H. Duckworth, ed. by M. C. Lyons and B. Towers (Cambridge: Cambridge University Press, 1962).

59 *The Fihrist of al-Nadim: The Tenth-Century Survey of Muslim Culture*, ed. and trans. by Bayard Dodge (New York: Columbia University Press, 1970), 2: 682–3. See also Ibn al Qifti, *Târikh al-hokamā*, Persian translation of

17th-cent. edn, ed. Bahman Dârayee (Tehran: University of Tehran Press, [1371] 1992), 179 ff.

60 C. Elgood, *Safavid Surgery* (Oxford: Pergamon Press, 1966), 23; 'Agili *Kholāṣat al-hekmat*, lithograph edn (Bombay, [1261] 1845), 4.

61 It is significant that even for refuting Galen's theory of the passage of blood between the two cavities of the heart, Ibn Nafis explicitly relied on Galen's anatomical dissection.

62 Cited in Gary Leiser, 'Medical Education in Islamic Lands from Seventh to the Fourteenth Century', *Journal of the History of Medicine and Allied Sciences* 38 (1983), 48–75, at 68. On Rāzi see also Lutz Richter-Bernburg, 'Abubakr Muḥammad al-Rhazi's Medical Works', *Medicina nei Secoli* 6 (1994), 377–92.

63 Albert Z. Iskandar, 'Galen and Rhazes on Examining Physicians', *Bulletin of the History of Medicine* 36 (1962), 362–5.

64 Campbell, *Arabian Medicine*, 12.

65 Ibn al Qifti, *Tārikh al-Ḥokamā*, 514. Al-Qifti cites only one book on anatomy, but Ibn abi Us.aybiʿa names another book of Masawayh on anatomy, *The Book of the Formation of Man and His Various Parts, on the Number of the Muscles, Joints, Bones, and Blood Vessels, and on the Causes of Pain* (Elgood, *Safavid Surgery*, 24).

66 Cited in Elgood, *Safavid Surgery*, 24.

67 Pormann and Savage-Smith, *Medieval Islamic Medicine*, 47; M. Meyerhof, 'Ibn An-Nafis (XIIIth cent.) and His Theory of Lesser Circulation', in *Studies in Medieval Arabic Medicine* (London: Variorum, 1984), 100–1.

68 Cited in Toby E. Huff, *The Rise of Early Modern Science: Islam, China and the West* (Cambridge: Cambridge University Press, 2003), 168.

69 Elgood, *Safavid Surgery*, 25; Huff, *The Rise of Early Modern Science*, 169; Conrad, 'Arab-Islamic Medicine', 712.

70 Huff, *The Rise of Early Modern Science*, (1993 edition), 1.

71 Techniques of surgery and surgical operations constitute a chapter in almost every compendium. See, for instance, the Zakhira of Jorjāni and the Canon of Ibn Sinā.

72 Ḥakim Mohammad, *Ẕakhirah-ye kāmela*, Persian manuscript ([1209] 1794), Library of the University of Tehran, no. 8825.

73 Elgood, *Safavid Surgery*, 19.

74 Albucasis, *On Surgery and Instruments: A Definitive Edition of the Arabic Text with English Translation and Commentary*, trans. M. S. Spink and G. L. Lewis (London: Wellcome Institute of the History of Medicine, 1973), 2 ff.

75 S. D. Goitein, 'The Medical Profession in the Light of the Cairo Geniza Documents', *Hebrew Union College Annual* 34 (1963), 177—cited in Franz Rosenthal, 'The Physician in Medieval Muslim Society', in *Science and Medicine in Islam: A Collection of Essays* (London: Variorum, 1991), 477.

76 Ibn al Qifti, *Tārikh al-ḥokamā*, 498–9.

77 Rosenthal, 'The Physician in Medieval Muslim Society', 477.

78 *Mofradāt-e Hendi (Simples from India)*, WMS. Per. 519.

79 J. Schacht and M. Meyerhof, *The Medico-Philosophical Controversy between Ibn Butlan of Baghdad and Ibn Ridwan of Cairo*, Faculty of Arts publication 13 (Cairo: Egyptian University, 1937), 77.

80 Leiser, 'Medical Education in Islamic Lands'.

81 Ibn al Qifti, *Tārikh al-ḥokamā*, 265–6.

82 David Waine, 'Dietetics in Medieval Islamic Culture', *Medical History* 43 (1999), 228–40: 233.

83 Fakhr al-Ḥokamā va Zubdat al-Ateebbā Ḥāji Mirzā Musā Savaji, *Dastur al-atebbā fi 'alāj al-vabâ*, lithograph edn (Tehran: Majles Library), 43–6.

84 Conrad, 'Arab-Islamic Medicine', 706.

85 Allāh Abādi, *Muḥeb al-Atebbā*, Persian MSS, WMS. Per 353, 1.

86 Elgood, *A Medical History of Persia*, 259.

87 Cyril Elgood, *Ṭibb-ul-Nabbi or Medicine of the Prophet*, Osiris 14 (1962), 33–192, at 40–1.

88 Pormann and Savage-Smith, *Medieval Islamic Medicine*, 74.

89 Ibn Qayyim al-Jawziyya, *The Medicine of the Prophet*, ed. and trans. Penelope Johnstone (Cambridge: Islamic Text Society, 1998), 63–8. See also Jalalu'd-Din Abd'ur-Rahman Al-Suyūṭī, *Medicine of the Prophet* (London: Ta-Ha, 1994), 100–1.

90 Mohammad Hādi al-'Alavi al-'Aqili-ye Shirāzi, *Kholāṣat al-ḥekmat* (Bombay, [1261] 1845), 7.

91 Karim b. Ebrahim, *Resālah-ye dallākiyya*, Persian manuscript, National Library, St Petersburg, no. 434, fols. 6a, 7b, 23b, 24, 27, 43a.

92 Ghazzāli, *Makātib-e Fārsi*, 64.

93 Ghazzāli, *Book of Knowledge*, section I, available at http://www.ghazali. org/works/bk1-sec-1.htm

94 Mohammad Ghazzāli, *Fazā'el al-ānām min rasāyel ḥujjat al-eslām (or makātib-e fārsi-ye Ghāzzāli)* (Persian writings of Ghazzāli), ed. Abbas Eqbāl (Tehran: Ebne Sina, [1333] 1954), 63.

95 Nancy Gallagher, *Medicine and Power in Tunisia, 1780–1900* (Cambridge: Cambridge University Press, 1983), 1.

96 Anne Marie Moulin, 'Disease Transmission in Nineteenth-Century Egypt', in H. Ebrahimnejad (ed.), *The Development of Modern Medicine in Non-Western Countries* (London/New York: Routledge, 2009), 44.

97 'Medical Education in Egypt', *British Medical Journal* (7 July 1894).

98 Conrad, 'Arab-Islamic Medicine', 717–18.

99 'Aqili, *Kholāṣat al-ḥekmat*, 6.

Select Bibliography

Bos, G., *Ibn al-Jazzār on Sexual Diseases and Their Treatment: A Critical Edition of Zâd al-musāfir wa-qut al-Ḥādir* (London: Kegan Paul, 1997).

Bos, G., *Ibn al-Jazzār on Fevers: A Critical Edition of Zâd al-musāfir wa-qut al-Hâḍir* (London: Kegan Paul, 2000).

Burnett, C., and D. Jacquart (eds), *Constantine the African and 'Alī ibn al-'Abbās al-Magūsī The Pantegni and Related Texts* (Leiden: Brill, 1994).

Conrad, L. I., '*Ṭā'ūn* and *wabā'*: Conceptions of Plague and Pestilence in Early Islam', *Journal of the Economic and Social History of the Orient* 25 (1982), 268–307.

Crussol des Epesse, B. T. de, *Discours sur l'oeil d'Esmā'il-e Gorgāni* (Tehran: Presses universitaires d'Iran; Institut Français de Recherche en Iran, 1998).

Dols, M. D., 'The Origins of the Islamic Hospital: Myth and Reality', *Bulletin of the History of Medicine* 61 (1987), 367–90.

Good, B. J., *Medicine, Rationality, and Experience: An Anthropological Perspective* (Cambridge: Cambridge University Press, 1994).

Gutas, D., *Avicenna and the Aristotelian Tradition: Introduction to Reading Avicenna's Philosophical Works* (Leiden: Brill, 1988).

Huff, Toby E., *The Rise of Early Modern Science: Islam, China, and the West*, (Cambridge: Cambridge University Press, 1993).

Jacquart, D., and F. Micheau, *La médecine arabe et l'occident médiéval* (Paris: Maisonneuve et Larose, 1990).

Maddison, F., and E. Savage-Smith, *Science, Tools and Magic*, 2 vols (Oxford: Oxford University Press, 1997).

Newman, A., '*Tashrīḥ-e Manṣurī*: Human Anatomy between the Galenic and Prophetical Medical Traditions', in Ž. Vesel et al. (eds), *La science dans le monde iranien à l'époque islamique* (Tehran: Institut Français de Recherche en Iran, 1998; 2nd edn, 2004), 253–71.

O'Leary, De Lacy, *How Greek Science Passed to the Arabs* (London: Routledge and Kegan Paul, [1949] 1979).

Peters, F. E., *Aristotle and the Arabs: The Aristotelian Tradition in Islam* (New York: New York University Press, 1968).

Pormann, P. E., 'La querelle des médecins arabistes et hellénistes et l'héritage oublié', in V. Boudon-Millot and G. Cobolet (eds), *Lire les médecins grecs ' la Renaissance: Aux origines dé l'édition médicale, Actes du colloque international de Paris (19–20 septembre 2003)* (Paris: De Boccard Edition-Diffusion, 2004), 113–41.

Savage-Smith, E., 'Attitudes toward Dissection in Medieval Islam', *Journal of the History of Medicine and Allied Sciences* 50 (1995), 67–110.

Savage-Smith, E., 'The Practice of Surgery in Islamic Lands: Myth and Reality', in Peregrine Horden and Emilie Savage-Smith (eds), *The Year 1000* (2000), 307–21.

Temkin, O., *Galenism: Rise and Decline of a Medical Philosophy* (Ithaca, NY: Cornell University Press, 1973).

5

History of Medicine in Eastern Europe, Including Russia

Marius Turda

Much has been done over the past three decades to strengthen the position of the history of medicine among other academic disciplines. In addition to the continuous preoccupation with national medical traditions, topics such as international eugenics, health organizations, and transnational welfare movements have also benefited from sustained analysis. In comparison to the traditional medical historiography that is largely based on the narration of individual achievements in any particular country, the new direction of research suggests the need for a re-classification of medical thinking about society based on synchronized readings of concurrent medical traditions across countries and regions. The history of medicine—proponents of this new historiographic approach suggest—must be constantly renewed, whether this be its subject-matter or conceptual techniques in order to cope with the increased artistry of new methodologies and challenges from other disciplines.

Vibrant as this scholarship undoubtedly is, it does not compensate for one major weakness: its restricted geographical focus. With the exception of Russian and Soviet histories of medicine, Eastern Europe is rarely mentioned in general histories of international medicine.[1] None of the books published in the prestigious Studies in the Social History of Medicine series, for example, deal with Eastern Europe. The reasons for this neglect are numerous, including the ideological segregation existing during communism, the linguistic complexity of the region, and the persistence of outdated notions about the history of medicine itself. Even the internationalization of Eastern European academia that accompanied the political changes of the 1990s, which permitted its rapid adaptation to fresh historiographies and methodology, had, at least initially, only a modest impact on the history of medicine in Eastern Europe. Sporadically, chapters dealing with Eastern European medicine have been published in edited volumes in the West,[2] complementing the singular efforts of a handful of scholars who have repeatedly argued for the importance of Eastern Europe in understanding wider European, as well as international, developments in the history of medicine.[3]

Nonetheless, a visible transformation of the scholarship started during the early twentieth-first century. Monographs and edited volumes published both in and about Eastern European countries now appear regularly, a trend not only driven by the emergence of a new generation of medical historians but, equally important, defining the crystallization of a new academic field in Eastern Europe, especially during the past decade.[4] A number of factors contributed directly to this process, including improved access to archives, the re-publication of interwar medical texts, the influx of Western scholarship, and, most importantly, Eastern European scholars studying abroad. Opening the archives, for instance, led to a careful analysis of historical documents that sought to understand the 'truth' behind some of the twentieth century's hitherto unapproachable topics, such as the participation of Eastern European physicians in the Holocaust. While these archival efforts have not necessarily resulted in the emergence of a conceptual consensus, supporters of this historiographic trend agreed on the crucial importance of medicine itself for reconstructing the national past.

Other avenues of research, namely authors who insisted on a comparative reading of medical traditions, also materialized after 1990. Compared with the first category of studies, this latter historiographic approach attempted to resist the dogmatic reductionism of document analysis and to transcend national interests by initiating a particular style of historical writing, one that proposed an interdisciplinary methodology informed by a detached narration of historical facts. The existing Eastern European history of medicine combines these different styles of writing, aiming to be conceptually and thematically innovative as well as attentive to hitherto unresearched topics. There is an equally substantial effort being made to place medical thinking in the larger contexts of national and international politics and culture. In pursuit of its new identity, current historical scholarship in Eastern Europe not only brings together significant themes and developments in medicine as part of social history, political demography, and cultural anthropology, but also forcefully engages with some of the most central topics pertaining to the national traditions of these countries. And although there still is a conceptual divide between this new generation of historians of medicine and other historians, the hegemonic status of the latter is clearly being challenged.

The aim of this chapter is to chart the broad contours of historical scholarship on medicine in Russia/Soviet Union and Eastern Europe. There are, of course, some significant differences between the two historical and geographical entities. However, when dealing with practical developments or clusters of ideas, the history of medicine in Eastern European countries, as much as in Russia, shares certain narratives, conceptual traits, and methodological conventions. To this end, I shall be employing 'Eastern Europe' to refer to the former communist countries in Eastern Europe, in particular Poland, Czechoslovakia, Hungary, Romania, Yugoslavia, and Bulgaria. The comparative conceptual strategy proposed here is intended not only to reveal much-needed research on neglected national case studies, but also to redefine wider debates in the history of medicine more generally. However, substantial research and analytical effort remains necessary to stimulate historiographic interest in these topics from a comparative perspective, at both regional and international levels.

History of Medicine in Russia/Soviet Union

Medicine was an intrinsic component of the Soviet programme of nation-building from the beginning of the Bolshevik Revolution. The depressing hygienic conditions of the civilian population during and following the First World War unquestionably contributed to a new appreciation of medicine as a source of social activism and national mobilization. Additionally, the effects of the typhus epidemics were so severe that V. I. Lenin, in 1919, did not hesitate to declare that 'either the louse conquers socialism or socialism conquers the louse'.[5] Neither succeeded completely, but this statement is indicative of the social radicalism for which the Soviet project of creating a new society and individual would later become known.

The most important manifestation of the Soviet approach to medicine was, therefore, to be found not merely in the establishment of medical institutions, but in the communist ideology itself. 'This ideology', as Mark G. Field remarked, 'saw illness and (premature) mortality as primarily the product of a sick or pathological society, i.e. capitalism, to be brought under control first by socialism, and then by communism.'[6] With the creation of the Commissariat of Health Protection in 1918, and then throughout the period of the New Economic Policy (1921–8), the Soviet regime set about challenging the validity of traditional Russian medicine, while criticizing the West for failing to understand the emerging 'proletariat' medicine. But this criticism was largely unjustified. Visiting the Soviet Union in the 1930s, the Swiss-American historian of medicine Henry E. Sigerist, for instance, stated unambiguously:

> I have come to the conclusion that what is being done in the Soviet Union today is the beginning of a new period in the history of medicine. All that has been achieved so far in five thousand years of medical history represents but a first epoch: the period of curative medicine. Now a new era, the period of preventive medicine, has begun in the Soviet Union.[7]

Other Western historians of medicine were, however, less inclined to eulogize Soviet medicine, preferring more critical evaluations instead. Following the pioneering studies published during the interwar period by Horsley Gantt, Arthur Newsholme, John A. Kingsbury, and Henry E. Sigerist,[8] a more analytical scholarship emerged in the 1960s and 1970s, exemplified especially by the works of Mark G. Field, Loren R. Graham, and Kendall E. Bailles.[9] During the 1980s and early 1990s, reflecting historiographic developments in Western European history of medicine, this scholarship diversified and new topics in Russian and Soviet medicine were proposed, including the professionalization of medicine, the history of public health, and social hygiene.[10] Scholars like Nancy Frieden,[11] Jeannete Tuve,[12] John Hutchinson,[13] and Susan Solomon,[14] among others, persuasively demonstrated how ideas of health and hygiene were instrumental in the formation of Russian and Soviet medical cultures, cultures which, these authors argued, were the result of a number of factors, including the historical tradition of community medicine (*zemstvo*), the financial exigencies of the emerging Soviet state and political apparatus, and the environmentalist ideology of the Bolshevik leadership (the pre-eminence of nurture over nature in shaping the new 'Soviet' man and woman).[15]

What is more, this new scholarship described how Russian and then Soviet physicians made use of their expertise to promote both political and social agendas; these physicians were, in fact, conditioned as much by the socio-political environment in which their ideas of social hygiene, public health, and preventive medicine were tested as they were by state mechanisms of power and control. As Susan Solomon has argued, with regard to the function social hygienists assumed during the 1920s:

> [t]he pivotal role of social hygiene in Soviet public health not only brought a new group of experts to prominence, it also broadened the scope and orientation of public health itself. In commissioning physicians to do research on issues of public health, the state medicalized a series of issues that had previously been treated as questions of law and order.[16]

Similarly, technical developments, such as those of the pharmaceutical industry, apart from qualifying as major medical achievements in their own right, were also—as Mary Schaeffer Conroy noted—the expression of a way of thinking about health that centred on the population and the ability of the Soviet state to sponsor scientific research and development, domestic production, distribution of medicine, and, of course, consumption of drugs.[17]

Following academia's gradual liberalization during the Perestroika and afterward, other areas of research have attracted attention by sharing a vision of medical history as a dynamic ensemble of ideas, individuals, and state agencies rather than as merely a sum of physicians and medical institutions. These new topics include gender and the politics of reproduction, the transfer of scientific knowledge between Soviet Russia and other European countries, and eugenics and epigenetics. The scholarship on gender, reproduction, and natalist policies in the Soviet Union and post-Soviet Russia has been in ascendancy since the late 1970s, paralleling broader development in the humanities, which centred on new theories of sexuality and power elaborated by Michel Foucault and others. Accordingly, scholars such as Gail Lapidus, Wendy Goldman, Rosalind Marsh, Michele Rivkin-Fish, Loren Graham and Pat Simpson have shown how, in its attempts to create a socialist body politic, the communist state manipulated both medical discourses on health and national discourses on the family, thereby interweaving the reproduction of the social organism with the reproduction of the nation while simultaneously emphasizing women's special role in this process of social engineering. The studies in this category are probably those that best accord with the idea that medicine under communism became an important locus for exercising state control and that medical knowledge lent scientific respectability to a variety of political and social projects.[18]

Other scholars have attempted to sort out the complex relationship between politics and medicine by marshalling evidence from the experience of medical research in their international contexts and showing how this experience permeated the national spheres of hygiene and health. This interaction between the international and national dimensions of the history of medicine is a valuable addition to the growing body of scholarship on the transfer, appropriation, and rejection of scientific knowledge in modern cultures. Drawing on these premises, several edited volumes brought Russian and Western scholarship together, thus successfully overcoming the rather conventional political narratives of Soviet studies. Take the contributions by Mark B. Mirsky, Vladimir M. Verbitski, and Tatyana S. Sorokina, for example, included in a volume edited by John H. Cule and John M. Lancaster. These three Russian historians of medicine discussed state medicine in Russia until 1918, obstetrics and gynaecology in the nineteenth century, and state preventive measures and state intervention in the provision of health care during the Moscow plagues of 1771 and 1772, respectively.[19]

More recently, contributions by Russian historians of medicine have increased in an indication of the growing commitment to a new range of scholarly debates, such as the relationship between medicine and the Holocaust and the history of eugenics. In this sense, Boris Yudin, for example, provided a convincing account of the controversies surrounding the ethical issues of medical research and human experiments in Russia and the Soviet Union during the first decades of the twentieth century;[20] Julia Gradskova, Elena Iarskaia-Smirnova, and Pavel Romanov engaged with issues of gender, social work, and child welfare;[21] while Yulia V. Khen revealed less discussed features of Russian eugenics.[22] These scholarly accomplishments are by no means isolated. Susan Gross Solomon's 2006 edited volume, for example, offered fresh perspectives and original scholarship on a range of topics pertaining to Soviet–German collaboration in medicine and public health between the wars.[23] Two of the contributions were by the Russian historians of medicine Marina Sorokina, who discussed the 200th anniversary of the Academy of Sciences of the USSR, and Nikolai Krementsov, who analysed the debate surrounding eugenics at the Seventh International Genetics Congress held in Edinburgh in 1939.[24] Both considered collaborations between Russian and European scientists, German in particular, both at the personal level and a reflection of wider international developments and scientific trends.

One corollary to the scholarship on international collaboration and transfer of knowledge is the history of eugenics and genetics.[25] Krementsov, for instance, had established himself as a historian of science during Stalinism and Soviet genetics, more specifically.[26] While Loren R. Graham had drawn attention to similar agendas shared by eugenics movements in Germany and Russia in the 1920s as early as the 1970s,[27] it was only in the past two decades that the wider eugenic discourses were subjected to sustained analysis, most notably in the works of Mark B. Adams.[28] The story of genetics in the Soviet Union, nevertheless, cannot be told in isolation from that of Lynsenkoism, the official Soviet science policy governing the work of geneticists in the USSR from about 1940 to 1960. The agriculturalist Trofim Lysenko (1898–1976) has attracted considerable attention from both Russian and Western scholars in the history of medicine.[29] The ideological battle between Lysenko's agrobiology (according to which environment predominated over heredity), proclaimed as 'socialist biology', and classical genetics began as early as 1936. This conflict impacted the evolution of medicine in both the Soviet Union and communist Eastern Europe, particularly after 1948. It was that year, at the meeting of the Lenin Pansoviet Academy of Agricultural

Sciences in Moscow, that Lysenko was given the authority by the Soviet Communist Party to destroy the study of genetics throughout the Soviet Union and Eastern Europe. The legacy of this episode in the history of Eastern European medicine is still largely undocumented, but there are signs of scholarly improvement.[30]

With the collapse of communism during the 1990s, and the conversion of Russian historians of medicine to non-Marxist interpretations of society and science, there is now a tendency to look anew at the medical heritages of the nineteenth and twentieth centuries. New contextual readings of these heritages, as those indicated above, show that the relationship between medicine, society, politics, and the state was much more complex than linear communist accounts had for decades suggested.[31] This is an area in which there is still much work to be carried out. Similarly, as we shall see in the following section, many of the manifestations of this aggregated scholarship can be detected in the new history of medicine emerging in Eastern Europe after 1989. This is why to investigate it may prove rewarding, as its growing conceptual diversity—as in the case of Russia/Soviet Union—invites us to rethink the existing geographical and cultural boundaries of the history of medicine. In turn, a more nuanced interpretation of the relationship between Eastern European medicine and its international context will certainly emerge once this context is properly documented, historically and scientifically.[32]

History of Medicine in Eastern Europe

Traditionally, studies on the history of medicine in Eastern Europe either have focused exclusively on the life and activities of important physicians—not surprisingly, perhaps, considering that in these countries history of medicine has been largely written by physicians[33]—or have ascribed to physicians their contribution to scientific knowledge in general.[34] Most of the scholarship produced during communism, moreover, was largely contaminated by dogmatic Marxism, making it difficult to assess its intellectual value. In this, of course, historians of medicine were no different from other categories of historians.[35]

Confronting the difficult access to archives, one initial direction of research concentrated on the role played by the Rockefeller Foundation in establishing institutes of hygiene and public health in Eastern

Europe between 1918 and 1940. Attempts were made by the victorious powers to establish a *cordon sanitaire* against communism and the resurgence of German imperialism following the First World War. Within this context, the Rockefeller Foundation offered an alternative vision of medical protection and financial support, one based on programmes of social hygiene and public health. The establishment of institutes of hygiene and public health during the interwar period was part of such programmes, in addition to offering training in modern methods of public health services to physicians and nurses. Numerous grants and fellowships, as well as direct financial contributions towards the costs of these new institutions, were being offered towards the creation of a group of professional experts who were to become—and many in fact did become—responsible for public health administrations in their native countries.[36]

Yet, in Eastern Europe, traditional medical practices and folk medicine, in addition to other methods employed by village healers, survived until the twentieth century. As scholars such as Aida Brenko, Željko Dugac, Mirjana Randić, and Mincho Georgiev have demonstrated with regard to the cases of Croatia and Bulgaria, at the beginning of the twentieth century traditional hygiene and healing were targeted by a new category of professionals educated in modern scientific medicine.[37] Moreover, following the Peace Treaties of 1920–1, countries benefiting territorially in the ensuing peace treaties, like Romania and Yugoslavia, had to address regional disparities and different institutional traditions in the newly annexed territories. These disparities existed, for instance, between the Romanian Old Kingdom and Serbia, which developed their health systems as independent nation-states, and Transylvania, Croatia, Bosnia, and Slovenia, which had been part of the Habsburg Empire prior to November 1918. In these circumstances, leading health reformers like the Croat Andrija Štampar (1888–1958), the Hungarian Béla Johan (1889–1983), and the Romanians Gheorghe Banu (1889–1957) and Iuliu Moldovan (1882–1966) played decisive roles in creating centralized systems for health and hygiene. Their conceptual approaches to nationalized hygiene and health systems became paramount in the interwar years when these doctors held important positions in the ministries of public health of Yugoslavia, Hungary, and Romania.[38] Even after Štampar was forced to resign and took over as the leading expert for the Health Organization of the League of Nations, his ideas remained prominent and, as an instance of cross-border transfers, notably strong among Bulgarian experts on public health.

The discursive contours of nationalism circulating within Eastern European medicine are also echoed in the eclectic historiography dealing with issues of gender and reproduction under communism. Initially most of this scholarship was produced by Western scholars,[39] but recently gender studies and women's history have benefited from intense local historical work, both strongly feminist and analytically comfortable with many subfields within the history of medicine. With the establishment of the journal *Aspasia* it seems that the hitherto largely absent Eastern European scholarly voices have finally found an appropriate forum for their social, cultural, and political interests.

However, the geographical diversity and multiplicity of historical traditions in Eastern European medicine during the twentieth century are perhaps best addressed by international teams of scholars rather than individuals. An example of this tendency is Kurt Schilde and Dagmar Schulte's edited volume on professional welfare in Eastern Europe.[40] The editors successfully assorted micro with oral history techniques, providing a convincing portrait of various episodes in the history of social health in Eastern Europe. Contributions to this volume cover aspects relating to social policies, as well as its agents and achievemens in Hungary, Poland, Bulgaria, Croatia, the Soviet Union and Romania, Slovenia, and Latvia. Milena Angelova, for instance, provides an overview of the activities of the Society for the Fight against Tuberculosis in Bulgaria between 1908 and 1944, while Silvana Rachieru and Dorottya Szikra and Eszter Varsa engaged with some of the challenges faced by social workers in interwar Romania and the settlement movement in Budapest during the 1940s, respectively. This wide geographic distribution of topics adopted by the new scholarship is a positive development, but can also gave rise to problems of conceptual communication: different components of the social history of medicine arguably talking quite different languages, be it the topic of public health, epidemics, hygiene, social protectionism, or eugenics. Sabine Hering and Berteke Waaldijk addressed this epistemological conundrum in their volume on the history of welfare in Eastern Europe between 1900 and 1960.[41]

The publication of these edited volumes offers new perspectives on some hitherto neglected topics in the history of welfare, social hygiene, and public health. Complementing this collaborative endeavour is another geared towards unearthing and editing forgotten sources on the history of public health and the history of medicine more generally. Romanian historians of medicine, such as Valentin-Veron Toma, Octavian Buda, and the Hungarian Gábor Palló, are particularly active in this field.[42] Others, like the Bulgarian Kristina Popova, have convincingly analysed the relationship between child welfare and national ideologies during the interwar period.[43] Ideas about the health of the nation were also evident in the work of those interwar health reformers preoccupied with improving the hygienic conditions of the peasantry, as demonstrated by Judit Bíró's 2006 collection of texts on rural public health in 1930s and 1940s Hungary.[44] She included excerpts from seminal works such as László Kerbolt's *The Sick Village* (1934) and Béla Johan's *Healing the Hungarian Village* (1939). Both Kerbolt and Johan, director of the National Institute of Hygiene in Budapest, argued for improved national health policies and provided assessments of working conditions, poverty, and diseases in the Hungarian villages. Predominantly focused on rural environments, precarious hygiene conditions, malnutrition, social diseases (such as alcoholism), sexually transmitted diseases (syphilis, in particular), high levels of infant mortality, the rejection of modern medicine, and a persistence of traditional methods of healing, they all constituted determinant factors in shaping the emergence of policies of health and social hygiene in interwar Hungary. With the Rockefeller Foundation's support, and under Johan's supervision, public health demonstrations were organized in Hungarian villages during the late 1920s with the aim of familiarizing the rural population with modern hygiene methods, regular health screening, and preventive medicine.[45]

Bíró's book, with its emphasis on the community and localism, also contributed to ongoing debates on the impact of state-controlled initiatives in public health and social hygiene on communities in rural parts of Eastern Europe during the interwar period. Central to medical theories developed by public health reformers about these regions was the idea that the biological condition of communities could also be improved with the help of external factors such as education and through a controlled environment to prevent and eradicate contagious diseases and parasites, as well as through sanitation and better housing.

Another direction of research powerfully illustrates this process: Eastern European countries were and are religiously and ethnically heterogeneous so, not surprisingly, the idea of a homogeneous national community figured prominently in the dominant health discourses elaborated between 1900 and 1945. In these circumstances, health and hygiene became part of a larger eugenic and biopolitical agenda, serving as a vehicle for transmitting a social and political message that transcended political differences and opposing ideological camps. The idea of the healthy nation was as diverse ideologically as it was geographically: it was adhered to by professionals, scientists, and political elites irrespective of their different political and cultural camps. In stark contrast to the Soviet Union, eugenics in Eastern Europe has only recently been revived as an academic topic. When its existence was acknowledged by local historians of medicine, it was generally dismissed as insignificant. Gheorghe Brătescu, for example, described eugenics in Romania as 'feeble'.[46] Similarly, in the 1970s, the Hungarian historian of medicine Endre Réti examined Darwin's influence on Hungarian medical thought in the first decades of the twentieth century, but marginalized the interest in eugenics of prominent Hungarian doctors. During the same period, Endre Czeizel, a historian of genetics, published several articles on the history of eugenics, but focused exclusively on the role played by Francis Galton and Karl Pearson in shaping the contours of the discipline, without mentioning the theoretical contributions made by Hungarian eugenicists.[47]

More recently, it was Maria Bucur who published the first book on an Eastern European eugenic movement, followed shortly by Magdalena Gawin's history of Polish eugenics and Gergana Mirčeva's discussion of Bulgarian eugenics.[48] In Eastern Europe, eugenics—as Darko Polšek, Attila Melegh, and Marius Turda have argued—also had distinctive national overtones, differentiated by each country's individual culture and social context. Exploring these specific permutations requires linguistic and analytical tools capable of capturing the multifarious nature of eugenic thinking. One must examine eugenic ideas and practices in their specific regional and national contexts on the one hand, while simultaneously integrating these phenomena into their international contexts on the other.[49] A new generation of historians of eugenics credits comparative methodological models, instead of the conventional scholarship's tendency to insist on the uniqueness of national cases, and suggests that the history of eugenics needs to be studied within a more integrative European and international framework. Rather than remaining mere appendices to specific national traditions, the commonly suppressed histories of the theory and practice of eugenics in Eastern Europe must necessarily be disclosed and discussed within their national historic contexts, and as local permutations of a larger, international, eugenic movement in interwar Europe.[50]

This new trajectory now includes such thorny topics as eugenic sterilization or the treatment of mental patients during the Second World War, both of which are only very recently touched upon by historians.[51] Worth mentioning in this context are Brigitta Baran and Gábor Gazdag, who focused on the scientific debates that led Hungarian psychiatrists like Károly Schaffer (1864–1939) and László Benedek (1887–1945) to engage in eugenic activities during the 1930s; they also revealed how some of these activities influenced public health policies and the treatment of mental patients during the Second World War. Equally important is their treatment of Schaffer and his school within the general development of European psychiatry during the first half of the twentieth century.[52] This recourse to historical memory is essential if, on the one hand, these countries are to be reconciled with their troubled past and if, on the other, the history of interwar eugenic movements is to be systematically analysed through their appropriate local, regional, national, and international contexts.

Conclusion

The time has finally come for the history of medicine in Eastern Europe and Russia/Soviet Union to be firmly situated within the international arena. To be sure, there is room for improvement, especially in terms of methodology and access to archival repositories. Above all, it is imperative that works of comprehensive synthesis are produced, studies that move away from narrow definitions of medical

history and are theoretically and analytically of genuine sophistica-
tion. As late as 1993, Ludmilla Jordanova pondered whether the
social history of medicine had achieved intellectual respectability as
an academic discipline. As she understood it, for this to happen the
discipline needed, first, to be based on 'a wide range of primary
sources known to active scholars, and a significant proportion of
these should be in the public domain, that is, highly accessible, if
possible published in some form'. Second, Jordanova continued, the
social history of medicine 'needs a basic map for the purpose of
intellectual navigation. However contentious such a map may be, it
provides the essential structure within which narratives are constructed, chronologies elaborated and frameworks refined.' Other
conditions required were 'a secondary literature' that 'is both sufficiently diverse and sufficiently large to act as a critical mass'; and,
finally, 'a mature field conducts sophisticated debates, which encourage interpretations to be refined and, if necessary, radically altered'.[53]

Though some nuances are surely missing from this description,
what Jordanova is arguing for—correctly I believe—is the meticulous
exploration of the interaction between medical texts and their social,
cultural, economic, and political contexts. Nowhere is this intellectual
programme more important than in Russia and Eastern Europe. The
history of medicine evolves on composite grounds: it reflects and is
affected by historical circumstances, both diachronically and syn-
chronically. Besides the task of mediating between the local canons
in Russia and Eastern Europe and their international framework,
there is a pressing need to tackle these phenomena in the framework
of the entangled history within these regions: namely, to look at
national medical traditions from a regional and cross-national perspective, and to thereby challenge the purported uniqueness and
mimetic competition of these national cultures.

History of medicine's importance to the general historiographic
traditions in these regions is yet to be acknowledged,[54] but the fact
that an increasing number of historians in Russia and Eastern Europe
are interested in the history of eugenics, medical anthropology, psychiatry, and criminal anthropology is already noticeable. Compared
with the pre-1989 period, this emerging scholarship claims not to be
vitiated by ideological manipulation and biased interpretations. It
remains, however, to be seen whether these new intellectual projects

will have the desired impact on the discipline of history, in general, and the history of medicine in particular. Current debates and contestations accruing around the meaning of national history in Russia and Eastern Europe are an eloquent example that scholars in these regions are finally able to produce different, almost competing, readings of the past. The history of medicine, too, is currently undergoing a remarkable transformation—one defined by society's need to engage with scientific advances and the ethical dilemmas they raise, on the one hand, and the inclusion of hitherto marginalized case studies on the other. The inclusion and juxtaposition of Russian and Eastern European histories of medicine with their well-known Western European counterparts thus lies at the heart of a more ambitious historiographic project that strives not only to yield original and timely archival research on these neglected national case studies, but also to redefine and diversify the overarching debate on the centrality of medicine in modern European history.

Notes

1 This is not to say that informative accounts of Eastern Europe medicine and health have not been produced by Western scholars, especially during the 1960s and 1970s, when reliable data were still available. Such studies include E. Richard Weinerman, *Social Medicine in Eastern Europe: The Organization of Health Services and the Education of Medical Personnel in Czechoslovakia, Hungary, and Poland* (Cambridge, MA: Harvard University Press, 1969); Michael Kaser, *Health Care in the Soviet Union and Eastern Europe* (London: Croom Helm, 1976); Michael Ryan, *The Organization of Soviet Medical Care* (Oxford: Blackwell, 1978); Gordon Hyde, *The Soviet Health System: A Historical and Comparative Study* (London: Lawrence and Wishart, 1974); and William A. Knaus, *Inside Russian Medicine: An American Doctor's First Hand Report* (New York: Everest House, 1981).

2 Chapters on Russia, Poland, and the Czech Republic are included in William C. Cockerham (ed.), *The Blackwell Companion to Medical Sociology* (Oxford: Blackwell, 2001); on Czechoslovakia and Croatia in Iris Borowy and Wolf D. Gruner (eds), *Facing Illness in Troubled Times: Health in Europe in the Interwar Years, 1918–1939* (Bern: Peter Lang, 2005); and on Hungary and Croatia in Iris Borowy and Anne Hardy (eds), *Of Medicine and Men: Biographies and Ideas in European Social Medicine between the World Wars* (Bern: Peter Lang, 2008).

3 Paul J. Weindling, *Epidemics and Genocide in Eastern Europe* (Oxford: Oxford University Press, 2000); Patrick Zylberman, 'Mosquitos and the Komitadjis: Malaria and Borders in Macedonia (1919–1938)', in Borowy and Gruner (eds), *Facing Illness in Troubled Times*, 305–43; Lion Murard and Patrick

Zylberman, 'French Social Medicine on the International Public Health Map in the 1930s', in Esteban Rodríguez-Ocaña (ed.), *The Politics of the Healthy Life: An International Perspective* (Sheffield: European Association for the History of Medicine and Health Publications, 2002), 197–218.

4 Petr Svobodný and Ludmila Hlaváčková, *Dějiny lékařství v českých zemích* (Prague: Triton, 2004); Károly Kapronczay and Katalin Kapronczay (eds), *Az orvostörténelem Magyarországon* (Budapest: Semmelweis Orvostörténeti Múzeum, 2005); and Radu Iftimovici, *Istoria universală a medicinii și farmaciei* (Bucharest: Editura Academiei Române, 2008).

5 Quoted in Mark G. Field, 'Soviet Medicine', in Roger Cooter and John Pickstone (eds), *Medicine in the Twentieth Century* (Amsterdam: Harwood Academic, 2000), 51–66, at 52.

6 Ibid.

7 Henry E. Sigerist, *Socialized Medicine in the Soviet Union* (New York: Norton, 1937), 308.

8 Horsley W. Gantt, *A Medical Review of Soviet Russia* (London: British Medical Association, 1928); Arthur Newsholme and John A. Kingsbury, *Red Medicine: Socialized Health in Soviet Russia* (Garden City, NY: Doubleday, 1933); Sigerist, *Socialized Medicine in the Soviet Union*; idem, *Medicine and Health in the Soviet Union* (New York: Citadel Press, 1947).

9 Mark G. Field, *Doctor and Patient in Soviet Russia* (Cambridge, MA: Harvard University Press, 1957); idem, *Soviet Socialized Medicine: An Introduction* (New York: Free Press, 1967); Loren R. Graham, *Science and Philosophy in the Soviet Union* (New York: Alfred Knopf, 1972); idem, *Between Science and Values* (New York: Columbia University Press, 1983); Kendall E. Bailes, *Technology and Society under Lenin and Stalin: Origins of the Soviet Technical Intelligentsia, 1917–1941* (Princeton: Princeton University Press, 1978).

10 Mark G. Field, 'The Hybrid Profession: Soviet Medicine', in Anthony Jones (ed.), *Professions and the State: Expertise and Autonomy in the Soviet Union and Eastern Europe* (Philadelphia: Temple University Press, 1991), 43–62.

11 Nancy M. Frieden, *Russian Physicians in an Era of Reform and Revolution, 1856–1905* (Princeton: Princeton University Press, 1981).

12 Jeanette E. Tuve, *The First Russian Women Physicians* (Newtonville, MA: Oriental Research Partners, 1984).

13 John F. Hutchinson, *Politics and Public Health in Revolutionary Russia, 1890–1918* (Baltimore: Johns Hopkins University Press, 1990).

14 Susan Solomon and John F. Hutchinson (eds), *Health and Society in Revolutionary Russia* (Bloomington: Indiana University Press, 1990).

15 Amir Weiner, 'Nature, Nurture, and Memory in a Socialist Utopia: Delineating the Soviet Socio-Ethnic Body in the Age of Socialism', *American Historical Review* 104 (4) (1999), 1114–55. See also Mark B. Adams, 'The Soviet Nature-Nurture Debate', in Loren R. Graham (ed.), *Science and the Soviet Social Order* (Cambridge, MA: Harvard University Press, 1990), 94–138; Daniel Beer, *Renovating Russia: The Human Sciences and the Fate of Liberal Modernity, 1880–1930* (Ithaca: Cornell University Press, 2008).

16 Susan Gross Solomon, 'The Expert and the State in Russian Public Health: Continuities and Change across the Revolutionary Divide', in Dorothy Porter (ed.), *The History of Public Health and the Modern State* (Amsterdam: Rodopi, 1994), 183–223, at 185.

17 Mary Schaffer Conroy, *The Soviet Pharmaceutical Business during Its First Two Decades, 1917–1937* (New York: Peter Lang, 2006).

18 Gail Lapidus, *Women in Soviet Society* (Berkeley: University of California Press, 1978); Wendy Goldman, *Women, the State and the Revolution: Soviet Family Policy and Social Life, 1917–1936* (Cambridge: Cambridge University Press, 1993); and the contributions by Janet Hyer, Susan Gross Solomon, and Christopher Williams in Rosalind J. Marsh (ed.), *Women in Russia and Ukraine* (Cambridge: Cambridge University Press, 1996); Michele Rivkin-Fish, *Women's Health in Post-Soviet Russia: The Politics of Intervention* (Bloomington: Indiana University Press, 2005); Pat Simpson, 'Bolshevism and "Sexual revolution": Visualising New Soviet Woman as an Eugenic Ideal 1917–1932', in Fae Brauer and Anthea Callen (eds), *Corpus Delecti: Art, Sex and Eugenics* (Aldershot: Ashgate, 2008), 209–38.

19 Mark B. Mirsky, 'State of Medicine in Russia (1581–1918)', in John H. Cule and John M. Lancaster (eds), *Russia and Wales: Essays on the History of State Involvement in Health Care* (Cardiff: History of Medicine Society of Wales, 1994), 15–29; Vladimir M. Verbitski, 'Ethical Problems in Nineteenth Century Russian Clinical Medicine Relating to Obstetrics and Gynaecology', ibid. 31–42; and Tatyana S. Sorokina, 'The Struggle against the Plague Moscow, 1771–1772', ibid. 43–65.

20 Boris Yudin, 'Human Experimentation in Russia/Soviet Union in the First Half of the 20th Century', in Volker Roelcke and Giovanni Maio (eds), *Twentieth Century Ethics of Human Research: Historical Perspectives on Values, Practices, and Regulations* (Stuttgart: Franz Steiner Verlag, 2004), 99–110.

21 Julia Gradskova, '"Nurseries Have Brought up Children": Maternity, Gender and Social Work in the Soviet Union in the 1930s to the 1950s', in Kurt Schilde and Dagmar Schulte (eds), *Need and Care: Glimpses into the Beginning of Eastern Europe's Professional Welfare* (Opladen: Barbara Budrich, 2005), 75–90; Elena Iarskaia-Smirnova and Pavel Romanov, 'Institutional Child Care in Soviet Russia: Everyday Life in the Children's Home "Krasnyi Gorodok" in Saratov, 1920s–1940s', ibid. 91–121.

22 Yulia V. Khen, 'Unknown Pages of Russian Eugenics', *Herald of the Russian Academy of Sciences* 76 (4) (2006), 385–91.

23 Susan Gross Solomon (ed.), *Doing Medicine Together: Germany and Russia between the Wars* (Toronto: University of Toronto Press, 2006).

24 Marina Sorokina, 'Partners of Choice/*Faute de Mieux?* Russians and Germans at the 200th Anniversary of the Academy of Sciences, 1925', in Solomon (ed.), *Doing Medicine Together*, 61–102; Nikolai Krementsov, 'Eugenics, *Rassenhygiene*, and Human Genetics in the Late 1930: The Case of the Seventh International Genetics Congress', ibid. 368–404.

25 For a Soviet perspective, see A. E. Gaissinovitch, 'The Origins of Soviet Genetics and the Struggle with Lamarckism, 1922–1929', *Journal of the History of Biology* 13 (1) (1980), 1–51.

26 Nikolai Krementsov, *Stalinist Science* (Princeton: Princeton University Press, 1997); *idem*, *International Science between the World Wars: The Case of Genetics* (London: Routledge, 2005).

27 Loren R. Graham, 'Science and Values: The Eugenics Movement in Germany', *American Historical Review* 82 (5) (1977), 1133–64.

28 Mark B. Adams, 'Eugenics in Russia, 1900–1940', in *idem* (ed.), *The Well-born Science: Eugenics in Germany, France, Brazil, and Russia* (Oxford: Oxford University Press, 1990), 153–216; *idem*, 'Eugenics as Social Medicine in Revolutionary Russia', in Solomon and Hutchinson (eds), *Health and Society in Revolutionary Russia*, 200–23; Alberto Spektorowski, 'The Eugenic Temptation in Socialism: Sweden, Germany, and the Soviet Union', *Comparative Studies in Society and History* 46 (2004), 84–106; Mark B. Adams, Garland E. Allen, and Sheila Faith Weiss, 'Human Heredity and Politics: A Comparative Institutional Study of the Eugenics Record Office at Cold Spring Harbor (United States), the Kaiser Wilhelm Institute for Anthropology, Human Heredity, and Eugenics (Germany), and the Maxim Gorky Medical Genetics Institute (USSR)', *Osiris* 20 (2005), 232–62.

29 Valery N. Soyfer, *Lysenko and the Tragedy of Soviet Science* (New Brunswick, NJ: Rutgers University Press, 1994); Nils Roll-Hansen, *The Lysenko Effect: The Politics of Science* (Amherst, NY: Prometheus Books, 2004).

30 William deJong-Lambert, 'Szczepan Pieniążek, Edmund Malinowski, and Lysenkoism in Poland', *East European Politics and Societies* 21 (3) (2007), 403–23; and William deJong-Lambert, 'The New Biology in Poland after the Second World War: Polish Lysenkoism', *Paedagogica Historica* 45 (2009), 403–20; Miklós Müller, 'Lysenkoism in Hungary', paper presented at the International Workshop on Lysenkoism, Harriman Institute, Columbia University, New York, 4–5 December 2009.

31 Irina Sirotkina, *Diagnosing Literary Genius: A Cultural History of Psychiatry in Russia, 1880–1930* (Baltimore: Johns Hopkins University Press, 2002).

32 Marius Turda, 'Focus on Social History of Medicine in Central and Eastern Europe', *Social History of Medicine* 21 (2008), 395–401; Marius Turda and Paul J. Weindling, 'Eugenics, Race and Nation in Central and Southeast Europe, 1900–1940: A Historiographic Overview', in Marius Turda and Paul J. Weindling (eds), *Blood and Homeland: Eugenics and Racial Nationalism in Central and Southeast Europe, 1900–1940* (Budapest: Central European University Press, 2007), 1–20; and Marius Turda et. al., 'Framing Issues of Health, Hygiene and Eugenics in Southeastern Europe', in Christian Promitzer et. al. (eds), *Health, Hygiene and Eugenics in Southeastern Europe to 1945* (Budapest: Central European University, 2011), 1–24.

33 Gh. Bratescu and Klaus Fabritius, *Biological and Medical Sciences in Romania* (Bucharest: Editura Ştiinţifică şi Enciclopedică, 1989; Lazar Stanojević

(ed.), *700 godina medicine u Srba—700 ans de médecine chez lez Serbes* (Belgrade: Srpska akademija nauka i umetnosti, 1971); Izet Mašić, *Korijeni medicine i zdravstva u Bosni i Hercegovini* (Sarajevo: Avicena, 2005); and Győző Birtalan, *Évszázadok orvosai* (Budapest: Akadémiai Kiadó, 1995). One should also mention here journals like *La Santé Publique*, *Archives de l'Union Médicale Balkanique* (published in Bucharest), and *Orvostörténeti Közlemények* (published in Budapest), which commissioned and published numerous articles written by physicians on the history of medicine from all communist countries.

34 The Croat health reformer Andrija Štampar is arguably the most known case. See M. D. Grmek (ed.), *Serving the Cause of Public Health: Selected Papers of Andrija Štampar* (Zagreb: Skola narodnog zdravlja Andrija Štampar, 1966); and Željko Dugac, 'New Public Health for a New State: Interwar Public Health in the Kingdom of Serbs, Croats, and Slovenes and the Rockefeller Foundation', in Borowy and Gruner (eds), *Facing Illness in Troubled Times*, 277–304.

35 There are of course exceptions in each country. For Romania, see Valeriu L. Bologa, *Din istoria medicinii româneşti şi universale* (Bucharest: Editura Academiei Republicii Populare Române, 1962).

36 For Hungary, see Gábor Palló, 'Make a Peak on the Plain: The Rockefeller Foundation's Szeged Project', in William H. Schneider (ed.), *Rockefeller Philanthropy and Modern Biomedicine: International Initiatives from World War I to the Cold War* (Bloomington: Indiana University Press, 2002), 87–105; for Romania, see Ecaterina Petrina, *The Impact of the Rockefeller Foundation on Romanian Scientific Development, 1920–1939*, PhD dissertation, Cornell University, 1997; for Yugoslavia, see Željko Dugač, *Protiv bolesti i neznanja: Rockefellerova fondacija u međuratnoj Jugoslaviji* (Zagreb: Srednja Europa, 2005); for Bulgaria, see Milena Angelova, 'Rokfelerovata fondatsiya i amerikanskata blizkoiztochna fondatsiya v Balgariya—initsiativi v poleto na sotsialnata rabota, 20–30te godini na XX vek', in Kristina Popova and Milena Angelova (eds), *Obshtestveno podpomagane i sotsialna rabota v Balgariya: Istoriya, institutsii, ideologii, imena* (Blagoevgrad: Yugozapaden universitet 'Neofit Rilski' Blagoevgrad, 2005), 112–25.

37 Aida Brenko, Željko Dugac, and Mirjana Randić, *Narodna medicina* (Zagreb: Etnografski muzej Zagreb, 2001); Mincho Georgiev (ed.), *Balgarska narodna medicina. Enciklopediya* (Sofia: Izdatelska kashta 'Petar Beron', 1999).

38 Henry E. Sigerist, 'Yugoslavia and the XIth International Congress of the History of Medicine', *Bulletin of the History of Medicine* 7 (1939), 99–147.

39 Alena Heitlinger, *Reproduction, Medicine and the Socialist State* (London: Macmillan, 1987); Nanette Funk and Magda Mueller (eds), *Gender Politics and Post Communism: Reflections from Eastern Europe and the Former Soviet Union* (New York: Routledge, 1993); Henry P. David (ed.), *From Abortion to Contraception: A Resource to Public Policies and Reproductive Behaviour in Central and Eastern Europe from 1917 to the Present* (Westport, CT: Greenwood Press, 1999); Susan Gal and Gail Kligman (eds), *Reproducing Gender: Politics, Publics, and Everyday Life after Socialism* (Princeton: Princeton University Press, 2000).

40 Kurt Schilde and Dagmar Schulte (eds), *Need and Care: Glimpses into the Beginnings of Eastern Europe's Professional Welfare* (Opladen: Barbara Budrich, 2005).

41 Sabine Hering and Berteke Waaldijk, *Guardians of the Poor: Custodians of the Public. Welfare History in Eastern Europe, 1900–1960* (Opladen: Barbara Budrich, 2006).

42 Valentin Veron-Toma and Adrian Majuru (eds), *Nebunia. O antropologie istorică românească* (Bucharest: Paralela 45, 2006); Octavian Buda, *Criminalitatea. O istorie medico-legală românească* (Bucharest: Paralela 45, 2007); Valentin Veron Toma, *Alexandru Sutzu: Începuturile psihiatriei ştiinţifice în România secolului al XIX-lea* (Bucharest: Dowiner, 2008); and Octavian Buda (ed.), *Despre regenerarea şi degenerarea unei naţiuni* (Bucharest: Tritonic, 2009).

43 Kristina Popova, *Natsionalnoto dete. Blagotvoritelnata i prosvetna deynost na Sajuza za zakrila na detsata v Balgariya 1925–1944* (Sofia: LIK, 1999).

44 Judit Bíró (ed.), *Hivatalos falukutatók: A vidéki Magyarország leírása 1930 és 1940 között* (Budapest: Polgart, 2006).

45 Gábor Palló, 'Rescue and Cordon Sanitaire: The Rockefeller Foundation in Hungarian Public Health', *Studies in History and Philosophy of Biological and Biomedical Sciences* 31 (2000), 433–45.

46 Gh. Brătescu, *Către sănătatea perfectă: O istorie a utopianismului medical* (Bucharest: Humanitas, 1999), 406–11.

47 Endre Réti, 'Darwin's Influence on Hungarian Medical Thought', *Medical History in Hungary* (Budapest, 1972), 157–67; Endre Czeizel, 'A biométerek és a mendelisták ellentéte', *Orvosi Hetilap* 113, 4 (1972), 213–17; Endre Czeizel, 'Az eugenika—létrejotte, kompromittálása és jövője', *Orvosi Hetilap* 113 (6) (1972), 331–4; Ferenc Pisztora, 'Benedek László élete, személyisége és életművének társadalom- és kultúrpsychiátriai, psychologiai és eugenikai vonatkozásai', *Ideggyógyászati Szemle* 41 (1988), 441–56.

48 Maria Bucur, *Eugenics and Modernization in Interwar Romania* (Pittsburgh: Pittsburgh University Press, 2000); Magdalena Gawin, *Rasa i nowoczesność. Historia polskiego ruchu eugenicznego, 1880–1952* (Warsawa: Wydawnicwo Neriton, 2003); Gergana Mirčeva, 'Balgarskiyat evgenichen proekt ot 20-te i 30-te godini na minaliya vek i normativniyat kod na 'rodnoto', *Kritika i humanizam* 17 (1) (2004), 207–21. See also Marius Turda, 'The Nation as Object: Race, Blood and Biopolitics in Interwar Romania', *Slavic Review* 66 (3) (2007), 413–41; and Ilija Malović, 'Eugenika kao ideološki sastojak fašizma u Srbiji 1930-ih godina XX veka', *Sociologija* 50 (1) (2008), 79–96.

49 Darko Polšek, *Sudbina odabranih: Eugenička nasljede u urijeme genske tehnologije* (Zagreb: ArTresor, 2004); Attila Melegh, *On the East-West Slope: Globalization, Nationalism, Racism and Discourses on Central and Eastern Europe* (Budapest: Central European University Press, 2006); Marius Turda and Paul J. Weindling (eds), *Blood and Homeland: Eugenics and Racial Nationalism in Central and Southeast Europe, 1900–1940* (Budapest: Central European University Press, 2007); Christian Promitzer et al. (eds), *Health, Hygiene, and Eugenics in Southeastern Europe to 1945*; and Marius Turda, *Modernism and Eugenics* (Basingstoke: Palgrave Macmillan, 2010).

50 Marius Turda, '"A New Religion": Eugenics and Racial Scientism in
    Pre-World War Hungary', *Totalitarian Movements and Political Religions* 7
    (3) (2006), 303–25; Marius Turda, 'Heredity and Eugenic Thought in
    Early Twentieth-Century Hungary', *Orvostörténeti Közlemények. Communica-
    tiones de Historia Artis Medicinae* 52 (1–2) (2006), 101–18; and *idem*, 'The
    Biology of War: Eugenics in Hungary, 1914–1918', *Austrian History Year-
    book* 40 (1) (2009), 238–64.
51 Marius Turda, '"To End the Degeneration of a Nation": Debates on
    Eugenic Sterilization in Interwar Romania', *Medical History* 53 (1) (2009),
    77–104; Béla Siró, 'Eugenikai törekvések az ideg- és elmegyógyászatban
    Magyarországon a két világháború között', *Orvosi Hetilap* 144 (35) (2003),
    1737–42; Magdalena Gawin, 'Polish Psychiatrists and Eugenic Steriliza-
    tion during the Interwar Period', *International Journal of Mental Health* 36 (1)
    (2007), 67–78; and Kamila Uzarczyk, 'War against the Unfit: Eugenic
    Sterilization in German Silesia, 1934–1944: *Sine Ira et Studio* (without
    Anger and Bias)', *International Journal of Mental Health* 36 (1) (2007),
    79–88. For the treatment of mental patients during the Second World
    War, see Vasyl Doguzov and Svitlana Rusalovs'ka, 'The Massacre of
    Mental Patients in Ukraine, 1941–1943', *International Journal of Mental
    Health* 36 (1) (2007), 105–11.
52 Brigitta Baran and Gábor Gazdag, 'The Fate of the Hungarian Psychi-
    atric Patients during World War II', *International Journal of Mental Health* 35
    (4) (2006–7), 88–99; and Brigitta Baran, István Bitter, Max Fink, Gábor
    Gazdag, and Edward Shorter, 'Károly Schaffer and His School: The
    Birth of Biological Psychiatry in Hungary, 1890–1940', *European Psychiatry*
    23 (6) (2008), 449–56.
53 Ludmilla Jordanova, 'Has the Social History of Medicine Come of Age?',
    Historical Journal 36 (2) (1993), 437–49, at 437.
54 For example, the most recent evaluation of Hungarian historiography
    does not even mention the contributions made by historians of medicine.
    See Gábor Gyáni, 'Trends in Contemporary Hungarian Historical Schol-
    arship', *Social History* 34 (2) (2009), 250–60.

Select Bibliography

Bernasconi, Sara, Heike Karge and Friederike Kind-Kovács (Hg.), *Beyond
    Medicine: History and Politics of Public Health in Twentieth Century Europe*
    (Budapest: Central European University Press, 2017).
Borowy, Iris, and Wolf D. Gruner (eds), *Facing Illness in Troubled Times: Health in
    Europe in the Interwar Years, 1918–1939* (Bern: Peter Lang, 2005).
Borowy, Iris, and Anne Hardy (eds), *Of Medicine and Men: Biographies and Ideas in
    European Social Medicine between the World Wars* (Bern: Peter Lang, 2008).
Bynum, W. F., and Roy Porter (eds), *Companion Encyclopedia of the History of
    Medicine*, 2 vols (London: Routledge, 1993).

Cooter, Roger, and John Pickstone (eds), *Medicine in the Twentieth Century* (London: Routledge, 2000).

DeJong-Lambert, William, *The Cold War Politics of Genetic Research: An Introduction to the Lysenko Affair* (Dordrecht: Springer, 2012).

Farley, John, *To Cast Out Disease: A History of the International Health Division of Rockefeller Foundation (1913–1951)* (Oxford: Oxford University Press, 2003).

Graham, Loren, *Lysenko's Ghost: Epigenetics and Russia* (Cambridge, Mass.: Harvard University Press, 2016).

Healy, Dan, *Bolshevik Sexual Forensics: Diagnosing Disorder in the Clinic and Courtroom, 1917–1939* (DeKalb: Northern Illinois University Press, 2009).

Porter, Roy (eds), *The Cambridge History of Medicine* (Cambridge: Cambridge University Press, 2006).

Promitzer, Christian, Sevasti Trubeta, and Marius Turda (eds), *Health, Hygiene, and Eugenics in Southeastern Europe to 1945* (Budapest: Central European University Press, 2011).

Rodríguez-Ocaña, Esteban (ed.), *The Politics of the Healthy Life: An International Perspective* (Sheffield: EAHMHP, 2002).

Savelli, Mat, and Sarah Marks, (eds), *Psychiatry in Communist Europe* (Basingstoke: Palgrave Macmillan, 2015).

Solomon, Susan Gross (eds), *Doing Medicine Together: Germany and Russia between the Wars* (Toronto: University of Toronto Press, 2006).

Solomon, Susan Gross, Lion Murard, and Patrick Zylberman (eds), *Shifting Boundaries of Public Health. Europe in the Twentieth Century* (Rochester, NY: University of Rochester Press, 2008).

Stauter-Halsted, Keely, *The Devil's Chain: Prostitution and Social Control in Partitioned Poland* (Ithaca, NY: Cornell University Press, 2015).

Turda, Marius, *Modernism and Eugenics* (Basingstoke: Palgrave Macmillan, 2010).

Turda, Marius, *Eugenics and Nation in Early 20th Century Hungary* (Basingstoke: Palgrave Macmillan, 2015).

Turda, Marius (ed.), *The History of Eugenics in East-Central Europe, 1900–1945: Sources and Commentaries* (London: Bloomsbury, 2015; 2017).

Woodward, John, and Robert Jütte (eds), *Coping with Sickness: Perspectives on Health Care, Past and Present* (Sheffield: EAHMHP, 1996).

6

Public Health and Medicine in Latin America

Anne-Emanuelle Birn

The countries of Latin America are enormously diverse demographically, geographically, politically, economically, and culturally, yet they share certain features, providing coherence to thinking about the history of health and medicine in regional terms. Subject to Iberian colonialism roughly from the late fifteenth to the nineteenth centuries, the countries that now constitute Latin America (Mexico, Spanish Central America, Cuba, Puerto Rico, and the Dominican Republic in the Caribbean, and ten of the thirteen countries in South America) share intertwining historical, linguistic, and cultural legacies.[1] Iberian imperialism included a particularly strong role for the Catholic Church, which heavily influenced medical and public health practices but never fully displaced traditional practitioners and healing ideologies, especially, but not only, in settings where significant Indigenous populations survived European conquest. Linguistic–cultural relations in Spanish Latin America (and with and within Portuguese Latin America) enabled limited interchange in the colonial era, for example through circulating materia medica, the work of Jesuits in medical geography, and colonial efforts at the control of epidemics.

With the exception of Cuba and Puerto Rico, contemporary Latin American republics achieved political independence in the nineteenth century; across northern and western South America the liberation movement was led and inspired by Simón Bolívar (1783–1830). In the case of Brazil, the exiled Portuguese monarchy created a displaced

Brazilian Empire in 1822, which lasted until 1889. Throughout the region, professional ties and conflict—typically regarding the spread of epidemic disease—were enhanced after the old order was toppled and rapidly accelerated in the nineteenth century with the rise of sea and rail transport and an increase in commerce.

After independence, European economic and cultural interests in the region persisted, broadening far beyond the former colonial powers to include, for example, English, French, and Dutch financial investments, and waves of immigrants from Southern and Eastern Europe, Asia, the Middle East, and beyond. Meanwhile, US political and economic power in the region mounted. These developments were reflected in medical ideas, organization, and practice. For example, post-revolutionary French medicine served as the predominant (but not the sole) model for the nineteenth- and early twentieth-century institutionalization and professionalization of health and medical fields; US medical influence accelerated after the Second World War, occasionally challenged by Soviet interests.

While Latin American health and medicine have long been viewed as derivative, more recent scholarship shows considerable regional innovation and the worldwide reverberation of a range of 'home-grown' medical ideas and practices, public health policies, and health care organizational models. Today, the region is characterized by enormous inequities, with seemingly insurmountable divides in health conditions and in medical and health services (related to research and professionalization) between elites, a precarious middling group, and large marginalized populations. Even so, certain locales (including Costa Rica and Cuba) have admirably addressed health inequalities. This chapter addresses these developments, diversities, and congruities through five historical eras and thematic perspectives and concludes with an analysis of historiographical approaches in the contemporary context, exploring the major challenges facing historians writing about Latin American health and medicine today, particularly the links between history and contemporary national and global health policy issues.

From a historiographical perspective, work on Latin American health and medicine followed a fairly traditional 'doctors and discoveries' trajectory through the 1960s, with two overlapping features distinguishing it from the Anglo-European literature: the very writing of medical history in the so-called periphery led to a far earlier recognition of the role of colonial authorities and institutions in shaping national and regional trends than among 'metropolitan' scholars; and some pioneering scholars addressed the role of Indigenous medical practice (if typically disparagingly) and syncretism in the shaping of Latin American medicine.[2] That said, these hagiographic approaches tended to overemphasize the one-way influence and importance of European medical developments. In the 1970s, a new generation of historians of health and medicine in various Latin American countries, marked by Marxist ideas and political movements, brought materialist and political economy explanations to the fore, paying special attention to imperialism and medicine; in subsequent decades the ideas of Michel Foucault and Pierre Bourdieu surfaced to shape more theoretical work that was sometimes short on empirical research, due to limited funding and archival access. By the 1990s, a new generation of historians of Latin American health and medicine emerged from throughout the Americas and beyond, leading to a flourishing of the field. Trained with sensibilities to the social history of medicine and to class, race/ethnicity, and gender/sexuality approaches, and benefiting from the reorganization of archives and opening up of the academic world following many years of repression and political and economic instability through much of the region, these historians have been producing some of the world's most exciting scholarship in the history of medicine and health, with less-than-deserved audiences due to language barriers.

Pre-Columbian Health Conditions and the Impact of the European Conquest

There is little surviving evidence concerning health and healing in pre-Columbian societies, though enduring practices of Kallawaya, Nahua, Aymara, and other Indigenous healers, together with anthro-archaeological and iconographic sources, as well as the various codices and natural histories compiled by European colonists, provide useful sketches. The Maya, for example, considered children to be a sign of good fortune and paid special attention to infant health. Aztec children even had their own medical god, Ixtlilton, a deity unknown elsewhere in the world. Various pre-Columbian populations are known for their adherence to hygienic precepts—such as bathing rituals following childbirth, widespread breastfeeding for the first several years of life, testing the milk of wet nurses, and monitoring the nursing mother's diet—and for treating ailments with a combination of magic and empiricism. Together these measures may account for a life expectancy estimated at approximately ten years longer than that of medieval and early-modern Europeans.

The Spanish and Portuguese (and later French, British, and Dutch) invasions and imperialist systems had a devastating demographic impact on Indigenous populations across the Americas. Most infamously, smallpox is believed to have been spread throughout Meso-America through distribution of infected blankets by the forces of Spanish conquistador Hernán Cortés (1485–1547), though mortality from forced labour was likely to have been far higher. All told, between one-third and one-half of local inhabitants of the region were killed in the late fifteenth and sixteenth centuries by warfare, forced labour and relocation, and epidemic mortality from measles, smallpox, and other infectious diseases, all caused or facilitated by the military, economic, and social aspects of the conquest.[3]

Unquestionably, pre-Columbian societies in Meso-America experienced colossal mortality from violence, occasional famine, and infectious diseases,[4] but the conquest stands out because of the magnitude of death as well as the enormous mortality differential between invaders and invaded. Iberian invaders used this differential to military and cultural advantage, trumpeting the presumed constitutional superiority of the invaders, understood today to be the result of immunity due to previous exposure to micro-organisms.

Colonial Era Medical Authority, Healers, and Epidemic Control

By the sixteenth century, Spanish authorities were carrying European medical practices to the viceroyalties in New Spain and Peru (in the eighteenth century further divided into viceroyalties of New Granada and Río de la Plata). Colonial Spanish and Portuguese administrations supported the founding of medical faculties in leading colonial cities, such as Lima and Salvador da Bahia, and, greatly abetted by the Catholic Church, built hundreds of hospitals across the continent separately serving colonists and native populations. Medical practitioners joined colonial ventures, initially hired by conquistadores to protect military forces. Since few medical elites were attracted by the low salaries and dangers of practice in the colonies, a range of popular healers and charlatans also migrated. As region after region came under European control, elite physicians began to be integrated into colonial authority structures. Immigrant and *criollo* medical authorities established strict rules about who could and could not practise medicine based on race, religious faith, sex, and social background. Despite certain well-publicized prosecutions for violators, these rules were often flouted.

Up and down the continent, a new hierarchy of medical practitioners was established, with titled physicians serving urban elites, Catholic hospitals providing charity care, and traditional healers and midwives—who began to meld the beliefs of a wide variety of Indigenous cultures with Galenic and herbalist practices from Europe—attending the majority of the population.[5] Religious missionaries—first Catholic, later joined by Protestant denominations—played a large role in building and running leprosaria and hospitals, intertwining medical and religious proselytization. Officially sanctioned physicians sought the power of the *Protomedicato* (medical board) to squeeze out illegal or impure healers but met with little success.[6] A fragmented and overlapping set of health authorities also emerged, with the viceroy and religious agencies overshadowing the regulatory role of the *Protomedicato* during epidemic times.[7]

In all settings, imperial medical activities met with long-standing healing traditions, in which women played vital roles. In Meso-America, *curanderas* and *brujas*—female spiritual healers—retained their authoritative community roles under Spanish colonialism and, like their male healer counterparts, integrated various Galenic concepts brought by the Europeans, such as the idea of hot and cold causes and therapies for disease, with Indigenous practices of spiritism, magic and divination, herbalism, and evil air healing. Where African slaves were imported as labourers, most notably in Brazil and the Caribbean, a variety of African spirito-healing practices were a major influence on the evolving medical syncretism.

Medical ideologies, institutions, and practices were central to the activities of conquest, subjugation, and economic exploitation that characterized the Euro-American imperial enterprise. Initially women healers were not considered important to the mission of 'civilizing' local populations, increasing labour productivity, and controlling epidemics, but over time they were recognized as important targets, interlocutors, and purveyors of imperial health efforts. In colonial Mexico and Central America, traditional midwives— *parteras*—maintained their primary purview over pregnancy, childbirth, and infant health even as Bourbon and, from the nineteenth century onwards, republican administrations attempted to regulate and displace them. Medical authorities blamed midwives for infant and maternal deaths and continuously pressed for midwifery training (and for a more circumscribed role for the midwife), licensing, or outright elimination. However, Mexican midwives were not covered by licensing regulations until 1945, and empirical midwives continue to practise in many Indigenous communities and beyond.[8]

One key reason for the survival of midwives in Mexico and elsewhere, despite persistent attacks on their legitimacy, was their comprehensive approach. Prenatal care involved observing the colour of nipples, the shape of the womb and the position of the foetus, and relieving physical ailments through massage and herbal remedies. Following childbirth, the midwife aided the new mother with household chores, offering both emotional and physical support. Within a few weeks after delivery (and sometimes during pregnancy and the early stages of childbirth), the new mother took one or more *temazcalli*, therapeutic steam baths, which served to cleanse her physically, ritually, and emotionally. Midwives and their patients believed that the baths increased the flow of milk, prevented illness, and helped adjust the balance of hot and cold influences.

Given the paucity of therapeutic measures in the European medical armamentarium, the Iberian invaders were eager to learn of Indigenous healing knowledge and the local pharmacopoeia, and began to sponsor catalogues of this knowledge. The earliest and most important of these was the *Codex Badianus* of 1552, an illustrated compendium of hundreds of medicinal herbs. Written in Nahuatl by Martin de la Cruz and translated into Latin by Juan Badiano (both Aztec men who had trained in a Mexico City Franciscan academy), it was produced for the Spanish Emperor. In Brazil, the Jesuits played a fundamental role in colonial medical care from 1554 until their expulsion two

centuries later, similarly learning from Indigenous botanical knowledge and mixing local and European healing practices.

Notwithstanding colonial medical investments, there is ample
evidence that sanitary and living conditions—and the associated
gastrointestinal and respiratory mortality—worsened markedly
under Spanish and Portuguese imperialism. The Mexica (Aztecs),
for example, kept the streets, markets, and plazas of their capital
Tenochtitlán conspicuously clean through regular refuse collection
and extensive sanitary and hygienic measures; waste water was carefully separated from the clean sources of Lake Texcoco, which surrounded the city.[9] But after Tenochtitlán was destroyed and rebuilt as
Mexico City under Spanish rule, Lake Texcoco was transformed into
a giant cesspool: landfill projects, heavy canal commerce, and inad-
equate sewage disposal led to frequent flooding and contamination,
with highly damaging health consequences.[10]

Throughout the colonial period and after, disease and death were
rife among Mestizos, and, especially, Indigenous and African-
descended populations due to a variety of factors: conflict; slavery or
indentured servitude; dangerous work in mines, building sites, and
plantations; dispossession from land, cultural heritage, and liveli-
hoods; crowded living conditions in towns; food shortages; trade and
travel; and ecological alterations (canalization, railways, and exploitation of forests) facilitating mosquito breeding sites and malaria. To
be sure, colonists also suffered widely from infectious and childhood
diseases, but occupational mortality and early death among Mestizo
labourers, African slaves, and Indigenous groups, coupled with stag-
geringly high infant mortality rates, meant that these groups on
average lived far shorter and sicklier lives than Iberian elites. Some
cities, such as Veracruz and Caracas, began to implement environmental and sanitary measures that were partially effective at controlling yellow fever and other disease outbreaks.[11] Many others struggled
with highly fatal outbreaks of a range of infectious diseases well into
the twentieth century.[12]

The most unifying episode of late Spanish medical colonialism was
linked to the very ailment that had been so destructive upon conquest:
smallpox. When English surgeon Edward Jenner (1749–1823)—
observing milkmaids around 1796—found that vaccination with cowpox (generally not deadly to humans) could prevent smallpox in

humans, he helped transform smallpox prevention into a far safer endeavour. In 1803, Charles IV, the Bourbon King of Spain, having lost a child to smallpox, sponsored an extraordinary expedition throughout the Spanish Empire. The small Balmis-Salvany group arrived in Puerto Rico in 1804, and then travelled on to Venezuela, Panama, Colombia, Ecuador, Peru, Chile, and Bolivia, administering smallpox vaccine throughout these territories on foot, horseback, and along waterways. Because there was no means of preserving the vaccine, it was administered live—arm to arm—preserved in the bodies of twenty-one Spanish orphans, with instructions for preparation passed along.[13] This first mass health campaign was a distant prelude to the World Health Organization's smallpox eradication campaign, conducted almost three centuries later.[14]

Nineteenth-Century Institutional Growth and Struggles Over Medical Pluralism

The wave of insurgencies and full-scale wars that undulated through Latin America between 1800 and 1825 brought independence to all of the region's Iberian colonies except Puerto Rico and Cuba (with Brazil becoming a republic in 1889). However, political turmoil, continued warfare within and between countries, and, in some settings, foreign occupation restricted the contours of nation-building. Following decades of instability, the region began to see greater trade, foreign investment, and economic development in the mid-nineteenth century, yet the social order and agrarian basis of most of the population remained largely unchanged from the colonial period. Moreover, the weak states of newly independent Latin America typically decentralized political power to local jurisdictions. In health terms, this situation meant that there was little effort to document or address problems, particularly in rural areas.

Even amidst the chaos of nineteenth-century independence struggles and unstable new republics, there was a burgeoning of national medical institutions throughout the region. In most Latin American countries, the sanitary authorities that had periodically mobilized to combat epidemic outbreaks during centuries of Spanish and Portuguese colonialism were transformed into permanent hygiene boards and departments. Infused with the new ideas and practices of

the day, national health agencies sought to implement modern measures and increase state purview over social welfare. These efforts took
place mostly in leading cities, with sanitation catering to elites, child
health aimed at the poor, and food and housing regulations moni-
tored fitfully. As the number and range of public health tools—from
Wassermann tests to mosquito larvae control—increased after 1900,
medico-civic professionals throughout Latin America advocated
greater attention to endemic problems. Still, health authorities in
many settings were hampered by limited state capacity and low
responsiveness to popular needs: the region's large rural populations
were typically allotted few systematic health improvements beyond
vaccination campaigns and epidemic disease control. By the second
half of the nineteenth century, attention to health and social welfare
increased in capitals and larger cities, with initially limited participation of most central governments. Since political administrations in
this period were often short-lived, charitable and religious agencies—
with considerable involvement of middle- and upper-class women—
provided the institutional base and continuity for measures to protect
health, particularly of women and children.

The institutional evolution of Mexican medicine is illustrative of
developments throughout Latin America in this era. Between Mexican independence in 1821 and the onset of the Mexican Revolution
almost a century later, the central government had a limited but
growing role in the provision and regulation of health and medical
services. Much authority rested in the hands of local governments,
which exercised their powers unevenly. Western allopaths and homo-
eopaths continued to serve mainly the wealthy classes of *criollos* and
urban Mestizos, although demand for their services, particularly in
cities and towns, arose from all sectors.[15] Mexico, like Brazil and most
of Latin America, followed a French model of medical education
well into the twentieth century. With the founding of the Medical
Sciences Establishment in 1833—precursor to the national Faculty of
Medicine—Mexican medical schools employed French texts and
methods, and the medical community discussed and adapted French
understandings of the medical themes, discoveries, and practices of
the day. The most brilliant and financially able students travelled to
Paris for graduate training and returned as leading researchers and

authorities. In the late nineteenth century, other influences, including German bacteriology and British, Danish, and North American tropical medicine, gained a foothold, but French ideas and practices retained a primordial role in medicine and social welfare. For example, infant health and welfare services borrowed and adapted heavily from French notions of puericulture and eugenics.[16] As late as 1928, a prestigious new medical journal entitled *Pasteur* was founded by the Franco-Mexican Medical Association.

Continuing their prior role, Catholic charity hospitals, together with a few new municipal institutions, served the poor, but their concentration in Mexico City and other urban settings, and their untoward reputation, made them a last resort for care. In times of illness or pregnancy, the majority of the urban and rural population relied upon midwives and traditional healers, both male and female, who resided in most communities. Depending on local cultural practices and mestizo or Indigenous influences, popular medicine comprised a mix of ideologies and practices, including spiritism, magic, and divination, herbalism, hot and cold influences, European allopathy and homoeopathy, evil air healing, and home remedies. In Peru, too, and throughout Latin America, the shortage of regular doctors meant that Indigenous, African, Asian, and other immigrant popular healers maintained a large presence.[17] Even so, physicians increasingly sought state support and the authority of their medical knowledge to squeeze out competing healing professions, including midwives. By the early twentieth century, titled physicians had gained greater power, acceptance, and wider diffusion among popular sectors.[18]

Health authorities in Mexico, as elsewhere, had few specific tools at their disposal beyond smallpox vaccination and environmental sanitation. It was principally during major epidemics, such as the 1833 cholera outbreak, that quarantine, fumigation, and isolation were exercised. National legislation expanded state control over hygiene and moral rectitude—for example, an 1864 law mandating inspection of prostitutes—but for the most part public health functioned locally or on an ad hoc basis.[19] Appointed sanitary commissions were responsible for monitoring housing conditions, cemetery hygiene, and street and market cleanliness, the latter following from practices of Aztec, Maya, Toltec, and other pre-Columbian cultures. While doctors discussed international medical developments, and various jurisdictions passed legislation, health officials were rarely given the resources or the authority to utilize these tools.

By 1900, larger towns—some under popular pressure—began to employ some of the new bacteriologically based public health measures: sanitation, food and milk inspection, diphtheria anti-toxin, and the sporadic collection of mortality statistics, in addition to more traditional functions such as housing reform and enforcement of wet-nurse and prostitute regulations. Public health officials in key ports, most notably Veracruz, were particularly concerned with outbreaks of plague, yellow fever, cholera, and other epidemic diseases,[20] wielded substantial implementation powers, and in turn faced considerable popular resistance, as when Rio de Janeiro sought to implement mandatory smallpox vaccination in 1904. Public health in rural Mexico received little routine attention, although certain national campaigns against smallpox and plague were able to reach even remote villages.

At a national level, responsibility for public health resided in the Superior Council of Public Health, founded in 1841, but it was only empowered to respond beyond Mexico City upon the request of municipal or regional jurisdictions. An 1891 sanitary code expanded the federal purview to include ports and borders, but it was unable to overturn the decentralized structure of routine public health functions. Still, over time, the purview of the Superior Council of Public Health expanded markedly. From 1885 to 1914, its President was Dr. Eduardo Liceaga, a revered public health leader, who reorganized the Council's responsibilities to include routine vaccination, the study of epidemics, and urban sanitation, and who oversaw the nation's first sanitary census. By 1904, the Council had over 6,000 employees, many of whom had received specialized training. The federal government stepped up infectious disease control, organizing a bacteriological laboratory along European lines and administering Pasteur's anti-rabies vaccine to thousands of people.[21] Liceaga was also lauded throughout the Americas for overseeing the elimination of yellow fever from Veracruz after a 1903–4 epidemic, employing a combination of sanitary measures, isolation of the sick, disinfection, and petrol-based insecticides. By 1914, even the *New York Times* had to recognize that the 'authorities of Mexico have given considerable attention to the study of sanitation and preventative medicine'.[22]

By no means did the ascendance of allopathy end the widespread presence of a variety of healers or the admixture of medical ideologies and practices in Latin America. In some settings, such as nineteenth-century Colombia, academic doctors' denigration of a widely followed Andean faith healer exploded into days of street violence. Yet the consolidating power of elite physicians in 1870s Bogotá did not lead to outright elimination of unofficial competitors; instead official doctors and popular healers settled into a more tolerant, long-term pluralism, whereby practices not officially sanctioned were popularized and survived side by side with allopathy.[23]

Yet the rivalry between professional doctors and 'traditional' practitioners may have been overplayed in some history of medicine literature, perhaps because earlier works were written by triumphant doctors and later assessments relied too heavily on officialist sources. In Peru, for example, nineteenth-century medical resentment was channelled into animosity between national and foreign doctors rather than against domestic competitors.[24] In Brazil, nineteenth-century attempts to create a hierarchy of legitimate practitioners reinforced the low social status of subaltern healers, including slaves, women, and African healers. Many flourished despite their clandestine status.[25]

In Costa Rica, traditional healers became a state-sanctioned popular medical corps that served as a practical counterpart to rising physician hegemony. Without a medical school until the mid-twentieth century, Costa Rica had to rely on an insufficient cadre of foreign-trained physicians (often with dubious credentials): experienced Indigenous empirics became a viable and much-needed—if at times fiercely contested—source of medical care, especially in rural areas. Because meeting popular demand for medical care made for good politics, the Costa Rican state privileged allopathic physicians without allowing them a medical monopoly. Even the arrival in the late nineteenth century of thousands of indentured Chinese labourers (to build railways) and tens of thousands of Jamaicans and other Afro-Caribbeans (to work on coastal fruit plantations) with their respective healers did not elicit state suppression since they served as (free) district physicians for these labourers.[26]

In sum, if the nineteenth century brought unprecedented institutional, scientific, and professional legitimacy to trained allopathic practitioners in Latin America, in parallel to Europeans and North

Americans, this was only part of the story. The economic and social conditions, cultural diversity, and weaker reach of the state in Latin America meant that a spectrum of popular healers would survive to a far greater extent than in Anglo-European settings, enabling the persistence, hidden or visible, of medical pluralism. By no means did pluralism translate into a single syncretic healing system, but the extensive borrowing back and forth among healing traditions has left footprints into the present.

Tropical Medicine, State-Building, and International Public Health

Medical institutionalization was a national effort, yet international public health activities intertwined with Latin American state-building efforts during the late nineteenth and early twentieth centuries. In this context 'international' was not an exclusively imperial, North–South category, but also involved regional efforts. Tropical medicine, the *sine qua non* health enterprise of European (and United States) empires, was also taken up in Latin America on local terms. Even as the Iberian empires were waning, colonial interests in much of the world were consolidating, made ever more lucrative by simultaneous revolutions in industry and raw material extraction, transport, and commerce. However, the colonial enterprise was marred by the threat of so-called tropical diseases that were (often erroneously) associated with the warm and wet climates of many colonial possessions. These ailments interrupted productivity and commerce, felled colonists and labourers, and served as a racialized rationale for imperialism itself, encouraging 'Northern' investments in medical research on such ailments as malaria, yellow fever, and onchocerciasis.

But tropical medicine was not only of concern to colonial powers. From the 1860s through the 1880s in Salvador da Bahia, a group of dedicated clinician-investigators—subsequently labelled the Tropicalistas—sought to counter European views of the deleterious impact of Brazil's racial heritage and climate (and implicitly culture) on health. Far from mimicking European research, the Bahian group 'invented' a kind of tropical medicine more than two decades before imperial English and French interests staked out the contours of this field. Unlike the physicians of Brazil's leading medical school in

Rio de Janeiro, who absorbed the racialist views of degeneration in the tropics that emanated from Europe, the Bahia school developed its own theory of combined bacteriological and social-environmental factors to explain decaying health—and the prevalence of diseases such as beriberi and hookworm in Brazil. The Tropicalistas' clinical observations and surgical experimentation on lower-class charity hospital patients furthered their theories of the intertwining of social conditions and parasitological manifestation. The Tropicalistas sought to create not just a Brazilianist medicine, but a Bahian variant— a pointed critique of the more rigid French-derived approach of the Rio school and of government policy on health matters. Yet the Tropicalistas were also heavily influenced by European developments: even as they contested disdainful views on Brazilian inferiority, they desperately sought the legitimacy that European science could grant them.[27]

In Argentina, Colombia, and other countries, too, local concerns with the economic impact of diseases such as yellow fever and malaria motivated national research that drew from South American as well as European ideas.[28] Around this time, a range of regional professional organizations within Latin America began to set common medical research and public health agendas, leading to considerable exchange of ideas and policies.[29] Nonetheless, a powerful driver of Latin American tropical medicine and international health came from the North. By the late nineteenth century, the United States' economic presence in Latin America was escalating, accompanied by tropical medicine concerns. The United States' 1898 war against Spain, although justified by the perennial threat of Cuba's yellow fever problem wreaking epidemic havoc on US shores, was underscored by American imperialist ambitions and resulted in its acquisition of Spain's remaining possessions in the Americas and the Pacific.[30] The lessons the Americans learned in Cuba, where mosquito-borne diseases killed more troops than firearms, would shape Pan-American health interests for many years to come.

Yellow fever had been afflicting ports from Buenos Aires to Halifax since the eighteenth century. The meat and hide economies of Argentina and Uruguay were particularly intent on keeping out yellow fever from Brazil, which might interrupt profitable exports. An 1887 Sanitary Convention signed by the trio detailed quarantine periods for ships bearing cholera, yellow fever, and plague and was in effect for five years before breaking apart. The following year, 1888, the Andean countries of Bolivia, Chile, Ecuador, and Peru signed the Lima Convention. But these efforts were short-lived and circumscribed due to mutual mistrust and poor enforcement.

It was a Cuban physician, Carlos Finlay (1833–1915), who set the stage for North American tropical medicine. At the International Sanitary Conference in Washington, DC, in 1878, Finlay proposed that yellow fever was transmitted through the bite of a mosquito. At the time, few believed him. In 1900, Walter Reed (1851–1902) was sent to Havana to head the American Yellow Fever Commission to control an outbreak at the US military garrison. There, Reed and his team confirmed Finlay's observation through experiments using mosquitoes fed on patients and then unleashed (fatally) on uninfected volunteers. Confirmation of the hardy *Aedes aegypti* mosquito (then *Stegomyia*) as the vector for yellow fever motivated large-scale sanitary assaults on mosquito breeding sites, in addition to quarantine of ships in infected ports. In occupied Cuba, US army surgeon William Gorgas (1854–1920) oversaw a series of measures—including daily inspection of homes and yards by legions of sanitarians, mandatory removal or covering of domestic water receptacles, severe fines on property owners for harbouring mosquito larvae, and isolation of every suspected case—that led to a dramatic decline in yellow fever.[31]

This development would enable the United States to accomplish the longtime imperial dream of building a canal across the Central American isthmus, an effort that French interests had to abandon in the 1880s after spending hundreds of millions of dollars and losing almost 20,000 labourers to malaria and yellow fever. When the United States took over building the canal in 1904, Gorgas became Chief Sanitary Officer. He redoubled the mosquito extermination effort he had led in Havana, with over 4,000 men divided in two brigades: one to eliminate *Aedes* around human settlements; and the other to clear jungles, drain swamps, and apply oil to *Anopheles* (the malaria mosquito) breeding sites. Massive use of screens, bednets, quinine, and even piped water for canal workers helped control yellow fever and malaria among workers,[32] enabling the canal to be built by 1914. However, these sanitary efforts overlooked—and the US occupation of Panama exacerbated—more pressing endemic problems for local populations, including malnutrition, diarrhoea, and tuberculosis.[33]

Ironically, the very completion of the canal raised the peril of new epidemics—such as cholera and plague—due to shorter shipping routes to and from Asia. This heightened the pressure to establish sanitary agreements. In Europe it took more than half a century to transcend inter-imperialist jealousies and resolve concerns over national sovereignty in order to establish a uniform system of disease notification, ship inspection, and maritime sanitation and found the Office International d'Hygiène Publique (Paris, 1907), followed by the League of Nations Health Organization after the First World War.

In the Americas, by contrast, international sanitary cooperation was more successful, motivated by immediate menaces. These concerns drove a group of governments in the region to found the Pan American Sanitary Bureau (PASB) in 1902 under the aegis of the US Public Health Service. Soon, almost all Latin American republics were represented at the organization's quadrennial conferences. The United States was particularly concerned that Latin American countries help draft, and thus comply with, enforceable sanitary codes. The PASB's early years were devoted to the establishment of region-wide protocols on the reporting and control of epidemic diseases, including yellow fever, plague, and cholera, culminating in a 1924 Sanitary Code, signed by all twenty-one PASB member countries. In its leadership and shaping of activities, the Bureau reflected North American hegemonic interests in Latin America, which covered investments in oil, fruticulture, mining and metallurgy, real estate, railways, banking, and other industries. Indeed, under its self-declared Monroe Doctrine of 1823, the United States had occupied ports and countries across the region whenever it sensed its economic and sanitary interests were threatened. Yet even as the PASB's agenda remained focused on sanitary and commercial concerns into the 1930s, it began to engage in other activities: sponsoring a widely disseminated public health journal, addressing maternal and child health concerns, and organizing an incipient system of technical cooperation.[34] After the Second World War, the PASB would officially become the Americas Office of the World Health Organization (WHO).

Just as these efforts were unfolding, a new agency appeared on the scene, one that would profoundly shape international health and influence the transition from European towards US medical influences in the Americas and far beyond. The Rockefeller Foundation

(RF) was established in 1913 by oil mogul-philanthropist John D. Rockefeller (1839–1937) 'to promote the well-being of mankind throughout the world'. After uncovering the important part played by public health in the economic advancement of the US South, the RF created an International Health Board (IHB, later International Health Division or IHD) to promote public health and modernize institutions, befriending dozens of governments around the world and preparing vast regions for investment and increased productivity. By the time of the IHD's dismantling in 1951, it had operated in over ninety countries, including almost every country in Latin America, with activities to control hookworm, yellow fever, malaria and other diseases, train professionals, and modernize and institutionalize government commitments to public health, all organized and overseen by its own officers stationed in the field.

Latin America served as a showcase for RF public health efforts. The RF's international work began with hookworm campaigns in the Caribbean and Central America,[35] based on its five-year campaign in the US South, in turn drawing from an effort by US army physician Bailey Ashford (1873–1934) in occupied Puerto Rico starting in 1903. Although RF officers believed that controlling hookworm-induced anaemia through a combination of prevention (education and promotion of latrine and shoe use) and treatment (with powerful antihelminthic drugs) would ignite demand for public health services throughout the Americas, reality was more complicated. Certainly, by the early twentieth century, there was already widespread interest in health services throughout the region, and most governments were pursuing public health institutionalization and a variety of disease-control efforts.

Still, most administrations were pleased to take advantage of the steady IHB interest and stream of funding (if in diminishing quantities over time) to build up infrastructure. In no arena were the effects of RF monies as visible as yellow fever, even though, paradoxically, this was a minor cause of death (if a major cause of quarantine and suspension of trade). In 1914, Gorgas, by this time Army Surgeon-General, convinced the RF that the soon-to-be-opened Panama Canal might facilitate the spread of yellow fever. Offering a chance for Rockefeller scientists to showcase their expertise internationally, yellow fever served as an expensive exception to the IHB rule of reasonably priced programmes with a ready cure. Recognition of the global, not just local, implications of yellow fever led to this exception.

In 1916, the IHB constituted a Yellow Fever Commission headed by Gorgas to make a reconnaissance trip through South America. Despite observations by Colombian and Brazilian doctors that yellow fever also existed in a sylvan form (known as 'jungle yellow fever'), the Commission's travel and subsequent eradication efforts focused on the 'key centres' theory—urban locales suspected of being endemic yellow fever loci, initially in the coastal cities of Ecuador, Peru, Colombia, Venezuela, and Brazil, and later Mexico. Following this criterion, the Commission initially found only Guayaquil to harbour yellow fever, and the IHB conducted a two-year disinfection campaign aimed solely at mosquito extermination, despite requests from both Ecuadorian officials and Commissioners to include improvement of water supply and sewage.

Adhering to equal single-mindedness, the IHB's yellow fever campaign moved on to Colombia, Peru, and Central America. The RF finally convinced the Mexican government to accept a campaign in 1921, leading to a massive four-year investment in the country that posed the greatest yellow fever danger to the United States due to its proximity and the volume of migration and trade. In Brazil, epidemic yellow fever was initially believed more problematic in the north than the south, but the disease's unexpected resurgence in Rio in the late 1920s—combined with the country's commitment to modernization—resulted in a massive two-decades-long RF–Brazilian government yellow fever campaign that eventually extended into rural areas.[36]

In addition to disease campaigns, the IHB/D supported development of local and national health departments, and conducted rural health demonstrations and training efforts for both specialists and rank-and-file public health workers. Field officers often complained about the dearth of well-trained medical graduates in Latin America, but the IHB sought to distance itself from medical education concerns, concentrating instead on those competent graduates eligible for its own fellowships. Beginning with an RF Medical Sciences Division survey of Brazilian medical schools in 1916, visiting RF experts made periodic assessments of medical education in a variety of Latin American countries.[37] They critiqued heavy reliance on clinicians as faculty, overcrowded classrooms, excessive French influence, and an insufficient role for experimental research, but the RF's involvement in Latin American medical education remained circumscribed until after the Second World War. The only Latin American medical school that the RF deemed worthy of assistance before this time was São Paulo's, which received a grant of nearly one million dollars in the 1920s to carry out Flexnerian reforms. São Paulo was also the lone Latin American site for an RF school of public health.

Still, the RF did not ignore Latin American public health training: it oriented its investment to individuals over institutions. Each year the IHD awarded dozens of public health fellowships to doctors, sanitary engineers, and nurses to study in the United States and return to their home countries to fill key positions. Between 1917 and 1950, 2,500 public health and nursing fellows were sponsored (including approximately 650 US fellows), with some 450 fellows from Latin America and the Caribbean. These fellows managed the relationship between the RF and individual countries, serving as interlocutors, as well as setting up research and graduate institutes to train subsequent generations of public health leaders. The IHD and returned fellows also helped set up in-country training stations for tens of thousands of middle- and lower-rank health workers. This enduring investment in Latin American public health education was considered by many to be the most successful aspect of US–Latin American cooperation.

In the early twentieth century, Latin America was a study in contrasts. Elites and a small middle class (and sometimes the military) began to enjoy the fruits of medical and public health progress particularly in urban settings. However, most of the population lived under comparable conditions—and attended similar types of healers—as they had during the nineteenth century or even the colonial period. Most national authorities at least rhetorically supported public health and medical modernization and at times offered patronage for modern research laboratories and new fields such as paediatrics and genetics; some universities were able to self-fund reforms and expansion. Ironically, through this period, Latin American countries were extensively involved in international efforts, with a steady presence at regional and European demographic, health, and medical congresses, but the contrast between state-building rhetoric and medical reality remained large.

Outside national capitals and important cities, implementation of even routine sanitary measures was left largely in local hands; some took these responsibilities seriously, but most had few resources and little authority to act beyond responding to epidemics and other crises. In many places, certainly the principal cities, private institutions, Catholic charity, and women's voluntary organizations filled the gap in public welfare, but funding instability and patronizing criteria for assistance limited their reach. By the interwar period, changes were afoot. Developments in mining, oil, railways, and other industries in Argentina, Brazil, Chile, Mexico, Peru, Venezuela, and elsewhere were accompanied by labour activism; unionized workers (typically excluding the vast majority toiling in agriculture) pressed for health benefits and social security. Protection systems proliferated,[38] though coverage was uneven and exacerbated inequality in many settings.

In countries as diverse as Costa Rica, Brazil, and Colombia, physicians staked a role in state-building efforts, claiming that they played a central part in enhancing not only population health but the nation's health. In Bolivia, for example, doctors hitched their hopes for greater legitimacy and allopathic professionalization—in a society where Kallawaya and other traditional healers predominated—on their participation in broader discussions of the nation's trajectory. Yet it was the ill-fated 1930s Chaco War (against Paraguay, and, by proxy, Argentina and foreign oil interests) that served as the turning point in the nation's political life and in its medical and public health approaches. Working-class mobilization and the formation of new leftist parties, spurred by the war's soaring death toll, helped end uncontested dominance by elite *criollos*, ushering in a period of 'military socialism' that served as a prelude to Bolivia's subsequent revolution.[39] Indeed, just as biomedicine was rising to its apex, the inextricable political contextualization of health and medical ideas and practices became ever more evident.

The Cold War and The Clash Between Technical and Social Approaches to Health

At the end of the Second World War, Latin American countries were poised for further change amidst post-war economic improvements, rising citizen expectations, and growth in public spending for health and social welfare. Even rural populations began gaining health services coverage, if in fits and starts and in stratified form. In 1947, Argentinean physiologist Bernardo Houssay (1887–1971), an RF grantee, became Latin America's first Nobel laureate in the sciences for his work in endocrinology. His prize simultaneously symbolized a coming-of-age of Latin American medicine and the role of US donors in this process. The support of the RF and other North American foundations for health and medical training, research, and institution-building in Latin America had increased during the war. And, crucially, a massive 1940s infusion of US State Department funding for health and other public infrastructure through the Institute of Inter-American Affairs (a patently propagandistic effort headed by one of the Rockefeller scions to garner support for the Allied Forces) created a palpable North American presence across the region.[40] However, as of 1946 a new geopolitical order was in place, and Latin America became one of the most important playing fields for the half-century Cold War rivalry between the US-led Western bloc and the Soviet-led Eastern bloc. Although only just beginning to receive attention by historians, several key themes are apparent.

One major theme has to do with the role of Soviet models of health and social welfare for Latin America's developing welfare states. Starting in the 1920s, Soviet accomplishments in social policy had become widely known and admired in Latin America. The 1930s and 1940s saw at least two dozen Latin American medical visitors to the Soviet Union—from Mexico, Argentina, Chile, Cuba, Brazil, Colombia, Venezuela, and Uruguay (and likely elsewhere)—instigated not by Comintern but by Latin Americans themselves. Up to several hundred other Latin American non-physician visitors made their way to the USSR by the 1950s. These observers—some self-funded, others sponsored by their governments—included both the curious and true believers. They carried out surveys of public health service organization, medical schools, and research institutes. Many of them published book-length accounts, which entered into lively debates throughout Latin America around how to shape institutions, services, and citizen rights in the health arena. During the same period, the PASB and the Montevideo-based International Institute for the Protection of Childhood followed Soviet developments closely. Later on, Chilean health policy expert Dr. Benjamin Viel's 1961 widely disseminated book on socialized medicine compared Chile's implementation of socialized medicine, a process begun in the late 1930s when Salvador Allende was Minister of Health, to the experiences of Great Britain and the Soviet Union, with the latter's organizational effectiveness much cited.

Of course by the late 1940s, Soviet exemplars were no longer the stuff of innocent debate. Western bloc nations, led by the United States, became increasingly concerned about the appeal of communism to the populations of so-called Third World countries, many of which had growing left-wing political movements by the 1950s. The US response was swift and large. First the Institute of Inter-American Affairs prolonged its funding of hospitals, sanitation systems, and DDT spraying against malaria into the early 1950s, replacing this initiative with an even broader bilateral programme called the International Cooperation Administration (in 1961, it became the US Agency for International Development). Latin America was one of the prime targets of the new US approach to bringing underdeveloped countries into the capitalist fold. Articulated by President Harry Truman in his 1949 inauguration speech, this entailed improving health and productivity and raising living standards through the provision of technical skills, knowledge, and equipment.[41]

The new health-related United Nations agencies, most notably the WHO and UNICEF, also became embroiled in Cold War ideology. With combating disease deemed a key element in the fight against communism, WHO began efforts against yaws, tuberculosis, and other ailments. Its Global Malaria Eradication Campaign was launched in 1955 and largely financed by the US government. In Mexico, Brazil, and other countries, the campaign displaced existing national approaches, honing in on technical, insecticide-based elimination of malaria's mosquito vector and sidestepping housing and work conditions and the social context of the disease.[42] However, the disease control ideological divide did not fall strictly on East–West lines: after rejoining the WHO in the late 1950s, the Soviets backed smallpox eradication; the campaign did not figure importantly in Latin America, as smallpox control had been increasingly achieved through national measures. The showdown between purely technical and socio-technical approaches to health did not take place until the 1970s, when WHO became the stage for a political struggle around primary health care. At the famed international conference held in Alma-Ata, USSR, in 1978 and through the 1980s, Latin America became an important showground for the promise and limits of primary care.

By the 1960s, the infrastructure approach was reoriented to a new concern: the control of population size/growth in underdeveloped countries as a means of lessening social and economic pressures that made communism an attractive political option. Once again Latin American countries, which were enjoying lengthening life expectancy yet retained traditional preferences for large families—as well as growing radical militancy, rapid urbanization, and high unemployment in dangerous proximity to the United States—made the region a top priority. Cold War reproductive health programmes even found an unlikely ally in the Catholic Church, whose anti-communism trumped its anti-contraception values in Peru and elsewhere.[43]

The influence of religious missionaries in Latin American health and hospital care was also renewed in this period. While most missionaries sympathized with North American anti-communism, evangelical medical missionaries, whose presence in the region soared as of the 1970s, did not always fit in neatly with (US) foreign policy goals. At the other end of the political spectrum, advocates of liberation medicine and left-wing Christian medical missionaries (especially from Scandinavia) often worked to counter official anti-communist foreign policy.

The Soviet role in Latin American health and medicine, about which little is known, seems to have centred less on infrastructure and in-country programmes than on fellowships and political support (with Cuba being a notable exception). As of the 1960s Moscow's Patrice Lumumba Friendship University hosted tens of thousands of medical students from the Third World, including large numbers of Latin American students, to train at its Faculty of Medicine. Medical student movements within Latin America, too, engaged with competing communist parties, in the Soviet Union, China, and then Cuba, which established a programme of medical solidarity that sent thousands of its doctors to work overseas. Preliminary evidence suggests that medical radicals in Ecuador, Venezuela, Mexico, and revolutionary movements across the region adroitly played off different parties to the Cold War against one another.

The two most prominent Latin American physician radicals were Argentinean Ernesto 'Che' Guevara (1928–67), who understood that widespread health gains could be realized only through socialist revolution, not advanced medical technology (leading him to play a pivotal role in Cuba's 1959 revolution and later in South American movements), and Chilean physician Salvador Allende (1908–73). Father of Latin American social medicine, the socialist Allende rose to prominence in the 1930s as a medical student leader, then health minister for the Popular Front, setting the wheels in motion for Chile's national health system.[44] In 1970, he was elected President, with a platform of nationalization and redistribution, including great attention to occupational and public health; the conservative physicians' association in Chile was among his fiercest opponents. Deposed in a US-backed military coup in 1973, Allende committed suicide, and medical radicals were among the thousands of people who were 'disappeared' or forced into exile or underground under dictatorships in Chile, Argentina, Uruguay, Brazil, Paraguay, and elsewhere.

Yet even as they faced severe repression, members of radical medical movements remained committed to the principles and policies of social medicine and social justice.[45] After the 1979 Sandinista revolution in Nicaragua, thousands of doctors and public health workers from throughout the Americas and beyond joined in the country's effort to implement primary health care to populations that had been overlooked for centuries, even amidst violent civil war. Brazil's collective health movement,[46] founded during the dictatorship, gave the scaffolding to decades of political struggle to realize a unified national health system and social redistribution measures. The Latin American Social Medicine Association (ALAMES), founded in 1984, strengthened analyses and solidarity at a regional level, supporting national and local political and scholarly efforts to the present.[47]

Amidst these dramatic developments, shaped (and funded) both by Cold War exigencies and by domestic political pressures for more attention to health and medicine, all Latin American countries enjoyed considerable institutional expansion in public health and medicine. This included the founding of new medical schools across the region and a huge increase in the number of trained medical personnel, the founding of national scientific funding agencies and the renewal of research institutes, the improvement of epidemiological surveillance and public health capacity, and expanded health services coverage. In Cuba and Costa Rica, such developments vastly decreased the inequities in health of previous eras, but in most settings inequalities persisted. In the late 1960s, US health policy analyst Milton Roemer famously noted that in order to determine health care coverage among Latin Americans, one merely needed to ask people's social class.

Just as the region's dictatorships and repressive regimes were starting to unravel in the 1980s (although conflict continued in parts of Central America and the Andean countries), a new set of challenges emerged that would once again batter health conditions. The oil shocks of the 1970s were an initial boon to oil producers Venezuela and Mexico, but importers were forced into debt, currency devaluation, and soaring inflation. Soon virtually all countries of the region, led by Mexico, began defaulting on their loans, while capital fled. In Latin America, per capita income declined by 7 per cent, consumption by 6 per cent, and investment by 4 per cent between 1980 and 1990. Hyperinflation reached an average of 1500 per cent by 1990. As country after country was 'rescued' by the World Bank and the International Monetary Fund, they were compelled to abide by a set of neoliberal, pro-market conditions: these policies included slashing government spending, privatizing social services, deregulating the economy, and liberalizing trade. The 1980s thus became a 'lost decade' for health and development, as public health services and institutions drastically deteriorated and health either stagnated or declined, with inequalities once again exacerbated. The end of the Cold War around 1990 once again brought the promise of change.

Conclusion

By the 1990s, political conditions throughout the region had stabilized, but economic woes persisted. Many countries that once had near-universal health systems now had partially or largely privatized health insurance, which drastically reduced access to services. The simplistic health transition theory—postulating a shift from infectious to chronic diseases as countries developed—was clearly disproven in Latin America, with soaring rates of both infectious and chronic diseases. In many settings, under-nutrition was resolved through the industrialization of cheap, energy-dense foods, with negative effects for small-scale farmers and a drastic impact on diabetes, now the leading cause of death in Mexico.

Yet certain developments, already present in previous eras, suggest that despite (or perhaps because of) global attention to terrorism and the 'clash of civilizations', the region is on more solid footing in health and medical terms. In addition to greater political (and in some places economic) stability, this at least partially stems from both an unprecedented decline in foreign interference in the region and an increase in collaboration across Latin America. One such effort is Cuba's Latin American School of Medicine (Escuela Latinoamericana de Medicina), founded in 1999 to train thousands of doctors from impoverished backgrounds from throughout the Americas and beyond who return home to serve their communities.[48] The Union of South American Nations, or UNASUR, was established in 2008 with the aim of fostering economic integration and within-region development aid. South-to-South cooperation, both within and beyond the region, is now a political priority in Brazil. Moreover, the elections in recent years of progressive governments at the local and national level in Brazil, Uruguay, Paraguay, Argentina, Chile, Venezuela, Honduras, Bolivia, and Ecuador, and other settings (some since elected out of office or deposed), variously led by doctors in the social medicine tradition, have resulted in renewed efforts at universal social and health policies, and even 'interculturalism', integrating traditional and Western medicine.

As evidenced by the issues touched upon here, the historiography of Latin American medicine and health is complex in geographic, cultural, social, and political terms. While stunted for a long time, the field has enjoyed a renaissance in recent years, making it one of the world's most dynamic history of medicine literatures.[49] Linking contemporary health policy and global health concerns to the writing of history poses certain challenges. Balancing local and national developments with regional and international influences and trends—clearly necessary for comprehensive analysis—is a near conceptual, archival, and temporal nightmare. Should each global health campaign be studied in each setting or can certain trends be generalized from a set of experiences? Comparative work is *de rigeur* but either deteriorates into superficiality or requires several lifetimes or even a (convenient) marriage of researchers. Establishing an equilibrium among works that rescue local scientific traditions, explore the 'cultures of health', address the making of medical and health policies, and track the trajectories of health personnel is no mean feat. Getting to know the past, inevitably, is a reflection of the present. Given the exciting, if often terribly destructive, politics of Latin America, its medical and health historiography is poised to be among the world's most engaging.

Acknowledgements

I am grateful to Raúl Necochea for his helpful comments on an earlier draft. My work on this chapter was supported in part by the Canada Research Chairs program.

Notes

1 Guyane, Guiana, and Suriname were colonized by, respectively, France, Britain, and the Netherlands.
2 Francisco Fernández del Castillo, *Antología de los escritos histórico-médicos del Doctor F. Fernández del Castillo* (México, D.F.: Facultad de Medicina, Universidad Nacional Autónoma de México (UNAM), 1982).
3 Robert McCaa, 'Spanish and Nahuatl Views on Smallpox and Demographic Catastrophe in the Conquest of Mexico', *Journal of Interdisciplinary History* 25 (3) (Winter 1995), 397–431; Noble David Cook, *Born to Die: Disease and New World Conquest, 1492–1650* (Cambridge: Cambridge University Press, 1998).
4 Suzanne Austin Alchon, *A Pest in the Land: New World Epidemics in a Global Perspective* (Albuquerque: University of New Mexico Press, 2003).
5 Joseph W. Bastien, 'Differences between Kallawaya-Andean and Greek European Humoral Medicine', *Social Science and Medicine* 28 (1989), 45–51.
6 Luz María Hernández Sáenz, *Learning to Heal: The Medical Profession in Colonial Mexico, 1767–1831* (New York: Peter Lang, 1997).
7 John Tate Lanning, *The Royal Protomedicato: The Regulation of the Medical Profession in the Spanish Empire* (Durham, NC: Duke University Press, 1985).
8 Ana María Carrillo, 'Nacimiento y muerte de una profesión: Las parteras tituladas en México', *Dynamis* 19 (1999), 167–90.
9 Bernard Ortiz de Montellano, *Aztec Medicine, Health and Nutrition* (New Brunswick, NJ: Rutgers University Press, 1990).
10 Donald B. Cooper, *Epidemic Disease in Mexico City, 1716–1813: An Administrative, Social, and Medical Study* (Austin: University of Texas Press, 1965).

11 Andrew Knaut, 'Yellow Fever and the Late Colonial Public Health Response in the Port of Veracruz', *Hispanic American Historical Review* 77 (1997), 619–44.

12 Adrián Carbonetti (ed.), *Historias de enfermedad en Córdoba desde la colonia hasta el siglo XX* (Córdoba: CONICET, 2007).

13 José Rigau-Pérez, 'La real expedición filantrópica de la vacuna de viruela: monarquía y modernidad en 1803', *Puerto Rico Health Sciences Journal* 23 (3) (2004), 223–31.

14 For further discussion of this, see Chapter 11 by Sanjoy Bhattacharya in this volume.

15 Claudia Agostoni, 'Médicos científicos y médicos ilícitos en la Ciudad de México durante el porfiriato', in *Estudios de Historia Moderna y Contemporánea de México* (Instituto de Investigaciones Históricas, UNAM, 1999), 13–31.

16 Alexandra Stern, 'Responsible Mothers and Normal Children: Eugenics, Nationalism, and Welfare in Post-Revolutionary Mexico, 1920–1940', *Journal of Historical Sociology* 12 (4) (1999), 369–97.

17 Marcos Cueto, Jorge Lossio, and Carol Pasco (eds), *El rastro de la salud en el Perú* (Lima: Instituto de Estudios Peruanos, 2009).

18 Ana Cecilia Rodríguez de Romo, 'Los médicos como Gremio de Poder en el porfiriato', *Boletín Mexicana de Historia y Filosofía de Medicina* 5 (2) (2002), 4–9.

19 Rosalina Estrada Urroz, 'Control sanitario o control social: la reglamentación prostibularia en el porfiriato', *Boletín Mexicana de Historia y Filosofía de Medicina* 5 (2) (2002), 21–5.

20 José Ronzón, *Sanidad y modernización en los puertos del Alto Caribe 1870–1915* (México, DF: Universidad Autónoma Metropolitana/Grupo Editorial Miguel Angel Porrúa, 2004).

21 Ana María Carrillo, 'Economía, política y salud pública en el México porfiriano, 1876–1910', *História, Ciências, Saúde—Manguinhos* 9 (suppl.) (2002), 67–87.

22 *New York Times* (26 April 1914).

23 David Sowell, *The Tale of Healer Miguel Perdomo Neira: Healing, Ideologies, and Power in the Nineteenth-Century Andes* (Wilmington, DE: Scholarly Resources, 2001).

24 Jorge Lossio. 'British Medicine in the Peruvian Andes: The Travels of Archibald Smith M.D. (1820–1870)', *História, Ciências, Saúde—Manguinhos* 13 (4) (2006), 833–50.

25 Marcio de Souza Soares, 'Cirurgiões Negros: saberes Africanos sobre o corpo e as doenças nas ruas do Rio de Janeiro durante a metade do século XIX', *Locus: Revista de História* 8 (2) (2002), 43–58.

26 Steven Palmer, *From Popular Medicine to Medical Populism: Doctors, Healers, and Public Power in Costa Rica 1800–1940* (Durham, NC: Duke University Press, 2003).

27 Julyan Peard, *Race, Place, and Medicine: The Idea of the Tropics in Nineteenth-Century Brazil* (Durham, NC: Duke University Press, 1999).

28 Adriana Alvarez, 'Malaria and the Emergence of Rural Health in Argentina: An Analysis from the Perspective of International Interaction and Co-operation', *Canadian Bulletin of Medical History* 25 (1) (2008), 137–60.

29 Marta de Almeida, 'Circuito Aberto: idéias e intercâmbios médico-científicos na América Latina nos primórdios do século XX', *História, Ciências, Saúde—Manguinhos* 13 (3) (2006), 733–57.

30 Mariola Espinosa, *Epidemic Invasions: Yellow Fever and the Limits of Cuban Independence, 1878–1930* (Chicago: University of Chicago Press, 2009).

31 Paul Basch, 'A Historical Perspective on International Health', *Infectious Disease Clinics of North America* 5 (1991), 183–96.

32 Paul Sutter, 'Tropical Conquest and the Rise of the Environmental Management State: The Case of U.S. Sanitary Efforts in Panama', in Alfred McCoy and Francisco Scarano (eds), *Colonial Crucible: Empire in the Making of the Modern American State* (Madison: University of Wisconsin Press, 2009), 317–26.

33 David McBride, *Missions for Science: U.S. Technology and Medicine in America's African World* (New Brunswick, NJ: Rutgers University Press, 2002).

34 Marcos Cueto, *El valor de la salud: una historia de la OPS* (Washington, DC: OPS, 2004); Anne-Emanuelle Birn, 'No More Surprising Than a Broken Pitcher? Maternal and Child Health in the Early Years of the Pan American Health Organization', *Canadian Bulletin of Medical History* 19 (1) (2002), 17–46.

35 Steven Palmer, *Launching Global Health: The Caribbean Odyssey of the Rockefeller Foundation* (Ann Arbor: University of Michigan Press, 2010).

36 Ilana Löwy, *Virus, moustiques, et modernité: la fièvre jaune au Brésil entre science et politique* (Paris: Éditions des Archives Contemporaines, 2001).

37 Marcos Cueto, 'Visions of Science and Development: The Rockefeller Foundation and the Latin American Medical Surveys of the 1920s', in *idem* (ed.), *Missionaries of Science: The Rockefeller Foundation and Latin America* (Bloomington: Indiana University Press, 1994), 1–22.

38 Patricio Márquez and Daniel Joly, 'A Historical Overview of the Ministries of Public Health and the Medical Programs of the Social Security Systems in Latin America', *Journal of Public Health Policy* 7 (1986), 378–94.

39 Ann Zulawski, *Unequal Cures: Public Health and Political Change in Bolivia, 1900–1950* (Durham, NC: Duke University Press, 2007).

40 André Luiz Vieira de Campos, *Políticas internacionais de saúde na era Vargas: o serviço especial de saúde pública, 1942–1960* (Rio de Janeiro: Fiocruz, 2006).

41 Marcos Cueto, 'International Health, the Early Cold War and Latin America', *Canadian Bulletin of Medical History* 25 (1) (2008), 17–41.

42 Marcos Cueto, *Cold War, Deadly Fevers: Malaria Eradication in Mexico, 1955–1975* (Washington, DC: Woodrow Wilson Center and Johns Hopkins University Press, 2007); Gilberto Hochman, 'From Autonomy to Partial Alignment: National Malaria Programs in the Time of Global Eradication, Brazil, 1941–1961', *Canadian Bulletin of Medical History* 25 (1) (2008), 161–92.

43 Raúl Necochea, 'Priests and Pills: Catholic Family Planning in Peru, 1967–1976', *Latin American Research Review* 43 (2) (2008), 34–56.
44 Maria Eliana Labra, 'Política e medicina social no Chile: narrativas sobre uma relação difícil', *História, Ciência, Saúde—Manguinhos* 7 (1) (2000), 23–46.
45 Howard Waitzkin, Cecilia Iriart, Alfredo Estrada, and Silvia LaMadrid, 'Social Medicine Then and Now: Lessons from Latin America', *American Journal of Public Health* 91 (10) (2001), 1592–1601.
46 Nísia Trindade Lima and José Paranaguá Santana, *Saúde coletiva como compromisso: a trajetória da abrasco* (Rio de Janeiro: Fiocruz, 2006).
47 Edmundo Granda, 'Algunas reflexiones a los veinticuatro años de la ALAMES', *Medicina Social* 3 (2) (2008), 217–25.
48 H. Michael Erisman, *Cuban Medical Internationalism: Origins, Evolution, and Goals* (Basingstoke: Palgrave Macmillan, 2009).
49 Anne-Emanuelle Birn and Raúl Necochea, 'Footprints on the Future: Looking Forward to Latin American Medical History in the Twenty-First Century', *Hispanic American Historical Review* 91 (3) (2011), 503–27.

Select Bibliography

Agostoni, Claudia, *Médicos, Campañas y Vacunas: La Viruela y la Cultura de su Prevención en México, 1870–1952* (México, DF: Universidad Nacional Autónoma de México, 2016).
Armus, Diego (ed.), *Entre médicos y curanderos: cultura, historia y enfermedad en la América Latina moderna* (Buenos Aires: Ed. Norma, 2002).
Armus, Diego, *The Ailing City: Health, Tuberculosis and Culture in Buenos Aires, 1870–1950* (Durham, NC: Duke University Press, 2011).
Benchimol, Jaime, *Dos micróbios aos mosquitos: febre amarela e a revolução pasteuriana no Brasil* (Rio de Janeiro: Fiocruz/UFRJ, 1999).
Birn, Anne-Emanuelle, *Marriage of Convenience: Rockefeller International Health and Revolutionary Mexico* (Rochester: University of Rochester Press, 2006).
Bohme, Susanna Rankin, *Toxic Injustice: A Transnational History of Exposure and Struggle* (Oakland, CA: University of California Press, 2015).
Cueto, Marcos, *The Return of Epidemics: Health and Society in Peru during the Twentieth Century* (Aldershot: Ashgate, 2001).
Cueto, Marcos and Palmer Steven, *Medicine and Public Health in Latin America: A History* (Cambridge University Press, 2014).
De Barros, Juanita, Palmer, Steven, and Wright, David (eds.), *Health and Medicine in the circum-Caribbean: 1800–1968* (New York: Routledge, 2009).
DiLiscia, María Silvia, *Saberes, terapias y prácticas indígenas, populares y científicas en Argentina (1750–1910)* (Madrid: Consejo Superior de Investigaciones Científicas, 2003).
Hochman, Gilberto, *The Sanitation of Brazil: Nation, State, and Public Health, 1889–1930*, transl. by Diane Grosklaus Whitty (Urban-Champaign: University of illinois Press, 2016).

Lambe, Jennifer, *Madhouse: Psychiatry and Politics in Cuban History* (Chapel Hill: University of North Carolina Press, 2017).

Magalhães, Rodrigo Cesar da Silva, *A erradicação do Aedes aegypti: Febre amarela, Fred Soper e saúde pública nas Américas (1918–1968)* (Rio de Janeiro: Editora Fiocruz, 2016).

Mckiernan-González, John, *Fevered Measures: Public Health and Race at the Texas-Mexico Border, 1848–1942* (Durham, N.C.: Duke University Press, 2012).

Necochea López, Raúl, *A History of Family Planning in Twentieth-Century Peru* (Chapel Hill: University of North Carolina Press, 2014).

Otovo, Okezi, *Progressive Mothers, Better Babies: Race, Public Health and the State in Brazil* (Austin: University of Texas Press, 2016).

Palmer, Steven, *From Popular Medicine to Medical Populism: Doctors, Healers, and Public Power in Costa Rica 1800–1940* (Durham, NC: Duke University Press, 2003).

Quevedo, Emilio, et al., *Café y gusanos, mosquitos y petróleo: el tránsito desde la higiene hacia la medicina tropical y la salud pública en Colombia, 1873–1953* (Bogotá: Universidad Nacional de Colombia, 2004).

Stepan, Nancy, *The Hour of Eugenics: Race, Gender, and Nation in Latin America* (Ithaca: Cornell University Press, 1991).

Trujillo-Pagan, Nicole, *Modern Colonization by Medical Intervention: U.S. Medicine in Puerto Rico* (Leiden: Brill Publishers 2013).

Zárate, C. M. Soledad, *Dar a luz en Chile, siglo XIX: De la 'ciencia de hembra' a la ciencia obstétrica* (Santiago: Ediciones de la Dirección de Bibliotecas, Archivos y Museos, 2007).

Zulawski, Ann, *Unequal Cures: Public Health and Political Change in Bolivia, 1900–1950* (Durham, NC: Duke University Press, 2007).

7

Science and Medicine in the United States of America

Edmund Ramsden

In the most celebrated of reflections on America, Alexis de Tocqueville (1805–59) expressed great optimism for its future as the embodiment of the democratic state. On his arrival in 1831, it seemed to him a society formed of all the peoples of the world, differing in language, belief, and character, yet forming a nation possessing 'happiness a hundred times greater than our own'.[1] What made this New World such an improvement on the Old? De Tocqueville saw in the United States a propitious combination of population and place—of the coming together of refined European values and traditions in a world of new possibilities. It was a land that was immense, fertile, and sparsely populated, allowing for freedom and independence. All seemed malleable and mobile as people were made and unmade, and landscapes transformed.

America gifted de Tocqueville the opportunity to express his liberal political ideals, arguing that its success was based on a community of common sensibility—that of personal interest, over and above that of the state. However, he also appended to his celebration of America a warning for its future. De Tocqueville saw the Americans as neglectful of the higher sciences, art, and literature. This resulted from a dedication to industry and trade and an ability to attract great minds from Europe.[2] However, perhaps more significantly, he expressed concern at the oppressive treatment of certain populations by the State. The freedoms extended to white populations in a federal system, allowing them to establish their own towns, cities, and laws, had not been extended to all. While African-Americans faced poverty and ill-health due to the poor environments in which they lived, Native Americans faced utter extermination.

While de Tocqueville was concerned with political systems and economies—sickness, health, and science getting only a passing mention—we can see many of his concerns reflected in the future work of historians of medicine. When Henry Sigerist described his first visit to America in 1932, he similarly wrote of his excitement at the immensity of the landscape, the heterogeneity of its peoples, and his optimism with regard to its future: 'Never before had I felt so clearly that I was envisaging history in the making.'[3] He observed how a nation that was once a medical backwater, dependent upon Europe for its ideas and education, was rapidly becoming a dominant force in world medicine. He sought explanations for this transformation. Yet he also expressed concern. While he may not have shared de Tocqueville's politics, Sigerist also identified the failure to secure the health and well-being of the population in its entirety, noting the significant inequalities in access to quality health care.[4]

Sigerist's history of medicine was socially embedded, grounded in the social and economic realities of contemporary society. Medicine offered a window onto American life, past, present, and future. In turn, an understanding of society and politics endowed the historian with the power to help remake health care.[5] For Sigerist and the many historians of medicine that have followed, the tensions, contradictions, conflicts, and speed of change in American society make it a particularly rich site for tracing the shifting meanings of sickness and methods of prevention and cure. Focusing on the fundamental elements of population and place, we have a nation that is diverse in terms of its peoples, cultures, and geography, allowing us to explore and compare the ways in which medicine is developed and applied in a number of different social, cultural, and physical contexts. We also have rapid growth, from a period in which European ideas, methods, and structures—British, French, and German—were adapted to the American context, to one in which the United States is at the forefront of large-scale initiatives in public health, disease control, and innovation in the biomedical sciences. And finally we have contradiction, most notably between profound faith in the technical capacities of medical science and equally profound dissatisfaction with the provision of health care.[6] The result is a nation particularly well suited for comparative analyses of health and medicine across peoples, place, and time.

The Identity and Character of Early American Medicine, Health, and Disease

The arrival of Europeans in the Americas brought diseases that decimated Native American populations. Colin Calloway describes a 'biological nightmare',[7] and Russell Thornton a 'holocaust',[8] as families, even entire tribes, were destroyed by smallpox, measles, plague, cholera, influenza, typhus, and yellow fever. These were illnesses against which native populations had no immunological resistance, having escaped the great epidemics of Europe and Asia. While now well known, it was not until the careful historical work of those such as Henry Dobyns that the demographic scale and historical significance of the devastation was fully appreciated.[9] While the North American continent has often been described as an empty wilderness or virgin land open to settlement by the European, it was, in effect, 'widowed'.[10] North America was relatively densely populated in 1492, with a population of somewhere between 5 to 10 million. By 1800, this had dwindled to a mere 600,000—a 'demographic disaster' that enabled its conquest by Europeans.[11]

The first European settlements also suffered disease, Virginia being described as a death-trap for colonists.[12] However, by the time of independence, Americans were celebrating the health of their nation's citizens, free as they were from the plagues of illness that swept across Europe. A nation's strength was to be measured in the health and vitality of its peoples, and for Benjamin Franklin (1706–90), independence had been inevitable—the reflection of the rapid population growth of America in contrast to that of Britain.[13] Such self-congratulation proved short-lived.[14] The problem of the American city loomed large in the minds of social reformers and physicians, earlier concerns with yellow fever and smallpox being replaced by the dread of cholera.[15] While concern with crowd diseases were also common in Europe and Asia, shifting trends in migration and the different climate and geography of the United States and its various regions meant the emergence of specific disease cultures and environments.[16]

Central to historical debates is the degree to which American medicine can be viewed as distinctive. Ronald Numbers suggests that an assumption of American exceptionalism has pervaded the literature. He notes how much has been made of the influence of the physical environment, the frontier culture, and the determination to eschew theory and specialization in favour of pragmatism and the general practitioner. The lack of distinction between physician and surgeon and the lack of a rigid medical aristocracy, for example, are seen to result from an American aversion to class distinction. This distinctiveness has been critically examined in a series of essays, edited by Numbers, focusing on New Spain, New France, and New England. While the authors accept that medicine was influenced by indigenous healers, there is also a consensus that American medical practices were directly related to older European traditions and 'changed remarkably little in transit'.[17]

Certainly, when we explore the development of American medicine in the nineteenth century, we can see varying degrees of influence of Britain, France, and Germany. Yet American practitioners were also selective and, in the new setting, medicine was adapted and altered.[18] In the first decades of the United States, therapeutic practices remained tied to traditional ideas of a balance or equilibrium of the body, demanding the physicians intervene through drugs or bloodletting.[19] American medical education was modelled on that of Edinburgh: it had a similar two-tier system, the practitioner attending general classes for a matter of months and the highest honour of MD being the privilege of those that were able and could afford to study intensively in Latin for two years. Yet while the British medical college was regulated by guild and government, distrust of elites and monopolies and an interest in the wealth that an open and competitive educational system could generate resulted in a more fluid medical marketplace in the United States.[20] The result was a proliferation of proprietary medical colleges that continued to reduce fees, requirements, and, thus, the standard of education and training. As a consequence, a variety of specialisms and alternatives to therapeutic activism could remain, emerge, and develop—optometry, chiropractics, osteopathy, psychology, and midwifery.[21]

This diversity and pluralism was only further reinforced with the growing influence of French medicine from the 1820s. Focusing on the professional interests of the physician, John Harley Warner argues that the turn away from rationalistic systems of practice towards clinical empiricism reflected fear and anxiety regarding the status of medicine in the United States.[22] With growing public concern surrounding the effectiveness of traditional therapeutics, compounded by the lack of licensing and regulation that lowered standards and allowed for alternative medicine, it seemed that the privilege bestowed upon the American medical man was being eroded. Empiricism would help consolidate legitimacy, status, and authority. It demanded moderation and the physician's ability to tailor treatment to take account of the specific characters of a patient—their age, race, gender, and occupation—as well as the social and physical environments in which they existed—climate, demography, and geography. Once again, this was no direct transfer from Europe to America, but the empiricist approach was wedded to a continued, if more muted, commitment to therapeutic activism.

Warner was one of the first to use this focus on empiricism to turn the attention of the historian to the variety of medical practices across the United States. He observed that historians have tended to generalize the experience of the Northeast to the rest of America.[23] With the questioning of universal rules of practice came a new emphasis on the local and new ideas about the differences between the medical needs and practices of African American and European, North, West, and South. The South has dominated the study of regional difference in American health and medicine—its climate and traditions of slavery and the plantation system having led to an historical tradition of Southern distinctiveness, almost a 'nation within a nation'.[24] While such environmentalist arguments have been disputed in history more generally, uniqueness is now being reclaimed through the case of disease. Malaria, yellow fever, and hookworm thrived in 'a modified West African disease environment'.[25] For Margaret Humphreys, the ongoing struggle with yellow fever, combined with rural poverty, meant that the objectives, attitudes, and achievements of southern public health officials were 'strikingly different' from their northern urban counterparts.[26] The South also had different populations and social structures. Anthropometric histories have revealed the health of the slave population to be extremely poor,[27] yet their resistance to yellow fever and malaria was used by apologists of slavery to

emphasize the medical distinctiveness of the black body and its suit-
ability to labouring in hot and humid environments.[28] As Warner
argues, this emphasis on the region's medical peculiarity was not simply
a reflection of racism, nationalism, and regional self-consciousness, but
an attempt to promote the status of the Southern medical practitioner
and compete with northern medical schools.

More recently, the work of Sharla Fett has added a further layer of
complexity by examining the distinctiveness of slave medicine—not
only due to African and West Indian remedies, but as the result of
attempts to confront the processes of dehumanization through
community-building and self-determination.[29] In turn, Todd Savitt
has extended our understanding of black medicine after 1865.
African Americans struggled to establish independent, and desperately needed, sources of medical education following emancipation.
Nevertheless, most black-owned proprietary institutions failed due to
a lack of funding, while the few successes remained dependent upon
white philanthropy and organized medicine.[30]

With the eclipse of the French model in the period of German
ascendancy after 1870, there took place a further standardization of
medical school, hospital, and experimental laboratory, and numerous
specialist societies emerged. The development of laboratory-based
medical science and the training of physicians in Germany brought
a significant improvement in medical education. New centres of
excellence, such as Harvard Medical College and the Johns Hopkins
School of Medicine, extended the length of degrees, demanded prior
education, and became tied to the university.[31] Yet, once again, there
was no straightforward transfer from one place to another. Thomas
Bonner argues that the mixed experiences of American students in
Germany, the tradition of egalitarianism, coupled with the competition between medical schools, led to a particularly aggressive
emphasis on laboratory instruction and clinical experience for all
students. There was also a great deal of division and debate over
what scientific medicine was, and how it was to be related to
practice and made useful to the populace. Warner argues that the
new experimental therapeutics based on physiological science divided
physicians—some seeking to understand the laws and principles that
governed health and illness, others seeking to retain an individualized
therapeutics based upon clinical empirical observation.[32] Indeed, this

tension can be seen to endure in the (much under-studied) differences between population medicine—the epidemiological, statistical, and biometric methods that allow for the study of disease in nature—and clinical medicine—based upon the laboratory and focused on the individual patient.

The Growth of American Medicine: Continuity and Fragmentation

Prior to World War I, Europe had imported students from the United States and exported medical experts, ideas, methods, and technologies. The world wars helped reverse this dependency.[33] Reconstruction in Europe demanded new and more effective hospitals, medical schools, and agencies of public health. These were provided through the support of American organizations and would reflect their visions of medical science and practice. In turn, the critical role of science in war enhanced belief in the power of medicine to rid the world not only of infectious, but also of chronic, disease, thus significantly extending the quality and length of life. When Vannevar Bush presented to the President his vision of federally funded 'big science' in 1945, he began by extolling the 'genius' behind the new drug, penicillin.[34]

As significant as the Public Health Service and its Laboratory of Hygiene was becoming, it grew slowly in the first half of the twentieth century.[35] With governmental finances severely restricted, much of the progress in medicine was supported by another largely American innovation—the philanthropic foundation. Their workings and influence have been subject to increasing historical analysis, the Rockefeller Foundation receiving the most attention.[36] A child of the Progressive Era, when medicine and sanitation were promoted as a means to national unity, order, and efficiency, Rockefeller philanthropy first turned its attention to the South.[37] From 1909, the Rockefeller Sanitary Commission for the Eradication of Hookworm combined scientific medicine and public health education—identifying the real causes of the disease, strengthening the dilapidated Southern boards of health, and using health demonstrations to promote preventative health behaviour and services.[38] While the aims of the Sanitary Commission have been associated with benevolent sanitary and health reform that broke down boundaries between North and South, urban and rural, private wealth and public agencies,[39] historians also see it driven by economic interest. That Rockefeller philanthropy soon applied its methods honed in the South to global populations reinforces this perspective. Many see the International Health Division as having promoted a capitalist, even colonial, medicine that commodified health, promoted technological solutions over prevention, economic gain over social equality, and generated medical dependency.[40] More recently, however, a more nuanced historical approach has emerged, focused on the complex, disparate, and often competing interests of foundation officials and local actors.[41]

While the actions of foundations were often limited and fragmented by continuous negotiation between its members, their structure also gave them certain advantages.[42] They could act and experiment in areas off-limits to government agencies.[43] Being governed by a small board also offered both flexibility, allowing for rapid change in goals or tactics, and continuity, or the ability to support a project or approach over a long period of time. As a result of their success, they left their mark not only on public health, but also on medical education.[44] Historians have explored how a vision of a scientific medicine was promoted and realized by leading figures in Rockefeller philanthropy, such as Abraham Flexner (1866–1959) and Alan Gregg (1890–1957).[45] Elizabeth Fee has focused on the early years of the Johns Hopkins School of Public Health and Hygiene, critical to the professionalization of public health in the United States.[46] There was much debate over what public health consisted of—a broad field or a specialty built on sanitary engineering and bacteriology, organized around germ theory or the amelioration of environmental conditions based upon scientific research or administrative practice. The Rockefeller Foundation ensured that it would be planned along scientific lines by scientifically trained elite. The biomedical sciences came to dominate at Johns Hopkins and soon throughout the United States—organized around the control of specific diseases, first infectious then chronic, at the expense of the social and political sciences.[47]

The lack of central government funds and organization meant that public health lacked visibility and definition.[48] It also allowed for the development of a diverse field, which combined a range of disciplines and professions and enabled new and innovative programmes to develop—in environmental health, social and behavioural science, health economics, population dynamics, and family planning. While further scholarship is required to address the range of agencies and organizations that acted in the absence of a coherent medical specialty, historians have identified a pattern of development that is reflective of American medicine as a whole,[49] that is, one of continued pluralism and an ever-increasing interest in the technical possibilities of scientific medicine over community and preventative activities. Just as the Rockefeller Foundation turned from reforming medical schools to supporting individual researchers and projects, leading to considerable eclecticism and incoherence, historians see government agencies as continuing this legacy. The generous government funding given to the National Institutes of Health was distributed across the United States according to a peer-review system, while other opportunistic agencies established their own research programmes, such as the Office of Naval Research.[50] This was then coupled to rapidly expanding biotechnology and pharmaceutical industries, again allied to academe.[51] The open marketplace so characteristic of American medicine continued, it seems, in biomedical research.[52]

Big science is America's solution to sickness—the consequence, perhaps, of its failure to realize a comprehensive national health care system. Understandably, the subject of health insurance has focused attention on the similarities and differences between American and European societies.[53] While the passing of the 1911 British Insurance Act helped trigger debate, even optimism, as did the 1946 National Health Service Act, it was not until 1965 that some form of compulsory health insurance was provided in the United States.[54] There are, of course, numerous reasons for this failure to reform medical care, many seeing it as stemming from individualistic ideals and a suspicion of government and pointing to the many derogatory references to 'socialized medicine'. Most also identify the financial and professional interests of physicians as a root cause.[55] Having struggled so severely to secure status and income, American physicians feared lowered wages and increased bureaucracy. These concerns were effectively exacerbated and operationalized through the American Medical Association, which manipulated anti-German feeling and Cold War rhetoric to present compulsory insurance as alien to American society.[56]

This process has been subject to intense focus by historians, as it is here that many see history as playing a critical role in advising policy, just as it was in the time of Sigerist. However, history is no longer used to assert the seemingly obvious benefits of universal health insurance. Contrary to Sigerist, historians now see its rejection as understandable, perhaps even inevitable, due to a decentralized political system, the weakness of worker unions, the unity of the business sector, and the strength of lobbying by health providers and insurers.[57] Yet those who merely associate American medicine with the private sphere are mistaken. As we have seen, American medicine has long combined private and public. The government pays for basic research and training and it patents, regulates, and purchases medical products. Similarly, while the United States may well rely on the private sector to distribute health care, the government has also assumed much of the cost of the provision of clinical services. Charles Rosenberg argues: 'American distinctiveness lies not in some unique devotion to the market and individualism, but in a widespread inattention to a more complex reality.'[58] There is a contradiction and tension here that can only be understood historically—the government has continuously filled the gaps in the system, despite near continuous political rhetoric that the state is best kept small.

The government first tried to intervene in health care provision as part of the New Deal, but strong opposition forced President Roosevelt to drop health reform from his proposed social security legislation. Seeking to prevent compulsory insurance, the American Medical Association did, however, acquiesce in regard to voluntary insurance. Many physicians were attracted to the idea of a stable and regular income during the Depression, just as hospitals were concerned to realize steady revenue and meet public demand. The result was a series of non-profit group initiatives—Blue Cross for hospital insurance and Blue Shield for physician insurance, and independent consumer cooperatives such as Kaiser Permanente.[59] This arrangement satisfied the interests of medical providers, employers, and workers. Shortages in hospital access were met by government through the Hill Burton Act of 1946. With the rising costs of health care provision (inevitable considering the tendency to equate specialization and technology with quality and to define disease according to availability of treatment), government turned to the private sector to invest in health provision, while increasingly providing for those least able to pay.[60] The result has been a large section of the population considered too wealthy for government support and too poor to meet spiralling insurance premiums.

Rosemary Stevens explores these tensions through the study of the American hospital. This is an institution torn between two competing roles—a social organization that represents charity and public purpose and an icon of capital, competition, and technological achievement.[61] For Stevens, the hospital embodies the central dilemma of national health policy: how to share the fruits of medical advance without establishing a large welfare state. The result is an 'idiosyncratically "American" institution', defined by technology, expertise, and entrepreneurship, by diversity reflective of the pluralism of American society, and by increased stratification according to class and race.[62] That the recent Obama health care legislation did not introduce a universal single payment system, but a complex and ongoing process of reform that includes insurance and pharmaceutical companies, ensures that history will continue to play a critical role in the controversy.

Race and Class: From Environment, To Contagion, to Genetic Medicine

When the sociologist Edward A. Ross (1866–1951) reflected on 'What is America?', he expressed a degree of pessimism not uncommon at the end of the Progressive Era.[63] America was defined, of course, by the people that inhabited it. It now seemed that the spirited, enterprising, and intelligent Northern European was being overwhelmed by the flood of immigrants from Southern and Eastern Europe. Ross was an outspoken eugenicist, a member of a movement that emphasised the association of certain classes and races with hereditary weakness and moral degeneracy. Yet, as Charles Rosenberg argues, the assumed inheritance of physique, character, and temperament was not dependent upon a notion of a discrete and particulate unit of heredity, but reflective of a much older tradition in which ideas of health and illness played a crucial role.[64] Disease was associated with certain moral sensibilities and failings. Degenerate characteristics and susceptibilities to illness acquired through poor habits were transmitted to the child, while diseases were spread by the immoral and unsanitary behaviour of certain groups. Through tracing the history of disease in

New York, America's 'hive of sickness and vice', particular plagues can be seen to have been associated with particular peoples, irrespective of the understanding of the mode of transmission.[65]

Even with the arrival of germ theory and the recognition that contagion crossed race and class lines, the perceived relationship between groups and particular diseases was redefined rather than removed. In her study of the polio epidemic of 1916, Naomi Rogers shows how the disease became more visible in the twentieth century following improved sanitation as children no longer acquired immunity through maternal antibodies.[66] Although it was the middle classes that were now more susceptible and the spread of the disease could be linked to cleanliness and order, scientists and health workers remained convinced that it was a "dirt disease" related to ignorance, poverty and overcrowding. Immigrant families from Southern and Eastern Europe were targeted by the public and by health officials. To retain this association between poverty, immigration, and disease, the fly was enrolled as an explanatory tool—a carrier of disease from working-class to middle-class homes.

Alan Kraut and Howard Markel have focused on this association between immigration and illness through the study of epidemics—a useful tool for analysing the various social responses to disease across time and space.[67] In his study of the typhus epidemic of 1892 in New York City, Markel examined how scientific debates over germ theory and public health were ignored in favour of targeting immigrants from Eastern Europe as problem populations. Russian Jews were stigmatized as carriers of disease, helping to justify the immigration restriction legislation of 1924.[68] It is useful to compare the treatment of various groups in relation to specific diseases and epidemics—trachoma becoming associated with Jewish populations, cholera with the Irish, and, more recently, AIDS with Haitians.[69] The Chinese were the first to be excluded from entering the United States on the basis of race. While these restrictions reflected broader cultural concerns over assimilation, they were reinforced by outbreaks of plague in Hawaii in 1899 and San Francisco in 1900. While San Francisco's Chinatown was known to be filthy and overcrowded, city officials did little to ameliorate the environment. Markel shows how they blamed the immigrants themselves. The result was a coercive, often brutal, self-defeating programme of quarantine involving violence, the forcible removal of families from their homes, the destruction of property, and the closure of businesses.

Such historical analyses highlight the tensions and contradictions in focusing on either population or place. In the case presented by Rogers, contagion is presented as a great equalizer, emphasizing the universality of disease, while environmental causes focused attention on the dirt and squalor of the working-class home and the incompetence of the working-class family. In the cases presented by Markel, it was the focus on contagious populations that resulted in the poor living conditions of immigrant communities being ignored by city officials. Often modes of explanation discriminate by combining the biological and the environmental. Gregg Mitman's study of asthma, for example, shows how theories of racial differences in susceptibility to allergens and belief in the unsanitary habits of African American and Latino families resulted in an 'ecology of injustice' that ignored appalling housing conditions.[70] This focus on specific populations as disease-ridden has only intensified with genetic medicine, particularly with its focus on chronic as opposed to acute illness.

Human genetics has been subject to intense historical interest in recent years. For some, the Second World War is a watershed in the history of heredity research; advances in population and medical genetics coupled to the atrocities committed in the name of eugenics transformed the science of heredity and its perceived applications. For most historians, however, there remain significant continuities between the new genetics and earlier attempts to improve the quality of the American population. Tracing the early history of molecular biology, Lily Kay has questioned the common assumption that applied science emerged out of basic research. She suggests the reverse: when the molecular biology programme was first defined in the 1930s, it was done in terms of its perceived technological and social potentials. The Rockefeller millions spent at Caltech reflected a concern with improving man's mental and physical attributes.[71]

Historians have, for the most part, sought to qualify what they see as exaggerated optimism over the power and benefit of genetic medicine.[72] As Diane Paul argues, diagnostic capabilities far exceed the therapeutic. The oft-celebrated phenylalanine diet for phenylke-tonuria (PKU)—a celebrated environmental solution to a recently defined genetic disease—is costly and imperfect.[73] Methods of gene therapy are as yet limited and have raised concerns over safety. The result is a turn to antenatal diagnostics and selective abortion; for this reason, many see genetic medicine as the thin end of the wedge, a slippery slope or back door towards broader eugenic programmes to improve the genetic quality of populations.[74] Such problems are only further compounded by the common associations made between a genetic disease and a particular community.

Once again, the diversity of the American population has proven particularly useful for analysing how different communities have very different experiences of genetic medicine. Keith Wailoo and Stephen Pemberton have traced the history of three risk diseases and the people most afflicted by them: cystic fibrosis among the white population; Tay-Sachs in relation to the Jewish American population; and sickle cell anaemia among the black population.[75] Different groups meant different promises and programmes. With regard to cystic fibrosis, the focus was on gene therapy, heralded as the new break-through in genetic medicine. Tay-Sachs resulted in a well-organized and community-driven programme of self-preservation focused on screening for marriage. Attempts to combat sickle cell anaemia were, in contrast, particularly troubled. While the failure of the government to act against sickle cell was at first seen to reflect their general neglect of African Americans, by the 1970s, following a mandatory screening programme and discrimination in health insurance, sport, and employment, there was a backlash against the perceived dangers and stigmatizing potential of genetic medicine. Even today, African Americans are less likely to utilize genetic screening techniques and to avail themselves of selective abortion.

The aversion of African Americans to genetic medicine is seen to be understandable when placed in historical context. For Wailoo, the notorious case of the Tuskegee Syphilis Experiment serves as an 'archetype' for understanding the relations between race and health care.[76] It began in 1932 when approximately 600 African American men in rural Alabama were recruited without their consent into a Public Health Service study of untreated syphilis. When the study ended in 1972, it concluded that the death rate of syphilitic men aged between 25 and 50 was 75 per cent greater than that of the general population. Not only did the authorities fail to treat those infected, but they deliberately prevented them accessing treatment when it became available. Seeking to explain the actions of the investigators, James Jones shows how the study drew from and fed into stereotypes about the sexual behaviour of African Americans.[77] Susan Lederer argues that patients were treated as experimental organisms, even cadavers—individuals for dissection identified, and their bodies obtained with the aid of local physicians.[78] Understandably, the experiment is a focal point for discussions of racism in science and medicine in America, and continues to trouble the relationship between the medical community and African Americans.

However, as Wailoo also argues, the implications of genetic medicine are complex and multifaceted and cannot be understood simply through the prism of biological racism.[79] In the 1920s, sickle cell anaemia was seen as a disease of 'Negro blood' that could spread through the wider population. It was used, therefore, as a means of arguing against inter-racial marriage. Once it was understood to be carried by a recessive allele in the 1940s, its social significance was radically altered. Out-breeding would now reduce its incidence. Wailoo argues that sickle cell anaemia has two very different identities, a consequence of new methods and technologies. By the 1950s, sickle cell had become an exemplar of genetic polymorphism—its role in protecting a carrier against malaria making it essential to the survival of a population. The lack of attention given to issues such as genetic diversity and polymorphism is the result of the preoccupation of historians with the relations between genetic medicine and eugenics. Only recently are we seeing work that addresses the ways in which genetic medicine was transformed, in the words of Susan Lindee, from 'medical backwater' to 'medical research frontier', and how various advocacy groups helped to drive this growing industry of blood-testing techniques, population-mapping studies, and screening programmes.[80]

Conclusion

Historians of medicine have long focused on disease, the more dramatic and visible the better, as a means of understanding tension, contradiction, continuity, and change in American society. In a classic example, Charles Rosenberg used cholera epidemics as a 'natural experiment' and 'sampling technique' as well as a subject—a 'randomly recurring stimulus against which the varying reactions of Americans could be judged'.[81] Similarly, in Katherine Ott's study of tuberculosis, the identity of the disease was not the same in 1870, 1900, or 1930.[82] Diseases are framed by the society in which they exist, and, as Keith Wailoo argues, it is by tracing their trajectory as social commodities that we reveal the general trajectory of American health care and biomedical research.[83] Others have focused on a disease across space as opposed to time, a cross-sectional 'snapshot' if you will, of the differential experience of health and sickness among the various groups that make up American society.

In such studies, historians have become increasingly aware of the methods, practices, and technologies that drive our social understanding of illness across time and space. New technologies not only make visible and give definition to specific diseases, but they can also redefine notions of health and illness more generally. Health and population surveys, for example, are extremely important to medical science, yet they have been largely neglected as a historical resource. Just as Margo Anderson used the history of the US census as a window through which to view American political, economic, and scientific life, in tracing the history of surveys we are offered insights into the shifting landscape of health and health research in the United States.[84] The Framingham Heart Study, for example, began in 1947 and pioneered the epidemiological study of chronic disease and contributed to our understanding of a 'risk' population.[85] Framingham was considered an ideal sample of the American population and had been studied before as a means of understanding an infectious disease—tuberculosis. It became a 'social laboratory' focused on a wide range of variables, normal as well as pathological. Like numerous other surveys, it not only mirrors the changes in American society and medicine, but actively contributes to them, allowing us to examine the effects of new measures and technologies, the continuous negotiation between interested parties over the questions asked and the application of data, and the experience of existing under the medical gaze.

A focus on such methods not only allows us to examine populations across time and space, but also to privilege the problem of place. This has become of increasing interest to historians of science and medicine in recent years. Tom Gieryn's suggestion that there exist 'truth-spots', for example, places associated with a particular form of knowledge production to which they lend credibility,[86] could also be usefully applied to the history of medicine—places associated with the study of health and disease. Attention has also been stimulated by work that recognizes the central role that health and medicine play in environmental history.[87] The idea of places of health and sickness, it is argued, allows us to traverse boundaries between humans and nature and between urban and rural environments. The tremendous upheavals of urban renewal, for example, in which physical and mental health concerns proved critical as a source of justification and criticism, should draw the attention of historians of American medicine.[88] The great multiplicity and change in peoples and places in the United States will continue to provide a rich field of research, while the complexity of relations between citizens and federal, state, and local government will always provide tensions and contradictions of interest to the historian of medicine.

Notes

1 Alexis de Tocqueville, *Democracy in America*, ed. J. P. Mayer with a new translation by George Lawrence (Garden City, NY: Doubleday, 1969).

2 Tocqueville, *Democracy in America*, (1969), 454–5.

3 H. E. Sigerist, *American Medicine* (New York: Norton, 1934), xvi.

4 Elizabeth Fee and T. M. Brown (eds), *Making Medical History: The Life and Times of Henry E. Sigerist* (Baltimore: Johns Hopkins University Press, 1997), 25.

5 H. E. Sigerist, *Medicine and Human Welfare* (College Park, MD: McGrath, [1945] 1971).

6 Charles Rosenberg, *Our Present Complaint: American Medicine Then and Now* (Baltimore, Johns Hopkins University Press, 2007).

7 Colin G. Calloway, *New Worlds for All: Indians, Europeans and the Remaking of Early America* (Baltimore: Johns Hopkins University Press, 1997), 25.

8 Russell Thornton, *American Indian Holocaust and Survival: A Population History since 1492* (Norman: University of Oklahoma Press, 1987).

9 Henry F. Dobyns, 'Estimating Aboriginal American Population', *Current Anthropology* 7 (1966), 395–416; *idem*, *Native American Historical Demography* (Bloomington: Indiana University Press, 1976); *idem*, *Their Number Become Thinned: Native American Population Dynamics in Eastern North America* (Knoxville: University of Tennessee Press, 1983). Another classic is A. W. Crosby, *The Columbian Exchange: Biological and Cultural Consequences of 1492* (Westport, CT: Greenwood Press, 1972).

10 Francis Jennings, *The Invasion of America: Indians, Colonialism, and the Cant of Conquest* (Chapel Hill: University of North Carolina Press, 1975), 15.

11 Calloway, *New Worlds for All*, 39–40; P. Baldwin, *Contagion and the State in Europe, 1830–1930* (Cambridge: Cambridge University Press, 1999).

12 Gerald N. Grob, *The Deadly Truth: A History of Disease in America* (Cambridge, MA: Harvard University Press, 2002), 52.

13 James H. Cassedy, *Demography in Early America: Beginnings of the Statistical Mind, 1600–1800* (Cambridge, MA: Harvard University Press, 1969); Dennis Hodgson, 'Benjamin Franklin on Population: From Policy to Theory', *Population and Development Review* 17 (1991), 639–61.

14 For anthropometric histories that have identified the decline in stature of the American population from the time of the Revolution due to ill-health, see: Richard, H. Steckel, 'Heights and Human Welfare: Recent Developments and New Directions', *Explorations in Economic History* 46 (2009), 1–23; Bernard Harris, 'Health, Height, and History: An Overview of Recent Developments in Anthropometric History', *Social History of Medicine* 7 (1994), 297–320.

15 Charles E. Rosenberg, *The Cholera Years: The United States in 1832, 1849, and 1866* (Chicago: University of Chicago Press, 1962).

16 K. David Patterson, 'Disease Environments of the Antebellum South', in Ronald L. Numbers and Todd L. Savitt (eds), *Science and Medicine in the Old South* (Baton Rouge: Louisiana State University Press, 1989), 152–72; John Duffy, *The Sanitarians: A History of American Public Health* (Urbana: University of Illinois Press, 1990).

17 Ronald Numbers (ed.), *Medicine in the New World: New Spain, New France, and New England* (Knoxville: University of Tennessee Press, 1987), 2, 157.

18 Lisa Rosner, 'Thistle on the Delaware: Edinburgh Medical Education and Philadelphia Practice, 1800–1825', *Social History of Medicine* 5 (1992), 19–42.

19 Charles Rosenberg, 'The Therapeutic Revolution: Medicine, Meaning, and Social Change in Nineteenth-Century America', *Perspectives in Biology and Medicine* 20 (1977), 485–506.

20 Paul Starr, *The Social Transformation of American Medicine* (New York: Basic Books, 1982).

21 Ronald Numbers, 'The Fall and Rise of the American Medical Profession', in Nathan Hatch (ed.), *The Professions in American History* (Notre Dame: University of Notre Dame Press, 1988); Martin Kaufman, 'American Medical Education', in Ronald Numbers (ed.), *The Education of American Physicians: Historical Essays* (Berkeley: University of California Press, 1980).

22 John Harley Warner, *Against the Spirit of the System: The French Impulse in Nineteenth-Century American Medicine* (Baltimore: Johns Hopkins University Press, 1998).

23 John Harley Warner, *The Therapeutic Perspective: Medical Practice, Knowledge, and Identity in America, 1820–1885* (Cambridge, MA: Harvard University Press, 1986), 3.

24 James O. Breeden, 'Disease as a Factor in Southern Distinctiveness', in Todd Savitt and James Harvey Young (eds), *Disease and Distinctiveness in the American South* (Knoxville: University of Tennessee Press, 1988), 1–28.

25 Patterson, 'Disease Environments', 158.

26 Margaret Humphreys, *Yellow Fever and the South* (New Brunswick, NJ: Rutgers University Press, 1992), 1. See also: John H. Ellis, *Yellow Fever and Public Health in the New South* (Lexington: University Press of Kentucky, 1992); and Jo Ann Carrigan, 'Yellow Fever: Scourge of the South', in Savitt and Young (eds), *Disease and Distinctiveness in the American South*.

27 Richard H. Steckel, 'A Peculiar Population: The Nutrition, Health, and Mortality of American Slaves from Childhood to Maturity', *Journal of Economic History* 46 (1986), 721–41.

28 Todd L. Savitt, 'Black Health on the Plantation: Masters, Slaves, and Physicians', in Numbers and Savitt (eds), *Science and Medicine in the Old South*; Savitt and Young (eds), *Disease and Distinctiveness in the American South*; Todd Savitt, *Medicine and Slavery: The Diseases and Health Care of Blacks in Antebellum Virginia* (Urbana: University of Illinois Press, 1978).

29 Sharla M. Fett, *Working Cures: Healing, Health, and Power on Southern Slave Plantations* (Chapel Hill: University of North Carolina Press, 2002).

30 Todd L. Savitt, *Race and Medicine in Nineteenth- and Early-Twentieth-Century America* (Kent, OH: Kent State University Press, 2007).

31 Numbers, 'The Fall and Rise'.

32 John Harley Warner, 'Ideals of Science and Their Discontents in Late-Nineteenth-Century American Medicine', *Isis* 82 (1991), 454–78. For an analysis of the strength of emphasis on scientific training and practical experience in the United States, see Thomas Neville Bonner, 'The German Model of Training Physicians in the United States, 1870–1914: How Closely Was It Followed?', *Bulletin of the History of Medicine* 64 (1990), 18–34.

33 William H. Schneider, 'The Men Who Followed Flexner: Richard Pearce, Alan Gregg, and the Rockefeller Foundation Medical Divisions, 1919–1951', in William H. Schneider (ed.), *Rockefeller Philanthropy and Modern Biomedicine: International Initiatives from World War I to the Cold War* (Bloomington: Indiana University Press, 2002), 7–60, at 10–11.

34 Vannevar Bush, *Science, the Endless Frontier: A Report to the President* (Washington, DC: United States Government Printing Office 1945), 5, Robert Cook-Deegan and Michael McGeary, 'The Jewel in the Federal Crown?: History, Politics, and the National Institutes of Health', in Rosemary A. Stevens, Charles E. Rosenberg, and Lawton R. Burns (eds), *History and Health Policy in the United States: Putting the Past Back In* (New Brunswick, NJ: Rutgers University Press, 2006), 176–201, at 179.

35 Fitzhugh Mullan, *Plagues and Politics: The Story of the United States Public Health Service* (New York: Basic Books, 1989).

36 E. Richard Brown, *Rockefeller Medicine Men: Medicine and Capitalism in America* (Berkeley: University of California Press, 1979); Jack D. Pressman, 'Human Understanding: Psychosomatic Medicine and the Mission of the Rockefeller Foundation', in Christopher Lawrence and George Weisz (eds), *Greater Than the Parts: Holism in Biomedicine, 1930–1950* (New York: Oxford University Press, 1998). For studies of other foundations relevant to health, see A. McGehee Harvey and Susan L. Abrams, *'For the*

168 *Edmund Ramsden*

Welfare of Mankind': The Commonwealth Fund and American Medicine (Baltimore: Johns Hopkins University Press, 1986); Clyde V. Kiser, *The Milbank Memorial Fund: Its Leaders and Its Work, 1905–1974* (New York: Milbank Memorial Fund, 1975).

37 John Ettling, *The Germ of Laziness: Rockefeller Philanthropy and Public Health in the New South* (Cambridge, MA: Harvard University Press, 1981); John Farley, *To Cast Out Disease: A History of the International Health Division of the Rockefeller Foundation (1913–1951)* (New York: Oxford University Press, 2004).

38 Elizabeth Toon, 'Selling the Public on Public Health: The Commonwealth and Milbank Health Demonstrations and the Meaning of Community Health Action', in Ellen Condliffe Lagemann (ed.), *Philanthropic Foundations: New Scholarship, New Possibilities* (Bloomington: University of Indiana Press, 1999), 119–30.

39 Ettling, *The Germ of Laziness*, viii.

40 Soma Hewa, *Colonialism, Tropical Disease and Imperial Medicine: Rockefeller Philanthropy in Sri Lanka* (Lanham: University Press of America, 1995).

41 Anne-Emanuelle Birn, *Marriage of Convenience: Rockefeller Health and Revolutionary Mexico* (Rochester, NY: University of Rochester Press, 2006); Schneider (ed.), *Rockefeller Philanthropy and Modern Biomedicine*; Ann Zulawski, *Unequal Cures: Public Health and Political Change in Bolivia, 1900–1950* (Durham, NC/London: Duke University Press, 2007).

42 Benjamin B. Page and David A. Valone (eds), *Philanthropic Foundations and the Globalization of Scientific Medicine and Public Health* (Lanham: University Press of America, 2007).

43 Adele Clarke, *Disciplining Reproduction: Modernity, American Life Sciences, and 'The Problems of Sex'* (Berkeley: University of California Press, 1998); Mathew Connelly, *Fatal Misconceptions* (Cambridge, MA: Belknap Press, 2008); Elizabeth Fee, 'Sin vs Science: Venereal Disease in Baltimore in the Twentieth Century', *Journal of the History of Medicine and Allied Sciences* 43 (1988), 141–64.

44 Kenneth M. Ludmerer, *Learning to Heal: The Development of American Medical Education* (Baltimore: Johns Hopkins University Press, 1985).

45 Barbara Barzansky and Norman Gevitz (eds), *Beyond Flexner: Medical Education in the Twentieth Century* (Westport, CT: Greenwood Press, 1992); Howard S. Berliner, *A System of Scientific Medicine: Philanthropic Foundations in the Flexner Era* (London/New York: Tavistock, 1985); Schneider, 'The Men Who Followed Flexner'.

46 Elizabeth Fee, *Disease and Discovery: A History of the Johns Hopkins School of Hygiene and Public Health, 1916–1939* (Baltimore: Johns Hopkins University Press, 1987); Elizabeth Fee and Roy M. Acheson (eds), *A History of Education in Public Health: Health That Mocks the Doctor's Rules* (Oxford: Oxford University Press, 1991).

47 See also James Colgrove, Gerald Markowitz, and David Rosner, *The Contested Boundaries of American Public Health* (New Brunswick, NJ: Rutgers University Press, 2008).

48 Elizabeth Fee, 'The Origins and Development of Public Health in the United States', in Roger Detels, et al. (eds), *Oxford Textbook of Public Health*, vol. 1 (Oxford: Oxford University Press, 1997), 35–54, at 49.

49 An example of a hugely influential organization in need of historical analysis would be the Metropolitan Life Insurance Company. There is also still considerable work to do on various foundations such as the Milbank Memorial, Josiah Macy Jr, and Rosenwald Funds.

50 Victoria A. Harden, *Inventing the NIH: Federal Biomedical Research Policy, 1887–1937* (Baltimore: Johns Hopkins University Press, 1986); Harvey M. Sapolsky, *Science and the Navy: The History of the Office of Naval Research* (Princeton: Princeton University Press, 1990). There is still considerable work to be done on both the Navy and Army in relation to medical and psychiatric research.

51 Eli Ginzberg and Anna B. Dutka, *The Financing of Biomedical Research* (Baltimore: Johns Hopkins University Press, 1989); John P. Swann. *Academic Scientists and the Pharmaceutical Industry: Cooperative Research in Twentieth-Century America* (Baltimore: Johns Hopkins University Press, 1988).

52 Cook-Deegan and McGeary, 'The Jewel in the Federal Crown?'.

53 There is a tendency to compare the United States with Britain in particular, the nations having important social, cultural, political, and scientific ties. The potentially useful comparison with Canada is rarely undertaken. See, for example, Theodore R. Marmor, 'Canada's Path, America's Choices: Lessons from the Canadian Experience with National Health Insurance', in R. Numbers (ed.), *Compulsory Health Insurance: The Continuing American Debate* (Westport, CT: Greenwood, 1982).

54 Gary Land, 'American Images of British Compulsory Health Insurance', in Numbers (ed.), *Compulsory Health Insurance*.

55 Jonathan Engel, *Doctors and Reformers: Discussion and Debate over Health Policy, 1925–1950* (Columbia: University of South Carolina Press, 2002); Ronald L. Numbers, *Almost Persuaded: American Physicians and Compulsory Health Insurance, 1912–1920* (Baltimore: Johns Hopkins University Press, 1978); Numbers (ed.), *Compulsory Health Insurance*.

56 Ronald Numbers, 'The Third Party: Health Insurance in America', in Morris J. Vogel and Charles E. Rosenberg (eds), *The Therapeutic Revolution: Essays in the Social History of American Medicine* (Philadelphia: University of Pennsylvania Press, 1979), 177–200.

57 Jonathan Engel, *Poor People's Medicine: Medicaid and American Charity Care since 1965* (Durham, NC: Duke University Press, 2006), xv–xvi.

58 Rosenberg, *Our Present Complaint*, 186–7.

59 Robert Cunningham III and Robert M. Cunningham Jr., *The Blues: A History of the Blue Cross and Blue Shield System* (Dekalb: Northern Illinois University Press, 1997); Michael R. Grey, *New Deal Medicine: The Rural Health Programs of the Farm Security Administration* (Baltimore: Johns Hopkins University Press, 1999); Rickey Hendricks, *A Model for National Health Care: The History of Kaiser Permanente* (New Brunswick, NJ: Rutgers University Press, 1993).

60 Stevens, Rosenberg, and Burns (eds), *History and Health Policy in the United States;* Lawrence D. Brown, *Politics and Health Care Organization: HMOs as Federal Policy* (Washington, DC: Brookings Institution, 1983).

61 Rosemary Stevens, *In Sickness and in Wealth: American Hospitals in the Twentieth Century* (New York: Basic Books, 1989), 4.

62 Ibid. 8.

63 Edward A. Ross, *What Is America?* (New York: Century, 1919).

64 Charles E. Rosenberg, *No Other Gods: On Science and American Social Thought* (Baltimore: Johns Hopkins University Press, 1976).

65 David Rosner (ed.), *Hives of Sickness: Public Health and Epidemics in New York City* (New Brunswick, NJ: Rutgers University Press, 1995).

66 Naomi Rogers, *Dirt and Disease: Polio before FDR* (New Brunswick, NJ: Rutgers University Press, 1992).

67 Alan M. Kraut, *Silent Travelers: Germs, Genes, and the 'Immigrant Menace'* (Baltimore: Johns Hopkins University Press, 1994); Howard Markel, *Quarantine! East European Jewish Immigrants and the New York City Epidemics of 1892* (Baltimore: Johns Hopkins University Press, 1997).

68 For an important study of the role of the medical inspection of immigrants as a technology of inclusion, rather than exclusion, see Amy L. Fairchild, *Science at the Borders: Immigrant Medical Inspection and the Shaping of the Modern Industrial Labor Force* (Baltimore: The Johns Hopkins University Press, 2003).

69 Howard Markel, *When Germs Travel: Six Major Epidemics That Have Invaded America since 1900 and the Fears They Have Unleashed* (New York: Pantheon Books, 2004).

70 Gregg Mitman, 'Cockroaches, Housing, and Race: A History of Asthma and Urban Ecology in America', in Mark Jackson (ed.), *Health and the Modern Home* (New York/London: Routledge, 2007), 244–65.

71 Lily E. Kay, *The Molecular Vision of Life: Caltech, the Rockefeller Foundation, and the Rise of the New Biology* (Oxford: Oxford University Press, 1993).

72 Joseph S. Alper, Catherine Ard, Adrienne Asch, Jon Beckwith, Peter Conrad, and Lisa N. Geller (eds), *The Double-Edged Helix: Social Implications of Genetics in a Diverse Society* (Baltimore: Johns Hopkins University Press, 2002); Dorothy Nelkin and Laurence Tancredi, *Dangerous Diagnostics: The Social Power of Biological Information* (Chicago: University of Chicago Press, 1989).

73 Diane Paul, 'A Double-Edged Sword', *Nature* 405 (2000), 515.

74 Troy Duster, *Backdoor to Eugenics* (London: Routledge, 1990).

75 Keith Wailoo and Stephen Pemberton, *The Troubled Dream of Genetic Medicine: Ethnicity and Innovation in Tay-Sachs, Cystic Fibrosis, and Sickle Cell Disease* (Baltimore: Johns Hopkins University Press, 2006).

76 Keith Wailoo, *Dying in the City of the Blues: Sickle Cell Anemia and the Politics of Race and Health* (Chapel Hill: University of North Carolina Press, 2001), 13.

77 James H. Jones, *Bad Blood: The Tuskegee Syphilis Experiment* (New York: Free Press, 1993).

78 Susan Lederer, 'Tucker's Heart: Racial Politics and Heart Transplantation in America', in Keith Wailoo, Julie Livingston, and Peter Guarnaccia (eds),

A Death Retold: Jesica Santillan, the Bungled Transplant, and Paradoxes of Medical Citizenship (Chapel Hill: University of North Carolina Press, 2006).

79 Keith Wailoo, *Drawing Blood: Technology and Disease Identity in Twentieth-Century America* (Baltimore: Johns Hopkins University Press, 1997), 137.

80 Susan Lindee, *Moments of Truth in Genetic Medicine* (Baltimore: Johns Hopkins University Press, 2005), 1.

81 Rosenberg, *The Cholera Years*, 4; Charles Rosenberg, 'Siting Epidemic Disease: 3 Centuries of American History', *Journal of Infectious Diseases*, 197 (2008), S4–S6.

82 Katherine Ott, *Fevered Lives: Tuberculosis in American Culture since 1870* (Cambridge, MA: Harvard University Press, 1996).

83 Wailoo, *Dying in the City*, 9.

84 Margo Anderson, *The American Census: A Social History* (New Haven, CT: Yale University Press, 1988).

85 Gerald M. Oppenheimer, 'Becoming the Framingham Study, 1947–1950', *American Journal of Public Health* 95 (2005), 602–10.

86 Thomas F. Gieryn, 'City as Truth-Spot: Laboratories and Field-Sites in Urban Studies', *Social Studies of Science* 36 (2006), 5–38.

87 Gregg Mitman, 'In Search of Health: Landscape and Disease in American Environmental History', *Environmental History* 10 (2005), 184–210; Dawn Day Biehler, *Pests in the City: Flies, Bedbugs, Cockroaches, and Rats* (Seattle: University of Washington Press, 2013); Michelle Murphy, Gregg Mitman, and Christopher Sellers (eds), *Landscapes of Exposure: Knowledge and Illness in Modern Environments, Osiris* 19 (2004); Michelle Murphy, *Sick Building Syndrome and the Problem of Uncertainty: Environmental Politics, Technoscience, and Women Workers* (Durham, NC: Duke University Press, 2006).

88 There is also work needed that addresses medical sociology, social psychiatry, and the relationship between medicine and the behavioural sciences more generally—see, for example, Samuel W. Bloom, *The Word as Scalpel: A History of Medical Sociology* (Oxford: Oxford University Press, 2002).

Select Bibliography

Derickson, Alan, *Health Security for All: Dreams of Universal Health Care in America* (Baltimore: Johns Hopkins University Press, 2005).

Fairchild, Amy L., Ronald Bayer, and James Colgrove, *Searching Eyes: Privacy, the State, and Disease Surveillance in America* (Berkeley: University of California Press, 2007).

Fee, Elizabeth, and Roy M. Acheson (eds), *A History of Education in Public Health: Health That Mocks the Doctor's Rules* (Oxford: Oxford University Press, 1991).

Fee, Elizabeth, and T. M. Brown (eds), *Making Medical History: The Life and Times of Henry E. Sigerist* (Baltimore: Johns Hopkins University Press, 1997).

Greene, Jeremy A., *Prescribing by Numbers: Drugs and the Definition of Disease* (Baltimore: Johns Hopkins University Press, 2007).

Grob, Gerald, *The Deadly Truth: A History of Disease in America* (Cambridge, MA: Harvard University Press, 2002).

Hoffman, Beatrix, *Health Care for Some: Rights and Rationing in the United States Since 1930* (Chicago, University of Chicago Press, 2012).

Leavitt, Judith Walzer, and Ronald L. Numbers (eds), *Sickness and Health in America: Readings in the History of Medicine and Public Health* (Madison: University of Wisconsin, 1997).

Numbers, Ronald (ed.), *Compulsory Health Insurance: The Continuing American Debate* (Westport, CT: Greenwood, 1982).

Numbers, Ronald, and Todd L. Savitt (eds), *Science and Medicine in the Old South* (Baton Rouge: Louisiana State University Press, 1989).

Rosenberg, Charles E., *Our Present Complaint: American Medicine, Then and Now* (Baltimore: Johns Hopkins University Press, 2007).

Starr, Paul, *The Social Transformation of American Medicine* (New York: Basic Books, 1982).

Stevens, Rosemary A., Charles E. Rosenberg, and Lawton R. Burns (eds), *History and Health Policy in the United States: Putting the Past Back In* (New Brunswick: Rutgers University Press, 2006).

Wailoo, Keith, *How Cancer Crossed the Color Line* (New York: Oxford University Press, 2011).

Warner, John Harley, and Janet A. Tighe (eds), *Major Problems in the History of American Medicine and Public Health* (Boston: Houghton Mifflin, 2001).

8

Medicine and Colonialism
in South Asia since 1500

Mark Harrison

In 1500, the region that we now know as South Asia was enjoying a period of relative stability. Although Vasco da Gama had reached the south-western coast of India two years previously it would be another decade before the Portuguese established a colonial presence in Goa. The Indian subcontinent was divided into numerous polities, none of which were especially powerful, and it was only after 1526 that it would gradually become united under the Mughal Empire—an entity that eventually controlled all but the southern tip of the subcontinent. Mughal rule added another layer to the cosmopolitan culture of South Asia but it did not alter radically the nature of medical practice there. By the time of the Mughal invasion, 'Islamic' medicine or *Unani ṭibb* had been established in parts of India for several centuries, having been introduced by Arab traders and earlier invaders from the north-west. Over time, it absorbed elements of local medical traditions, principally *Ayurveda*, which was practised largely, but not exclusively, by Hindu physicians called *vaidyas* or *vaids*. It was an ancient tradition passed on partly by word of mouth and partly through Sanskrit texts; its centre of gravity lay in the north of the subcontinent but its practitioners were widely disseminated. In parts of southern India, the dominant medical tradition—also largely a Hindu tradition—was *siddha*, a form of medicine influenced by tantrism and alchemy, which made extensive use of chemical therapies.

All these traditions viewed disease as an imbalance of bodily substances (like humours in the Western tradition), which they saw as existing in dynamic equilibrium with the environment.[1] This enabled elements of all three traditions to be blended together and patients often visited practitioners of a different ethnicity from their own. However, in the first instance, most Indians would have sought medical advice or treatment from a diverse array of local healers and wisefolk, ranging from holy men and shamanic healers to bone-setters and persons skilled in the use of medicinal plants.[2] In bazaars, practitioners also had access to a wide range of drugs, some of which came from as far afield as China and East Africa.

Over the next five centuries this medical culture began to change, albeit slowly, as the influence of European medical practitioners, traders, and governors began to be felt. As more and more of India fell under the sway of colonial rule, the pace of change accelerated as Indian traditions began to respond to the challenges posed by a different medical system. From the nineteenth century, the consolidation of the British colonial state also brought the first medical interventions in the lives of its Indian subjects: sometimes in the form of preventive medicine, sometimes through curative facilities such as hospitals and dispensaries. As exposure to Western medicine increased, many Indians began to avail themselves of opportunities to acquire knowledge of it, and by 1900, thousands were graduating in Western medicine every year. By the end of British rule in 1947, Western medicine was firmly established as the dominant form of medicine and would remain so after independence. But Indian medical traditions did not die. Most adapted to the presence of another medical system and some even began to expand overseas, following the diaspora that began under colonial rule and which has continued ever since.

These centuries of change have captured the imagination of many historians who have attempted variously to chart the histories of Indian medical traditions and assess the interventions made by the colonial powers. There is now an extensive corpus of literature on all these aspects of the subcontinent's recent medical history and the task of reviewing it is daunting. Nevertheless, this chapter attempts to sketch some of the main themes in historical scholarship, focusing particularly on those issues that have generated the most controversy. It cannot pretend to be an exhaustive survey but it may suffice to provide a flavour of the debate, some indication of where scholarship is heading, and where much remains to be done.

Rival Traditions?

The impact of colonial rule on Indian medical traditions has been the subject of considerable debate. Until recently it was assumed that the advent of formal colonial rule had had a negative, if not disastrous, impact upon Indian medical traditions. During the sixteenth and seventeenth centuries there were attempts to proscribe forms of unlicensed medical practice in Portuguese territories, for example. However, it is now generally recognized that these efforts failed; and not surprisingly, in view of the practical difficulties involved. Official attempts to constrain local practitioners were also undermined by Portuguese physicians who often sought experience with Indians before they were employed in European hospitals. Nearly all visitors agreed that Indians possessed superior knowledge of how to treat local diseases,[3] and it was for this reason that they were employed as assistants in most of the hospitals erected for the treatment of Europeans.[4]

However, respect for Indian medical knowledge ought not to be exaggerated. With the exception of some missionary scholars based in the Danish settlement of Tranquebar,[5] most Europeans had a confused idea of Indian medicine and often conflated different types of practitioner.[6] Insofar as admiration for Indian medicine existed, it lauded the therapeutic efficacy of Indian treatments rather than the principles underlying them.[7] By the early nineteenth century, even this grudging respect had largely evaporated. The Native Medical Institution, founded in Calcutta in 1822 to teach elements of both European and Indian medicine, was wound up in 1835. From that point on, the state supported institutions for the teaching of Western medicine only, the first being the Calcutta Medical College, founded in 1835. This transition is said to be symptomatic of a more general shift in opinion, away from an 'Orientalist' form of governance—in which the form and even some of the content of Indian traditions was recognized by the state—to the vigorous imposition of Western values upon Indian society.[8] Following this onslaught, it was assumed that Indian medical traditions went into a steep decline that did not begin to reverse until the devolution of political power in 1919. These reforms enabled Indians to make policy on health and medicine for the first time, albeit only at provincial levels of government.[9]

Few historians deny that the early nineteenth century saw a shift in official attitudes towards Indian medicine but the withdrawal of state funding from the Native Medical Institution did not have such a negative impact as once imagined. Rather, it appears that Indian traditions retained much of their popularity throughout the nineteenth century and underwent a period of critical self-examination that left them reinvigorated and resurgent. This renewal often took place in the context of religious revivalism and political nationalism, being stimulated only partly by the challenge posed by Western medicine.[10] The main impetus for the reform of *Unani* medicine, for example, may have emanated from a long-established Arabic tradition of scientism rather than competition with or emulation of Western practitioners.[11] Either way, *Ayurvedic* and *Unani* medicine remained important cultural forces throughout the nineteenth century and this was sometimes implicitly recognized by the state during periods of emergency, such as epidemics, when it was forced to rely on traditional practitioners to augment government services.[12]

The process by which Indian traditions of medicine adapted to the challenges and opportunities of colonial modernity has been examined in recent works by Guy Attewell and Kavita Sivaramakrishnan. Both stress the vital role of print media in the dissemination of new medical ideas, including Western notions of health and disease, which were gradually being incorporated into Indian medical traditions. Like some other scholars, they emphasize the porous nature of Indian medicine and the lack of any distinct alignment with religious belief. Many practitioners of *Ayurveda*, for example, were to be found among Sikhs as well as Hindus, while Hindus also practised *Unani ṭibb*. The patient base of these different medical traditions was equally broad and inclusive.[13] Again, both studies reinforce the emerging picture of gradual adaptation rather than radical change.

While provincial administrations began to recognize Indian medicine after 1919, and while it was supported by central government after 1947, there was no need actively to revive Indian medical traditions because they were already thriving. They had positioned themselves skilfully to take advantage of their difference from Western medicine by emphasizing their links with spiritual traditions and their advocacy of holistic as opposed to reductive treatments.[14] Yet, practitioners of traditional medicine also adopted elements from Western medicine to inspire greater confidence among patients. As a result, some *Ayurvedic* and *Unani* practitioners began to train in colleges rather than serve apprenticeships, to acquire knowledge of Western physiology and anatomy, and to treat patients in hospitals as well as in their homes. Like practitioners of Western medicine, they also began to obtain their drugs from the booming Indian pharmaceutical industry and many lost the ability to identify these plants in the wild.[15] Although Western drugs—especially those produced by Western pharmaceutical companies—were aggressively marketed in India, *Ayurvedic* medicines and other traditional preparations were mass-produced and mass-marketed too.[16] All this had begun to happen before independence from Britain, suggesting that while colonial rule affected the development of these medical traditions, it did not have a powerfully detrimental effect.

Epidemics and Colonial Politics

For much of the 1980s and 1990s, the historiography of medicine in India was dominated by the study of epidemics. At first, attention focused upon the great mortality caused by malaria and more episodically by diseases such as smallpox, cholera, and plague.[17] But later on, historians turned their attention to the political and social ramifications of epidemics, drawing their inspiration from historians of Europe and America who used them as 'windows' through which to observe societies under strain.[18] It was assumed that epidemics brought to the surface social tensions that were otherwise masked by a veneer of normality. By the mid-1980s the historiography of epidemics acquired an additional dimension as members of the Subaltern Studies collective began to take an interest in the popular protests provoked by state responses to epidemics. The original aim of the collective was similar to that of E. P. Thompson and other British social historians, in that it hoped to rescue the voice of India's downtrodden masses from the 'condescension of posterity'.[19] Up to that point, colonial historiography had been content either to criticize British rule or to record the history of India's liberation struggle. However, in doing so, attention remained firmly fixed upon the role of elites, such as leaders of the Indian National Congress. The important role of workers and peasants in the liberation struggle was largely overlooked.

Drawing on the work of the Italian Marxist Antonio Gramsci, David Arnold set out to write the history of epidemics from the viewpoint of these largely forgotten peoples. He showed how traumatic events such as the spread of cholera from its place of origin in deltaic Bengal were viewed by many peasants as symptomatic of the political chaos and dislocation caused by territorial annexation.[20] However, Arnold's chief interest was in social responses to measures devised by the colonial government to control the spread of epidemic diseases. This led him to analyse not only cholera epidemics but the day-to-day work involved in the prevention of smallpox through vaccination and, later, attempts to contain the plague epidemic that erupted in western India in 1896.[21] Arnold's work on smallpox made much of the invasive and secular character of vaccination and the fact that it was apparently rejected by many Indians on cultural grounds. His study of the response to the arrival of plague also highlighted the tendency of the authorities to ignore Indian cultural sensibilities. This was perhaps most evident in policies such as the forcible medical inspection of women, and the violation of caste and other religious taboos through enforced hospitalization and segregation. These draconian measures elicited a powerful backlash, recalling the trauma of the Indian Mutiny/Rebellion and marking the beginning of so-called 'extremist' nationalism.

Although Arnold examined the responses of the colonial state and the role played by nationalist politicians, he emphasized the spontaneous nature of much popular protest: the mass flight from cities such as Bombay, the strikes of mill-hands and factory workers, and attacks on hospitals and government officials. In doing so, he made use of both official reports—reading them 'against the grain' in an attempt to weed out colonial bias—and vernacular newspapers, accessible in translated extracts in reports on the 'native press'. However, these sources rarely provide the historian with the authentic voice of subaltern protest; after all, most peasants and factory workers were illiterate and unable even to write their name. More importantly, perhaps, they do not allow us to generalize about the nature of 'Indian' responses to epidemic disease. As Raj Chandavarkar pointed out in a perceptive essay on plague panics in India, there was no unified or homogeneous response to either the disease or the measures designed to contain it.[22] He argued that the popular backlash provoked by plague measures had less to do with the state impinging upon 'popular culture' than with the peculiar political and economic circumstances surrounding the epidemic. Resistance to measures such as hospitalization was not simply a function of caste or other religious sensibilities but reflected the fact that Indians, like many Western peoples, preferred to remain with their families and that they were suspicious of the intentions of medical practitioners.

Epidemics are rarely unified events and various communities experience them differently. This is true in any society but especially, perhaps, in a vast, predominantly rural country like British India. Nor do epidemics necessarily tell us much about the nature of social relations. They are, by definition, atypical events and may give a misleading impression of the degree of hostility towards the state or Western medicine. Unfortunately, we still lack the *longue durée* histories that might enable us to draw reliable conclusions about attitudes to state medicine and outbreaks of epidemic disease. We simply do not know how Indian communities adjusted to the endemic or frequent epidemic presence of cholera or plague, for example. This is not a problem unique to the historiography of South Asia, however. It is perhaps unrealistic to expect a major monograph on the history of cholera in British India when none exists for Great Britain itself, at least beyond the first epidemic of 1831–2.

But the historiography of epidemics has not perished altogether. Although there is no grand history of cholera or plague in the making, there is growing interest in the relationship between epidemics and religious pilgrimages: both Hindu pilgrimages within India and the annual pilgrimage of Muslims to Mecca and Medina. These were intensely problematic issues for the colonial state but it was forced to grapple with them under the spotlight of international concern. The International Sanitary Conference convened at Constantinople in 1866 established India as the source of the cholera pandemics that had recently afflicted Europe and much of the rest of the world.[23] The immediate cause of the 1865–6 pandemic was an outbreak of cholera in Mecca, which was widely attributed to pilgrims from India. However, large gatherings of pilgrims at religious fairs in India, such as the *melas* held at Hardwar and other sacred sites on the River Ganges, were also seen as hubs from which cholera radiated throughout India. As such, there was an expectation that the British government would take measures to reduce the likelihood of epidemics, including the improvement of sanitation at pilgrimage sites and, if necessary, the proscription of pilgrimage altogether. However, intervention in such a sensitive area carried great risks and the colonial authorities, centrally and locally, aimed to strike a balance between appeasing international opinion and maintaining social order.[24] Arrangements for the sanitary regulation of pilgrimage inevitably produced a great deal of friction; nevertheless, it appears that sanitary measures at such gatherings led gradually to the acceptance of Western notions of hygiene.[25]

After 1866, the way in which the British authorities dealt with epidemic disease was scrutinized internationally and other countries took measures to reduce the risk of infection from India. The quarantines imposed by European countries and international boards of health at Constantinople and Alexandria are therefore of great interest to historians who wish to view British India in the wider context of international politics. Most agree on the vital importance of quarantine in Anglo-Indian medical policy and that the state did its best to minimize disruption of trade and communication with the rest of the world. It is also agreed that official medical doctrine in India reflected this overriding consideration, maintaining that cholera was rarely, if ever, a contagious disease. However, while most studies emphasize the determination of the Government of India to remove or reduce quarantine,[26] Sheldon Watts claims that it did so largely at the behest of the government in London. In his view, London was determined to see the removal or relaxation of quarantine at all costs.[27] However, recent work confirms that the Anglo-Indian government had an agenda in Central and Southern Asia that was sometimes at odds with that of the home government, and that this manifested itself clearly in debates over quarantine.[28]

Sanitary Reform: A Lost Opportunity?

The dominance of quarantine in official deliberations sometimes overshadowed the more mundane aspects of public health policy. However, in the mid-Victorian period, sanitary reform was becoming more important, being regarded as the touchstone of an enlightened and civilized state. Many British medical officers and civil servants therefore believed that it was their duty to bestow the benefits of sanitation upon the population of India, seeking to replicate the process of reform in Britain itself. By the end of the century, it was widely assumed that imperial rule meant sanitary progress, and so the official narrative stood for the remainder of British rule.[29] But supporters of the liberation struggle often took a different view. While some progress was acknowledged, it was held that the vast majority of the Indian population, particularly in rural areas, obtained few medical or sanitary benefits from British rule.[30] After 1947, it also became clear that many of the grandiose claims made about the Empire's sanitary achievements were unsupportable.[31]

Historians differ in their explanations of these generally accepted limitations. In one of the first major interventions of the post-independence period, Hugh Tinker asserted that sanitary reform flourished only in those areas where effective control of public health remained in British hands. Starting with the transfer of power to elected municipalities in the 1870s, devolution, in his view, had generally been disastrous for public health because most Indian politicians took little interest in such matters.[32] At the opposite extreme are those who support Radhika Ramasubban's contention that sanitary improvement was confined only to small enclaves of the colonial state and that the British 'lost the historic opportunity for initiating sanitary reform'. In her view, they were not simply indifferent to the health of the Indian population but actively scuttled all initiatives put forward by Indians.[33] This position has subsequently been endorsed by many scholars, among them David Arnold and Anil Kumar.[34] Arnold, for example, blames the Government of India for devolving responsibility for day-to-day sanitary work on municipal authorities that were poorly financed and inexperienced.[35] Other historians have also pointed to the weakness of newly formed municipalities such as those in the jute-manufacturing towns of Bengal.[36]

It is generally acknowledged that colonial health policy privileged the needs of Europeans and key sectors of Indian society—such as the army—upon which the state depended for its security. However, some historians believe that it is impossible to account for the limitations of public health solely by reference to the priorities of the colonial government. Roger Jeffery, for example, has pointed to the difficulties of implementing sanitary improvements in a vast country with limited resources. He remains unconvinced that there was 'any conceivable

alternative' to the policies developed under British rule.[37] The funding of sanitary reform depended to some extent on different systems of
taxation. Local authorities in parts of India such as the North West
Provinces and Oudh (present-day Uttar Pradesh), which raised revenue using trade taxes (*octroi*), were particularly vulnerable to fluctu-
ating economic conditions and tended to have significantly lower
levels of public health funding than provinces, such as Bengal, which
depended mainly on property taxes.[38] The narrow, property-owning
franchise in Indian municipalities also meant that landed interests
often acted as a drag on sanitary reform.[39]

But by which criteria ought colonial public health measures to be
judged? It is all very well to write of the limitations of colonial health
policy but is there a 'normal' process of modernization against which
developments in India can be judged? Can we criticize the colonial
administration for devolving much of the responsibility for public
health to local governments when the same bodies—rather than
central government—bore the responsibility for public health in
Britain? There was certainly much debate in both official and nationalist circles about the relative balance of responsibilities between
local, provincial, and central government. However, until the emergence of socialized health care in the Soviet Union, very few people
advocated State involvement in public health of the kind envisaged by
Ramasubban. Indeed, attitudes towards State intervention in public
health shifted markedly over time but not necessarily in the same
direction. As colonial rule drew to a close, the State began to fracture
in ways that meant that responsibility was shared more widely than
previously. As the case of smallpox vaccination shows, it was spread
across a variety of agencies from central government down to local
and district boards, in the middle of which were the new provincial
health departments, some of which were headed by Indians after
1919. Although alliances were often formed between different agencies at times of crisis, they tended to work against each other in a way
that compounded some of the scientific and technical problems that
reduced the effectiveness of vaccination.[40] As Sanjoy Bhattacharya
has argued, these complex structures and the tensions they engendered persisted well beyond 1947. The impetus behind the vaccination programme increased with the involvement of the World
Health Organization from the 1960s, but the disjointed nature of

public health intervention remained until the disease was eradicated from India in 1975.[41]

The measures taken against smallpox reveal the difficulty of reconciling contrary tendencies in South Asia's transition to modernity. The desire for devolution complicated the response to a problem for which there appeared to be a technical solution. But in the case of malaria—the greatest cause of mortality in South Asia year on year—it became increasingly evident that there was no simple technical fix. Although the discovery of the mosquito vector of malaria parasites raised great hopes at the beginning of the twentieth century, experiments with mosquito control in even limited areas proved disappointing.[42] The same was true of prophylaxis with quinine, although it proved valuable in the treatment of malaria. According to some historians, the blame for the failure of malaria control rests firmly with the colonial government. Malaria ranked low on the government's list of priorities: unlike plague or cholera, it did not stir civil unrest or compromise trade and communications with the rest of the world. Above all, perhaps, any effective response to the problem was negated by the huge cost entailed by measures such as drainage and the fact that they were likely to conflict with other priorities such as irrigation for agricultural development.[43]

Most historians acknowledge the limited progress made during the period of British rule,[44] but in the absence of any detailed, large-scale study of malaria in British India we ought to be wary of generalization. Even the first half of the twentieth century, which has formed the subject of most studies of malaria in South Asia, is thinly covered. We currently lack studies of epidemic areas such as Sindh, for example, and while excellent work has been done examining the links between malaria epidemics, famine, and irrigation,[45] we need more detailed research on the relationship between malaria and agricultural development. The political aspects of the problem have also been largely ignored, except insofar as they were bound up with the international health movement from the 1930s.[46] Further work on anti-malaria policies is required before we will be able to evaluate the government's response to the problem of malaria or its role in aggravating it.

The case of malaria reminds us of how much basic work remains to be done on the history of public health in India. Indeed, colonial health policies have often been considered without regard to their impact on mortality or morbidity. In the 1970s and 1980s, Ira Klein, Tim Dyson, and others began to analyse mortality trends in British India but few historians have taken their work further.[47] Judith Richell's detailed study of disease and demography in Burma is one of the few exceptions.[48] She concludes that public health made little impact upon mortality, an observation borne out by a recent study of smallpox vaccination in the province, which shows that the practical difficulties of implementing vaccination in Burma far exceeded those encountered in the presidencies of British India.[49] This raises the question of how far Richell's conclusions apply to other provinces where mortality began to decline in the 1920s. In a chapter devoted to the subject in a recent monograph, the historian Sumit Guha has argued that India's 'mortality transition' was due primarily to better weather conditions. In his view, climatic stability enabled the Indian population to maintain a 'moderate' level of malnutrition, whereas the more unstable weather patterns of previous decades had resulted in severe famines.[50] He claims that the oscillation between adequate nutrition and severe malnutrition was a major factor in the severe mortality crises of the later nineteenth century.[51] Other recent studies also attribute mortality decline, in part, to better nutrition,[52] but cannot be regarded as conclusive. Indeed, if the persistent debate over mortality decline in Western countries is anything to go by the controversy over what happened in India has only just begun.

Some aspects of India's epidemiological history have scarcely been examined at all, particularly certain chronic diseases that became significant causes of death in the course of the twentieth century. From the turn of the century, crusading public health workers began to highlight the growing problem of respiratory diseases in Indian towns, particularly among textile mill workers.[53] Neither the epidemiological nor the political ramifications of tuberculosis and other respiratory diseases have been examined in detail, nor have other diseases hitherto regarded as confined to Western civilization. David Arnold's recent study of diabetes stands as a notable exception,[54] but we need similar studies of cancer, for example, which became increasingly prominent in epidemiological studies from the 1940s.[55]

Controlling Bodies and Minds

Since the late 1980s many historians have commented on medicine's use as a tool of social control and its hegemonic role in establishing the dominance of Western culture. David Arnold can reasonably be said to have inaugurated this trend, blending together insights from Foucault and Gramsci.[56] Since then, scholarship has highlighted the medical elements within racial theories, for example,[57] and the role of medical institutions in expressing and consolidating colonial power. But institutions such as leprosy colonies and lunatic asylums arguably did little to cement colonial rule. While there was a growing desire to confine 'lepers' from the 1890s, in most parts of India (Orissa excepted) relatively few people were incarcerated in leprosaria.[58] Lunatic asylums also aimed to incarcerate disruptive elements but the numbers involved were again negligible.[59] Nor were these institutions particularly successful in moulding their inmates to fit colonial expectations of civilized life. Disciplinary regimes, dietaries, and treatments often had to be negotiated with inmates, forcing concessions from the authorities.[60] Indeed, colonial authority was often diluted by the fact that many of these institutions were run on a day-to-day basis by Indian staff with agendas very different from those of their British superiors.[61] Medical authority was imposed with rather more success in India's jails, however. From the 1830s, jails were increasingly subject to medical regulation as part of a broader programme of prison reform and in response to the staggering death rate among inmates. Indeed, jails offered tremendous scope for clinical experimentation and trials with new vaccines, trials that contributed substantially to the legitimacy of key medical technologies such as inoculation against plague.[62]

One medical institution that stands out from all the others is the so-called 'lock hospital', the sole purpose of which was to cure women suspected of having 'venereal diseases'. These 'hospitals' were established in or adjacent to military cantonments from the late eighteenth century, the aim being to reduce the likelihood that soldiers would be infected and thus rendered unfit for duty. It would appear that the Indian lock hospitals were among the first of their kind and that they established a precedent later built upon in Britain, with the passage of the controversial Contagious Diseases Acts in the 1860s. Similar legislation was passed in India shortly afterwards, placing on a firmer foundation the measures that had existed on and off in cantonments for many decades. The Acts were repealed in the 1880s following protests from women's groups and Christians offended by state-sanctioned immorality, but in India the use of lock hospitals continued under the guise of other legislation, marking a continuity of attitudes and approaches throughout the period of British rule.[63] The impact of the Contagious Diseases Acts in the Indian context is open to question, however. Some claim that the Acts bore lightly on the communities they affected and were not especially oppressive,[64] while others stress the opportunities that the Acts presented to subordinate staff for extortion and bribery.[65]

Either way, lock hospitals were untypical of British medical institutions, even custodial ones, in that most hospitals were intended to reach out to Indian communities in a way that demonstrated the benevolence of colonial rulers. Hospitals and dispensaries for the poor (attended predominantly by untouchables and Indian Christians) were said to highlight the apparent indifference of Indian elites by contrast with the humane ethos of a Christian power. The same was true of hospitals for women. A 'lying-in' or maternity hospital was established in Madras in the 1840s and quickly became a model of its kind, contrasting with the harshness with which Hindu women (particularly widows) were treated by their own communities.[66] Together with the growth of municipal and company-owned dispensaries from the 1830s, such institutions were part of a concerted effort to 'civilize' the Indian people. Their foundation coincided with public health initiatives that had a similar aim, notably the extension of vaccination against smallpox.[67] Medicine can thus be said to have a played a major role in a new vision of colonialism that evolved in the final years of Company rule, and which expanded massively with the transfer of government to the Crown in 1858.

By the mid-nineteenth century, it is clear that many prominent Indians were also beginning to see hospitals and dispensaries as a way of enhancing their position within their communities. Detailed work has only just begun on the establishment and running of philanthropic hospitals like the Jamsetji Jeejeebhoy Hospital in Bombay, but it is already clear that the number of such institutions and the growing popularity of hospitals for particular religious and caste groups should lead us to question some of the more sweeping, pessimistic assertions formerly made about Indian cultural resistance to Western medicine.

Like any other people, Indians responded to the opportunities provided by hospitals in a balanced and rational manner, weighing up their merits and defects. Although suspicion of hospitals often increased at times of excitement, such as during epidemics, the overall trend was towards a growth in hospital use, though less among women than men. At first, Indians tended to be selective about which services they used. There was a marked preference for some surgical techniques, like cataract removal, and for certain therapies—such as quinine treatment for malaria—which had widely acknowledged benefits. However, in time, demand for all kinds of services spread within the context of an increasingly diverse and pluralistic medical marketplace. By the twentieth century, demand for hospital care was outstripping supply. State funding was never adequate to finance an effective hospital system, even in large urban areas such as Delhi, while Indian and European philanthropic efforts were unable to fill the gap.[68] From 1910, the Government of India admitted that it would be unable to provide medical care for the majority of the Indian people, particularly in rural areas, and pinned its hopes on training more Indians in Western medicine. This meant ceding more power to Indian doctors in those hospitals that had been established, and from the 1920s, Indian practitioners lobbied successfully to become consultants.[69]

The rise of Indian-influenced hospital medicine is a story that has yet to be told; we also have very few accounts of medical practice and health care in rural areas, the only real exception being studies of missionary medicine. Missionaries employed medical care as a means of winning the trust of Indians in the hope that they would eventually convert to Christianity. Mission clinics were seldom successful in achieving their ultimate goal of conversion but in many remote areas, such as the tribal regions of India, and in locations such as the North West Frontier, they were often the only Western medical institutions and performed an important role, especially in cataract surgery and dispensing drugs.[70] Private or semi-private initiatives to provide medical care for women, through missionary clinics and such bodies as the semi-official Dufferin Fund, established by the wife of the viceroy in 1888, also had some localized success among Christian and low-caste women. However, they found it hard to persuade high-caste Hindus and Muslims to allow their women to enter Western establishments, even if staffed entirely by female doctors, midwives, and nurses.[71]

Conclusion

Missionary medicine, state medicine, and Indian medical traditions have all attracted considerable interest among historians of South Asia. It has been impossible to do justice to the numerous works on these subjects in a single chapter but this essay may provide a guide to readers approaching the subject of medicine in South Asia for the first time. It has mapped the contours of existing scholarship and identified some of the main themes and issues that have animated it. It has also pointed to important lacunae that remain to be filled. Would-be students of South Asian medicine and health care will find much in the primary sources that eludes them here and, if nothing else, the silences in this chapter may serve to indicate the vast opportunities that await any scholar willing to take up the challenge.

Notes

1 Francis Zimmerman, *The Jungle and the Aroma of Meats: An Ecological Theme in Hindu Medicine* (Berkeley: University of California Press, 1987).

2 Being oral cultures, most of these are lost to the historian, except through occasional references in some European texts. Some impression of these may be obtained from Sudhir Kakar, *Shamans, Mystics and Doctors: A Psychological Inquiry into India and its Healing Traditions* (New Delhi: Oxford University Press, 1982).

3 M. N. Pearson, 'First Contacts between Indian and European Medical Systems: Goa in the Sixteenth Century', in D. Arnold (ed.), *Warm Climates and Western Medicine* (Amsterdam: Rodopi, 1996), 20–41; M. N. Pearson, 'The Thin End of the Wedge: Medical Relativities as a Paradigm of Early Modern Indian-European Relations', *Modern Asian Studies*, 29 (1995), 141–70.

4 Pratik Chakrabarti, '"Neither of meate nor drinke, but what the Doctor alloweth": Medicine amidst War and Commerce in Eighteenth-Century Madras', *Bulletin of the History of Medicine*, 80 (2006), 1–38; Pratik Chakrabarti, 'Medical Marketplaces beyond the West: Bazaar Medicine, Trade and the English Establishment in Eighteenth-Century India', in P. Wallis and M. Jenner (eds), *Medicine and the Market in Early Modern England* (London: Palgrave, 2007), 196–215.

5 C. S. Mohanavelu, *German Tamilology: German Contributions to Tamil Language, Literature and Culture during the Period 1706–1945* (Madras: South India Saiva Siddhanta Works Publishing Society, 1993).

6 Dominick Wujastyk, 'Change and Continuity in Early Modern Indian Medical Thought', *Journal of Indian Philosophy*, 33 (2005), 95–118.

7 Mark Harrison, 'Medicine and Orientalism: Perspectives on Europe's Encounter with Indian Medical Systems', in B. Pati and M. Harrison (eds), *Health, Medicine and Empire: Perspectives on Colonial India* (Hyderabad: Orient Longman, 2001), 37–87.

8 Poonam Bala, *Imperialism and Medicine in Bengal* (New Delhi: Sage, 1991); Anil Kumar, *Medicine and the Raj: British Medical Policy in India 1835–1911* (New Delhi: Sage, 1998), 17–22.

9 Kumar, *Medicine and the Raj*, 22.

10 B. D. Metcalfe, 'Nationalist Muslims in British India: The Case of Hakim Ajmal Khan', *Modern Asian Studies*, 19 (1985), 1–28; K. N. Panikkar, *Culture, Ideology, Hegemony: Intellectuals and Social Consciousness in Colonial India* (New Delhi: Tulika, 1995), 145–75; Neshat Quaiser, 'Politics, Culture and Colonialism: Unani's Debate with Doctory', in Pati and Harrison (eds), *Health, Medicine and Empire*, 317–55.

11 Seema Alavi, *Islam and Healing: Loss and Recovery of an Indo-Muslim Medical Tradition* (Basingstoke: Palgrave, 2008).

12 J. C. Hume, 'Rival Traditions: Western Medicine and Yunani-Tibb in the Punjab, 1849–1899', *Bulletin of the History of Medicine*, 51 (1977), 214–31.

13 Guy Attewell, *Refiguring Unani Tibb: Plural Healing in Late Colonial India* (Hyderabad: Orient Longman, 2007); Kavita Sivaramakrishnan, *Old Potions, New Bottles: Recasting Indigenous Medicine in Colonial Punjab 1850–1945* (Hyderabad: Orient Longman, 2006).

14 Jean M. Langford, *Fluent Bodies: Ayurvedic Remedies for Postcolonial Imbalance* (Durham, NC: Duke University Press, 2002).

15 Projit Bihari Mukharji, 'Medicine and Modernity in Colonial Bengal, c.1775–1930', PhD thesis, University of London, 2006; Poonam Bala, ' "Defying" Medical Autonomy: Indigenous Elites and Medicine in Colonial India', in P. Bala (ed.), *Biomedicine as a Contested Site* (Lanham: Lexington Books, 2009), 29–44.

16 Madhuri Sharma, 'Western Medicine and Indian Responses: A Case Study of Banaras Region, c.1890–1947', PhD thesis, Jawaharlal Nehru University, 2007.

17 Ira Klein, 'Urban Development and Death: Bombay City, 1870–1914', *Modern Asian Studies*, 20 (1986), 725–54.

18 Ian Catanach, 'Plague and the Indian Village, 1896–1914', in P. Robb (ed.), *Rural India: Land, Power and Society under British Rule* (London: Curzon Press, 1983), 216–43; *idem*, 'Poona Politicians and the Plague', *South Asia*, 7 (1984), 1–18; *idem*, 'Plague and the Tensions of Empire: India, 1896–1918', in D. Arnold (ed.), *Imperial Medicine and Indigenous Societies* (Manchester: Manchester University Press, 1988), 149–71; Ira Klein, 'Plague, Policy and Popular Unrest in British India', *Modern Asian Studies*, 22 (1988), 723–55.

19 Ranajit Guha, 'On Some Aspects of the Historiography of Colonial India', in R. Guha (ed.), *Subaltern Studies I: Writings on South Asian History and Society* (Delhi: Oxford University Press, 1982), 1–8.

20 David Arnold, 'Cholera and Colonialism in British India', *Past and Present*, 113 (1986), 118–51.

21 David Arnold, 'Smallpox and Colonial Medicine in Nineteenth-Century India', in *idem* (ed.), *Imperial Medicine*, 45–65; *idem*, 'Touching the Body: Perspectives on the India Plague, 1896–1900', in R. Guha (ed.), *Subaltern Studies V: Writings on South Asian History and Society* (Delhi: Oxford University Press, 1987), 55–90; *idem Colonizing the Body: State Medicine and Epidemic Disease in Nineteenth-Century India* (Berkeley: University of California Press, 1993).

22 Rajnarayan Chandavarkar, 'Plague Panic and Epidemic Politics in India, 1896–1914', in T. Ranger and P. Slack (eds), *Epidemics and Ideas: Essays on the Historical Perception of Pestilence* (Cambridge: Cambridge University Press, 1994), 203–40.

23 Valeska Huber, 'The Unification of the Globe by Disease? The International Sanitary Conferences on Cholera, 1851–1894', *The Historical Journal*, 49 (2006), 453–76.

24 Mark Harrison, 'Quarantine, Pilgrimage, and Colonial Trade: India 1866–1900', *Indian Economic and Social History Review*, 29 (1992), 117–44; Manjiri Kamat, '"The Palkhi as Plague Carrier": The Pandharpur Fair and the Sanitary Fixation of the Colonial State; British India, 1908–1916', in B. Pati and M. Harrison (eds), *Health, Medicine and Empire: Perspectives on Colonial India* (Hyderabad: Orient Longman, 2001), 299–316; Biswamoy Pati, '"Ordering" "Disorder" in a Holy City: Colonial Health Interventions in Puri during the Nineteenth Century', in Pati and Harrison (eds), *Health, Medicine and Empire*, 270–98; Amna Khalid, '"Subordinate" Negotiations: Indigenous Staff, the Colonial State and Public', and Saurabh Mishra, 'Beyond the Bounds of Time? The Haj Pilgrimage from the Indian Subcontinent, 1865–1920', in B. Pati and M. Harrison (eds), *The Social History of Health and Medicine in Colonial India* (London: Routledge, 2008), 31–44, 45–73.

25 Amna Khalid, 'The Colonial Behemoth: The Sanitary Regulation of Pilgrimage Sites in Northern India, c.1867–1915', DPhil thesis, University of Oxford, 2008; Saurabh Mishra, 'Pilgrimage, Politics and Pestilence: The Haj from the Indian Subcontinent, 1860–1920', DPhil thesis, University of Oxford, 2008.

26 Harrison, 'Quarantine, Pilgrimage and Colonial Trade'.

27 Sheldon Watts, 'From Rapid Change to Stasis: Official Responses to Cholera in British-Ruled India and Egypt: 1860 to c.1921', *Journal of World History*, 12 (2001), 321–74.

28 Sanchari Dutta, 'Plague, Quarantine and Empire: British-Indian Sanitary Strategies in Central Asia, 1897–1907', in Pati and Harrison (eds), *The Social History of Health and Medicine*, 93–112.

29 Ronald Ross, *Memoirs* (London: Murray, 1923), 17.

30 R. Palme Dutt, *India Today* (London: Gollancz, 1940), 79.

31 J. B. Harrison, 'Allahabad: A Sanitary History', in K. Ballhatchet and J. B. Harrison (eds), *The City in South Asia* (London: Curzon Press, 1980), 167–96.

32 H. R. Tinker, *The Foundations of Local Self-Government in India, Pakistan and Burma* (London: Pall Mall Press, 1954), 73.

33 Radhika Ramasubban, *Public Health and Medical Research in India: Their Origins and Development under the Impact of British Colonial Policy* (Stockholm: SAREC, 1982); Radhika Ramasubban, 'Imperial Health in British India, 1857–1900', in R. MacLeod and M. Lewis (eds), *Disease, Medicine, and Empire: Perspectives on Western India and the Experience of European Expansion* (London: Routledge, 1988), 38–60.

34 Kumar, *Medicine and the Raj*; Kabita Ray, *History of Public Health: Colonial Bengal 1921–1947* (Calcutta: K. P. Bagchi and Sons, 1998); J. C. Hume, 'Colonialism and Sanitary Medicine: The Development of Preventive Health Policy in the Punjab, 1860–1900', *Modern Asian Studies*, 20 (1986), 703–24.

35 David Arnold, 'Medical Priorities and Practice in Nineteenth-Century British India', *South Asia Research*, 5 (1985), 167–83.

36 Subho Basu, 'Emergence of the Mill Towns in Bengal 1880–1920: Migration Pattern and Survival Strategies of Industrial Workers', *Calcutta Historical Review*, 18 (1995), 97–134.

37 Roger Jeffery, *The Politics of Health in India* (Berkeley: University of California Press, 1988), 92.

38 Mark Harrison, *Public Health in British India: Anglo-Indian Preventive Medicine 1859–1914* (Cambridge: Cambridge University Press, 1994), 176–7.

39 Sandip Hazareesingh, *The Colonial City and the Challenge of Modernity: Urban Hegemonies and Civic Contestations in Bombay (1900–1925)* (Hyderabad: Orient Longman, 2007); Mridula Ramanna, *Western Medicine and Public Health in Colonial Bombay 1845–1895* (Hyderabad: Orient Longman, 2002); Mridula Ramanna, 'Randchodlal Chotalal: Pioneer of Public Health in Ahmedabad', *Radical Journal of Health*, 11 (1996), 99–111; V. R. Muraleedharan and D. Veeraraghavan, 'Disease, Death and Local Administration: Madras City in early 1900s', *Radical Journal of Health*, 1 (1995), 9–24.

40 Sanjoy Bhattacharya, Mark Harrison, and Michael Worboys, *Fractured States: Smallpox, Public Health and Vaccination Policy 1800–1947* (Hyderabad: Orient Longman, 2005).

41 Sanjoy Bhattacharya, *Expunging Variola: The Control and Eradication of Smallpox in India 1947–1977* (Hyderabad: Orient Longman, 2006).

42 W. F. Bynum, 'An Experiment that Failed: Malaria Control at Mian Mir', *Parassitologia*, 36 (1994), 107–20.

43 Sheldon Watts, 'British Development Policies and Malaria in India 1897–c.1929', *Past and Present*, 165 (1999), 141–81.

44 V. R. Muraleedharan, 'Malady in Madras: The Colonial Government's Response to Malaria in the Early Twentieth Century', in D. Kumar (ed.), *Science and Empire: Essays in Indian Context (1700–1947)* (New Delhi: Oxford University Press, 1991), 101–14; V. R. Muraleedharan, 'Rural Health Care in Madras Presidency: 1919–39', *Indian Economic and Social History Review*, 24 (1987), 324–34.

45 M. B. McAlpin, 'Famines, Epidemics and Population Growth: The Case of India', in R. I. Rotberg and T. K. Rabb (eds), *Hunger and History: The Impact of Changing Food Production and Consumption Patterns on Society* (Cambridge: Cambridge University Press, 1985), 153–68; Simon Commander, 'The Mechanics of Demographic and Economic Growth in Uttar Pradesh, 1800–1900', in T. Dyson (ed.), *India's Historical Demography: Studies in Famine, Disease and Society* (London: Curzon Press, 1989), 49–72; S. Zurbrigg, 'Re-thinking the Human Factor in Malaria Mortality: The Case of Punjab, 1868–1940', *Parassitalogia*, 36 (1994), 121–35; Elizabeth Whitcombe, 'Famine Mortality', *Economic and Political Weekly*, 28 (1993), 1169–79; Elizabeth Whitcombe, 'The Costs of Irrigation: Waterlogging, Salinity and Malaria', in D. Arnold and R. Guha (eds), *Essays on the Environmental History of South Asia* (New Delhi: Oxford University Press, 1995), 257–59; Kohei Wakimura, 'Famines, Epidemics and Mortality in Northern India', in P. Robb, K. Sugihara, and H. Yanagisawa (eds), *Local Agrarian Societies in Colonial India: Japanese Perspectives* (London: Curzon Press, 1996), 280–310.

46 Sunil S. Amrith, *Decolonizing International Health: India and Southeast Asia, 1930–65* (London: Palgrave, 2006).

47 Ira Klein, 'Death in India, 1871–1921', *Journal of Asian Studies*, 22 (1973), 639–59; T. Dyson (ed.), *India's Historical Demography: Studies in Famine, Disease and Society* (London: Curzon Press, 1989).

48 Judith L. Richell, *Disease and Demography in Colonial Burma* (Singapore: NUS Press, 2006).

49 Atsuko Naono, *State of Vaccination: The Fight against Smallpox in Colonial Burma* (Hyderabad: Orient Blackswan, 2009).

50 Sumit Guha, *Health and Population in South Asia from Earliest Times to the Present* (London: Hurst, 2001), 68–94.

51 Mike David, *Late Victorian Holocausts: El Niño Famines and the Making of the Third World* (London: Verso, 2001).

52 Sheila Zurbrigg, 'Re-thinking Public Health: Food, Hunger, and Mortality Decline in South Asian History', in I. Qadeer, K. Sen, and K. R. Nayar (eds), *Public Health and the Poverty of Reforms: The South Asian Predicament* (Delhi: Sage, 2001), 174–97.

53 Mark Harrison and Michael Worboys, 'A Disease of Civilisation: Tuberculosis in Britain, Africa and India, 1900–39', in L. Marks and M. Worboys (eds), *Migrants, Minorities and Health: Historical and Contemporary Studies* (London: Routledge, 1997), 93–124.

54 David Arnold, 'Diabetes in the Tropics: Race, Place and Class in India, 1880–1965', *Social History of Medicine*, 22 (2009), 245–62.

55 R. Doll, P. Page, J. A. Waterhouse and D. M. Parkin, *Cancer in Five Continents* (Geneva: International Union Against Cancer, 1966).

56 Arnold, *Colonizing the Body*.

57 Mark Harrison, *Climates and Constitutions: Health, Race, Environment and British Imperialism in India, 1600–1850* (Delhi: Oxford University Press, 1999).

58 Sanjiv Kakar, 'Leprosy in Colonial India, 1860–1940: Colonial Politics and Missionary Medicine', *Medical History*, 40 (1996), 215–30; Biswamoy

Pati and Chandi P. Nanda, 'The Leprosy Patient and Society: Colonial Orissa, 1870s–1940s', in Pati and Harrison (eds), *The Social History of Health and Medicine*, 113–28.

59 Waltraud Ernst, *Mad Tales from the Raj: The European Insane in British India, 1800–1858* (London: Routledge, 1991); *eadem*, 'Colonial Policies, Racial Politics and the Development of Psychiatric Institutions in Early Nineteenth-Century British India', in W. Ernst and B. Harris (eds), *Race, Science and Medicine, 1700–1960* (London: Routledge, 1999), 80–100.

60 Jane Buckingham, *Leprosy in Colonial South India: Medicine and Conflict* (Basingstoke: Palgrave, 2002); Sanjiv Kakar, 'Medical Developments and Patient Unrest in the Leprosy Asylum', in Pati and Harrison (eds), *Health, Medicine and Empire*, 188–216.

61 James Mills, *Madness, Cannabis and Colonialism: The 'Native-Only' Lunatic Asylums of British India, 1857–1900* (London: Macmillan, 2000).

62 Sanchari Dutta, 'Disease, Medicine and Hygiene in the Prisons of British India: Bengal, 1860–1910', DPhil thesis, University of Oxford, 2007.

63 Philippa Levine, *Prostitution, Race and Politics: Policing Venereal Disease in the British Empire* (London: Routledge, 2003); Kenneth Ballhatchet, *Race, Sex and Class under the British Raj: Imperial Attitudes and Policies and their Critics, 1793–1905* (London: Weidenfeld and Nicholson, 1980); Douglas M. Peers, 'Soldiers, Surgeons and the Campaigns to Combat Sexually Transmitted Diseases in Colonial India, 1805–1860', *Medical History*, 42 (1998), 823–54.

64 Ronald Hyam, *Empire and Sexuality: The British Experience* (Manchester: Manchester University Press, 1991).

65 Erica Wald, 'Vice, Medicine, the Military and the Making of Colonial India, 1780–1880', PhD thesis, University of Cambridge, 2009; Levine, *Prostitution*, Chapters 3–4; Harrison, *Public Health*, 74–6.

66 Sean F. Lang, 'Maternal Mortality and the State in British India, c.1840–c.1920', PhD thesis, Anglia Ruskin University, 2007.

67 Nils Brimnes, 'Variolation, Vaccination and Popular Resistance in Early Colonial South India', *Medical History*, 48 (2004), 199–228; Bhattacharya, Harrison, and Worboys, *Fractured States*, Chapter 1; Arnold, 'Smallpox and Colonial Medicine'.

68 Samiksha Sehrawat, 'Medical Care for a New Capital: Hospital and Government Policy in Colonial Delhi and Haryana, c.1900–1920', DPhil thesis, University of Oxford, 2006.

69 Mark Harrison, 'Introduction', in M. Harrison, M. Jones, and H. Sweet (eds), *From Western Medicine to Global Medicine: The Hospital beyond the West* (Hyderabad: Orient Blackswan, 2009).

70 David Hardiman, *Missionaries and Their Medicine: A Christian Modernity for Tribal India* (Manchester: Manchester University Press, 2008).

71 Maneesha Lal, 'The Politics of Gender and Medicine in Colonial India: The Countess of Dufferin's Fund, 1885–1888', *Bulletin of the History of Medicine*, 68 (1994), 29–66.

Select Bibliography

Arnold, David, *Colonizing the Body: State Medicine and Epidemic Disease in Nineteenth-Century India* (Berkeley: University of California Press, 1993).

Attewell, Guy, *Refiguring Unani Tibb: Plural Healing in Late Colonial India* (New Delhi: Orient Longman, 2007).

Bhattacharya, Sanjoy, Mark Harrison, and Michael Worboys, *Fractured States: Smallpox, Public Health and Vaccination Policy in British India, 1800–1947* (Hyderabad: Orient Longman, 2005).

Dyson, T. (ed.), *India's Historical Demography: Studies in Famine, Disease and Society* (London: Curzon Press, 1989).

Hardiman, David and Mukharji, Proji Bihari (eds.), *Medical Marginaility in South Asia: Situating Subaltern Therapetuics* (London: Routledge, 2012).

Harrison, Mark, *Public Health in British India: Anglo-Indian Preventive Medicine 1859–1914* (Cambridge: Cambridge University Press, 1994).

Hodges, Sarah (ed.), *Reproductive Health in India: History, Politics and Controversies* (New Delhi: Orient Longman, 2006).

Kumar, Deepak and Basu, Raj Sekhar (eds.), *Medical Encounters in British India* (New Delhi: Oxford University Press, 2013).

Mills, James, *Madness, Cannabis and Colonialism; The 'Native Only' Lunatic Asylums of British India, 1857–1900* (London: MacMillan, 2000).

Mukharji, Projit, *Doctoring Traditions: Ayurveda, Small Technologies, and Braided Sciences* (Chicago: Chicago University Press, 2016).

Pati, Biswamoy, and Mark Harrison (eds), *Health, Medicine and Empire: Perspectives on Colonial India* (Hyderabad: Orient Longman, 2001).

Pati, Biswamoy, and Mark Harrison (eds), *The Social History of Health and Medicine in Colonial India* (London: Routledge, 2009).

Sherawat, Samiksha, *Colonial Medical Care in North India: Gender, State, and Society c.1840–1920* (New Delhi: Oxford, 2013).

Sivaramakrishnan, Kavita, *Old Potions, New Bottles: Recasting Indigenous Medicine in Colonial Punjab, 1850–1945* (New Delhi: Orient Longman, 2006).

9

History of Medicine in Sub-Saharan Africa

Lyn Schumaker

Africa's medical traditions exhibit an impressive reach and thera-peutic variety. They have spread globally, especially in Latin America and the Caribbean. There they infuse folk medicine and spirit-healing—in Caribbean *vodun* and in Latin American offshoots of central African *lemba* and West Africa's cult of Ogun. The faith healing of North American evangelical churches is also partly based on the medicine of African slaves. African medicine speaks to modern audiences through drumming and dance, and through its broader conception of responsibility for health, implicating the social group, the commu-nity, even the state, in the cause and cure of human distress. Many forms of African medical practice emphasize human interdependence with nature and the desire to achieve balance, blending concerns about human health and the health of the environment, a strikingly modern approach in an era of concern about climate change.

In Africa, racial, economic, and political factors have determined the availability of medicine and its institutional organization. In the colonial period African healers responded to the criminalization of witchcraft accusations by going underground or presenting a less controversial public face as herbalists. Meanwhile Western and Indian practitioners migrated into higher niches created by racially based medical governance in settler-dominated colonies and early white-ruled nations such as South Africa. Despite the end of colonialism and, later, apartheid, a racially and class-biased political economy still largely determines African health. The colonial legacy of medical experimentation and coercive disease campaigns causes even well-intentioned research and health interventions to trigger negative responses in the twenty-first century, as in South Africa's debate over the use of anti-retroviral therapy against HIV/AIDS.

In Africa's historiography of medicine, one can perceive two quite different strands: one originating in the discipline of history of medicine, largely confined to the history of Western medicine in Africa; the other originating in African history, dealing with a broader spectrum of medical practices, often delving into the meanings given by Africans to human experiences such as birth and death, well-being and suffering. This chapter aims to bring together these two historiographical strands to envisage a future history of medicine that is Africa-centred in its definitions and interests, not just its geographical focus. I begin with African medicine and its historical development. Africa's so-called 'traditional medicine' is actually a dynamic array of healing practices and theories, differing widely across the continent, often incorporating scientific and religious imports. It is the main source of medical treatment for the continent's population today, as in the past. The second section outlines African medicine's interaction with world religions, such as Christianity, Islam, and Hinduism, absorbing their healing practices and interpreting their meanings according to African beliefs. The third section discusses colonial medicine, the subject of much recent scholarship. Africa's experience of colonial medicine has challenged the traditional view of colonial/imperial hegemony—colonial medicine's impress upon Africa's peoples was often minimal. Nevertheless, valuable insights have come through study of the variable acceptance of colonial medicine in Africa and how it strengthened or breached the racial cleavages of colonial societies, offered meaning in the face of epidemics, and enforced or ameliorated colonial labour regimes.

The fourth section looks at post-colonial medicine, suggesting that 'contemporary medicine' is a better way of capturing developments across Africa since the mid-twentieth century. Each African country has its own chronology, varying widely in indigenous healing practices, political formation, and economic factors that shape its experiences of medicine. The final section discusses the historiography of medicine in Africa, pointing out its gaps and failures as well as its accomplishments. It directs attention to the underlying conditions of the production of research—funding priorities and publication targets that maintain the dominance of the history of Western medicine as a subject, while marginalizing the medical traditions of Africa and the developing world.

Africa's Medical Traditions

Historically, European observers have always made assumptions about Africa's healing practices that placed them outside European definitions of medicine. Explorers called the African healer a 'witch doctor', a term that emphasized superstition over knowledge. They also interpreted African medical knowledge as religious in character, with the exception of plant-based remedies, which in the early days of exploration were thought appropriate to the ills that might befall travellers.

Even relatively enlightened colonial observers, such as the Southern Rhodesian medical doctor Michael Gelfand, perpetuated similar assumptions when shifting the terminology from 'witch doctor' to 'traditional healer' or 'native doctor'. These terms were intended to show respect to the practitioners of ancient medical traditions, which, though unwritten, were based on complex knowledge of African illnesses. By emphasizing unchanging tradition, however, this terminology denied African medicine a past or a future, making it a medicine without history for a 'people without history'. Once exploration gave way to settlement and administration, the story of Western medicine dominated those few colonialist histories that examined medical issues. In the more general discipline of history, the assumption that Africans had no history was remedied by a post-independence, nationalist-driven campaign to produce pre-colonial histories. In the history of medicine, however, there have until recently been few challenges to the picture of traditional healing as a static body of knowledge and traditional healers as preservers of heritage. African healers themselves often use tradition as a strategy to vie for recognition and resources from the post-colonial state or international organizations.

Traditional medicine is traditional, however, only insofar as it originated in Africa. Change has been ubiquitous from the beginning and African healers are some of the most enquiring practitioners in the world. Among early practitioners of African medicine were healer-chiefs who enlarged the frontiers of human settlement and, when confronting Africa's often difficult environments, protected their followers using herbal, social, and spiritual tools. As African frontiers expanded, they constantly revised their understandings of the environment—perhaps one reason why pragmatism and experimentation characterize healers' work today. This point is missed by scholars who describe traditional medicine as 'closed' in contrast to Western science's supposedly 'open' nature, an argument strikingly similar to white colonial racial views.[1]

The influence of Africa's healing traditions has been deep and globally far-reaching, despite their failure to attract the popular attention received by Chinese acupuncture or Indian meditation in the West. The diaspora of African medicine is an area in need of much more exploration. While Janzen's study of the movement of the pre-colonial Lemba cult of affliction from Africa to the New World constitutes a constructive beginning, more recent work on the cultural legacy of central African slaves in the Americas unfortunately subsumes healing within religion.[2] Nevertheless, African healing arts prosper when associated with highly successful African religions such as Ogun worship and the Orisha tradition, which have over forty million adherents in West Africa and Latin America, as well as increasing popularity in North America.

Many kinds of African healing are based on notions of 'balance', with a pharmacopoeia to address imbalances in environments and persons. Hot-cold and wet-dry axes are employed by healers both in areas influenced by Islamic medicine and in types of healing that long predate Islam, while the roots of Hippocratic humoral medicine in Egypt may reflect universal human concerns originating in Africa. In Africa, however, concern about balance transcends the purely medical, such that it might be described as one of the human senses.[3]

African medical traditions emerged with special reference to environmental survival and to a precarious balance between healing power and political power. *Ngoma*, the drum, is an ancient symbol of political leadership *and* of healing ability. Political leadership was closely associated with the ability to keep healthy both a society and the land it utilized, addressing reproductive and productive health. Africa has experienced a relentless process of aridification, a climatic trend making many of its environments an uncertain foundation for human life.

The low density of population over much of the continent led to deep concerns about fertility. Medicines and protective rituals surrounded every aspect of reproductive life including birth, sex, and the nurturing of women and children. Similarly, land, crops, and animals were protected through medication by healers, invocation of the ancestors, and chiefly rituals. Along with male and female chiefs, women acting as mediums, healers, and central figures in the household often carried particular responsibilities. Healers and ritual specialists diagnosed human and environmental problems and used ritual speech to per-suade people to change their behaviour or to invoke spiritual forces. African healers and ritual specialists, today as in the past, are valued because of their ability to contact and influence the forces that control life, death, and nature. In Africa these forces are seen as both good and bad—there is no essential dualism separating good from evil forces. As Sandra T. Barnes has pointed out, in 'African cosmologies where Ogun is a central figure, destruction and creation are two aspects of a unity that cannot be broken into opposing parts', and balance, so important in Africa, must be achieved through dynamic pairings, such as protection/destruction.[4] Healers are often feared because they might use these forces for anti-social purposes, pros-pering at the expense of their communities through sorcery. Never-theless, chiefs are expected to use sorcery to protect their people. Within this context illnesses tend to be divided into three classes: 'natural' diseases or 'diseases of God', often remedied with herbal treatments; 'diseases of man', caused by humans using sorcery to attack others; and illnesses caused by offending ancestral spirits or illnesses that characterize the early stage of becoming a healer, when a healing spirit is making contact. These categories can overlap, or an illness may change category as it develops, with long-term ill-nesses or illnesses that affect more than one part of the body likely to be blamed on witchcraft or spirit attack.

Africa's ancient and widespread practice of *ngoma* healing plays a prominent role in contemporary private practice in many parts of Africa. In *ngoma* healing sessions, complaints of a physical, psycho-logical, or social nature must be voiced in order to bring about healing. The afflicted person joins a community of sufferers and learns to manage the illness through accommodation with the afflict-ing spirit, sometimes undergoing an apprenticeship that leads to becoming a fully fledged healer. *Ngoma* has been globally significant since its move to the New World with African slaves. Its contemporary influence on African healing churches is also reflected among their offshoots in America and Europe, while South African *sangomas* have adapted *ngoma* for new audiences among the urban black poor and wealthier European and South Asian groups.[5]

Healing can become a family business passed on from generation to generation, with rural members of the extended family supplying urban healers with the raw materials for plant- and animal-based medicines from rural 'home' areas. Trainee healers learn forms of ritual speech that invoke spirits or create new states of being in patients or social groups. Words are used to activate medicines, and the rhythm of drums, too, can act as a kind of speech—particular rhythms call spirits or produce effects in the patient's body. Singing out the complaint and dancing the affliction are therapeutic practices that call attention to the performative aspects of healing and its languages, and not only in Africa. Becoming a patient in any cultural setting requires a change of social status usually accomplished through ritualistic forms of speech or writing, including the diagnostic speech of the Western doctor or the medical 'papers' needed to confirm important life transitions (birth and death certificates). Early Western observers of African medicine often failed to appreciate the ritualistic and performative aspects of their own medical language except in obviously religious contexts such as evangelical healing. This led many to mistakenly view African medicine as essentially religious in character.

African Medicine and World Religions

African medicine has been treated as religion because of its intertwining with the continent's many types of animistic belief. However, there is nothing special in this—religion and medicine also overlap in other parts of the world. When confronting African medicine, however, Islamic reformers and Christian missionaries have solidified its association with religion by interpreting African spirits as Satanic, demanding complete reliance on Christian or Islamic faith healing or the exclusive use of scientific medicine. In some cases, however, the African healing practices they interpret as pagan were based on earlier, now Africanized, Christian or Islamic rituals and spirits.

Swahili medicine is a prime example. Research over the past two decades has revealed the African roots of Swahili culture, which thrived in both the interior and the coastal areas of eastern Africa wherever fishing and farming societies intermingled. Traders from the Swahili coast gradually ventured north into Arabia and Persia, taking high-status Persian names and returning with highly attractive foreign goods. By 800 CE they also brought Islam.[6] Interactions between Islam and the earlier spirit therapies of the region can be read 'archaeologically' in the layering of different varieties of spirits and their changing status as their healing power increased or diminished with shifts in the political power of the groups with which they were associated. Thus when people in eastern Africa seek explanations for affliction, it is among this historically changing array of spirits that many find meaning, solace, and cures. For example, 'European' spirits are no longer relevant after the end of European colonialism, while pagan spirits have recently become less anti-Islamic and Islamic spirits have become more orthodox in response to the increasing status of orthodox Islam. Exceptions are *kimasai* and *mijikenda*, both from non-Islamic groups (Maasai and Mijikenda) that enjoy some celebrity in Swahili society. Meanwhile Islamic practitioners vary widely in the theories and practices they employ—humoral concepts and orthodox Islamic medical concepts can be mixed with ideas drawn from witchcraft beliefs, spirit healing, and Western biomedicine. Indeed, earlier types of Islamic medicine included ideas of spirit possession and attack (by *majini, shetani*) and their cure. Recent types of Islamic medicine reject all forms of spirit explanation and mystical cures.[7]

Both Islamic and Hindu forms of Indian medicine followed Indian migrants to the continent, for example in South Africa from the 1860s. Indian medicine, both *Unani ṭibb* (Islamic) and *Ayurvedic* (Hindu), shares with African medicine humoral ideas about using medicines and diet to achieve balance. Indian shops in cities like Durban historically marketed both African and Indian medicines, while itinerant Indian traders carried African and Indian medicines to rural Africans during the decades of segregation. Early Indian migrants sought indigenous African substitutes for Indian plant-based medicines, while African and Indian healers and patients experimented with both types of healing.[8]

Although Christianity is very old in North Africa and the Horn of Africa, and the central African Kingdom of Kongo converted as early as 1491, most studies of mission medicine focus on the nineteenth- and early-twentieth-century missions that were chiefly responsible for the introduction of scientific medicine and hospital care. These missionaries joined early European traders, hunters, and explorers during the period when disruption caused by the slave trade and early colonial exploitation, such as red rubber extraction, created a context in which Africans were open to new forms of religion and in need of healing.

By the late nineteenth and early twentieth centuries, scientific medicine became central to mission activity partly due to its growing status in the metropoles. The preference for scientific medicine among mainstream mission churches also reflected fears that spiritual healing might encourage African spirit beliefs. Initiated by Terence Ranger, research on missionaries' struggles over the appropriate relationship between healing and scientific medicine have prospered, with the picture extended and complicated by subsequent work.[9] For example, Charles Good examined the geographical and technological limitations missionaries faced in Malawi's difficult terrain, finding that evangelization of the faith and of scientific medical beliefs proceeded unevenly in ways that may have encouraged medical pluralism.[10] Other recent work shows how African catechists played key roles in debates over African healing practices,[11] while in other cases African nurses and medical auxiliaries actively translated mission medicine using local African ritual and secular language, fitting it to African conceptual systems in ways that white mission staff neither understood nor controlled.[12]

Although mission medicine proved popular in most parts of Africa—often more popular than government services where they existed—some Africans broke from mainstream churches, founding African churches that practised faith healing. These addressed the failure of mission ritual and mission medicine to deal with the full range of spiritual and physical afflictions recognized by Africans, especially witchcraft. Schism over the role of Christianity in healing continues today, for example in the case of Archbishop Milingo in Zambia, whose use of faith healing at a time of crisis in the country's health and economy in the 1980s proved so controversial that the Catholic Church removed him from the country.[13]

Colonial Medicine

Megan Vaughan's *Curing Their Ills* in 1991 was a milestone in the understanding of Western medicine in Africa.[14] It juxtaposed government medical and psychiatric services, disease campaigns, mission medicine, and tropical medicine, revealing the diverse settings and relationships within which they acted. Vaughan's book contributed to a growing picture of medicine as a morally complex activity, revising earlier critiques that it was simply an instrument of colonial power. A chapter on mission medicine in John and Jean Comaroff's *Of Revelation and Revolution* also contributed to this new understanding, portraying the ambiguities of mission medical practices that brought different people together, cutting across the racial cleavages of colonial society.[15]

Initially, during colonial conquest, tropical medicine focused on European health. Its greatest successes came with the 'scramble for Africa's diseases', resulting in good careers for metropolitan researchers but mixed benefits for African populations exposed both to disease and to early colonial experiments in preventive and curative measures. Racially based theories of disease sometimes labelled 'native' populations as reservoirs of infection—as in the case of malaria among humans (believed to be caught from too close proximity to African women and children), or sleeping sickness among animals (tolerated by Africa's wild antelope but deadly to European cattle). Nevertheless, the argument that a 'sanitation syndrome' was the chief cause of segregation in colonial cities has been disputed—it was one among many factors, social, economic, and political—and timing was of the essence, racial medical theories having the most impact when epidemics coincided with crucial phases of city development. Racial segregation in medical institutions has also proved to be more complex than initially thought, with much good work being done on South Africa.[16]

The influence of tropical medicine declined in the 1920s as attention shifted to the health of indigenous peoples and to diseases that stood in the way of development. This included a public health focus on water-borne diseases, industrial diseases like tuberculosis, and maternity services and child health. Malaria remained important because colonial doctors began to recognize its impact on Africans, especially on children's survival. The shift to African health spurred government-funded military-style 'disease campaigns', focused on diseases like sleeping sickness, yaws, and syphilis. Africans sometimes found mass medical examination and treatment stigmatizing or causing fears of infertility when vaccination targeted children. However, campaigns could also be seen as cleansing, on the model of pre-colonial witchcraft cleansing by chiefs and later colonial witch-cleansing movements.[17] Early studies of syphilis and tuberculosis in Africans bolstered arguments for white rule and segregation by supporting theories of African physical inferiority or promiscuity or dangerous cultural practices, often distracting from economic conditions that were more important.[18] Similar theories would emerge in scientific discourses during the HIV/AIDS epidemic.[19]

Colonial industries also organized medical services for workers, which varied enormously in quality. Mining companies typically sent ill or disabled workers 'home' to rural areas instead of providing treatment, one of the reasons for the rapid spread of tuberculosis to rural areas in the colonial period. Historians of the political economy of disease have examined migration to mines and plantations in considerable depth on a regional basis. Despite its potential as an approach for understanding global interconnections in disease history, however, little work has followed up Burke and Richardson's pioneering study of links between nineteenth-century phthisis, tin-mining, and Cornish labour migration to South Africa.[20]

The tiny specialism of colonial and imperial psychology, meanwhile, has become something of a boom industry.[21] Colonial psychologists, few in number and often embedded in settler societies, developed theories of the 'African mind' that justified European control, projecting colonial violence onto Africans or using Freudian interpretations of African child development to explain the failure of Africans to embrace European work regimes.[22] Others medicalized African dissent or explained it as 'mass hysteria'.[23] But others used Freudian psychoanalysis to question simplistic racial or cultural views of African subjectivity.[24] Scholars have also examined institutionalization along models familiar from European studies of madness.[25] Meanwhile recent work has revealed how limited was the reach of psychiatry; Julie Parle explores the meanings of mental affliction in the family and community, as well as the asylum, enriching the analysis by including witchcraft and suicide.[26] An important gap in this literature is the history of cross-cultural psychology during the 1960s, unexplored despite its impact on attempts to develop culturally sensitive forms of psychological testing for education, employment, and clinical treatment in the crucial period around African independence.

Post-Colonial Medicine?

After independence new African states saw medicine as central to modern nationhood, increasing funds for hospitals and medical schools, which, like big dam projects, reflected modernity and national pride. Primary care services were extended into rural areas to make up for colonial shortfalls, displacing mission medicine. Africanization of health care staff, already begun in the late colonial period, intensified after independence even in countries that already supported a substantial number of Western-trained African doctors; since the late nineteenth century African doctors had worked in Nigeria and South Africa, while Malawi's first president, Hastings Kamuzu Banda, had worked as a doctor in Scotland. In most places the first African nurses, usually male, had been trained at colonial mission stations, but after independence training increasingly moved to urban nursing colleges.[27] The politics of race, gender, and class that shaped the careers of female nurses working in hospitals could be enormously complex, with South Africa perhaps best represented in the scholarship.[28] Despite the lack of publicity for their work in the West, post-colonial African doctors have been involved in crucial stages of disease research on the continent, pinpointing the emergence of East Africa's HIV epidemic, for example.[29]

The term 'contemporary' may be more appropriate than 'post-colonial' for capturing the history of national experiences on the continent since the mid-twentieth century. Ethiopia, for example, experienced colonialism only briefly and nurtured medical traditions that have yet to be given full historical treatment.[30] South Africa was independent well before 1950 (though for the black majority, white rule arguably shared much with direct European colonialism). 'Post-colonial' also diverts attention from continuities with the colonial period—in Africanization programmes, for example. It also obscures the similarities of today's health crises to the overlapping demographic and environmental crises of the early colonial period caused by wars, harsh labour regimes, and resource pillaging. Today, neoliberal reforms, resource wars, and global trade conditions have ravaged African health care services and harmed natural resources and small-scale agricultural production on which health ultimately depends. As in the period around World War I, these conditions exacerbate epidemics even when they do not directly cause them. Market reforms in the 1990s, for example, demanded the introduction of fees for health care in the midst of Africa's emerging HIV epidemic.

Thus it is vital to focus on economic change as well as political breakpoints when devising a chronology of medicine for Africa. Colonial law transformed the organization of traditional practitioners, forcing them out of the political sphere and privatizing their practice, but colonial commerce at the same time transformed traditional medicine's pharmacopoeia, its packaging, and marketing. Today, neoliberalism has been similarly transformative. Market reforms and the reorganization of health care services have stimulated the expansion of traditional medicine and the blossoming of mass production and larger trading networks. This has been accompanied by a brisk informal trade in Western pharmaceuticals and medical procedures, due to the breakdown of government regulation and the pressures on hospital staff salaries that lead the highly qualified to seek jobs abroad while others sell hospital drugs to supplement shrinking incomes or set up independent, unregulated surgeries.

South Africa's quite different political trajectory, with its early transition to white rule and jockeying for power between different white factions, is a case that also defies easy post-colonial interpretations. The country's racially based distribution of health care reached its peak under apartheid, when medical researchers led the world in heart transplant technology, an achievement built on the wealth of resources spent on medical care for the white minority, and neglect of the African majority. Majority rule has not, however, ended the uneven distribution of medical benefits. Class differences, largely aligned with race, determine access and quality of health care. The weight of this history is still felt in the twenty-first century, for example, in South Africa's debate over the use of anti-retroviral therapy against HIV/AIDS. This debate is not only framed by questions about the trustworthiness of Western scientific understandings of HIV but also about how state funding for health care should be fairly distributed—into relatively expensive treatment for HIV or into primary care and prevention.

Global Asymmetries and Inconvenient Histories

The writing of history of medicine in Africa began with an imperial/ colonial bias: medical historians, including colonial doctors, assumed medicine was a civilizing force pitted against the suffering and super- stition intrinsic to Africa. They told a story of Western medicine's triumphs over disease already familiar from Europe's own 'great man' medical history. When Prins evaluated the historiography in 1989, he applauded new work that engaged with African concerns, but despite some successes large areas of African experience remain invisible.[31] Today the priorities of the broader discipline of history of medicine still limit what research can be done in Africa, making it easier to study Western medicine at the expense of the many other topics that are possible in this richly diverse continent. Nevertheless, new work is eroding disciplinary and methodological boundaries and demonstrat- ing how history of medicine could strengthen its ethical and intellec- tual reach by making Africa and other marginal regions of the world more central to its project.

What Prins applauded was a generation of African-studies-trained scholars who placed medicine in its historical and social contexts. This was exemplified by the work of John Janzen and Steven Feierman, who used a mix of anthropological and historical approaches to African health-seeking in plural medical contexts.[32] Similarly, Harriet Ngubane and Murray Last and Gordon Chavunduka provided a sociological analysis and some of the first historical accounts of African medicine, although Last and Chavunduka's contribution was framed by the Western concept of professionalization.[33] These works estab- lished a methodological dialogue between anthropology and history that has characterized the best of the subsequent literature.

Prins also highlighted work focused on the complex interactions among Africa's peoples, pathogens, and politics, led by John Ford's study of colonial sleeping sickness campaigns.[34] This has resulted in a still growing literature on environment and health, and regional epidemic histories.[35] Prins also noted work in the political economy of health and disease, especially Randall Packard's study of tuberculosis in South Africa.[36] In light of Roy Porter's groundbreaking articles on the role of the patient in Britain, Prins also expected future historians of Africa to produce more patient-centred histories. This hope has been only partially fulfilled. Another key assessment of medicine's African historiography was Megan Vaughan's 1994 discussion of problems of methodology and approach—in particular, the failure to question Western medicine's 'theory of itself' as an objective, culturally neutral process.[37] At the level of practice, she argued, Western medicine may not be all that different from other types of healing, amenable to the same approaches applied to African healers.

Colonial mission medicine proved a tempting example. Subsequently scholars looked at mission doctors and nurses in detail, examining their assumptions about African patients and their conflicts with healers. Nurses, both European and African, as well as medical auxiliaries, are often central to the interactions between Western and African healing practices described in these studies. Work that ventures out from the mission enclave to capture wider African perspectives is rare, however. Hunt's study of birth in the Congo sets a high standard. She begins with pre-colonial African understandings of birth and its dangers, and its unexpected metaphorical role in the making of masculinity through boys' initiation rituals. This provides a firm basis for examining the subsequent medicalization of birth by colonial missions and government and its impact on Congolese notions of citizenship and the state.[38] Also innovative is Good's study of the Universities' Mission to Central Africa in Malawi, capturing the mission's interactions with African communities through its use of technologies of transport, as well as medicine.[39]

Vaughan also called for more studies of medical research, as did Maureen Malowany, the latter emphasizing the importance of detailed examination of what medical researchers think and how they experiment and promote their findings.[40] Today numerous scholars are examining trajectories of discovery and intervention in disease history, with notable work in veterinary medicine, which has received little attention in the past.[41] Recent work on medical research stations also breaks new ground by employing the memories of African researchers as a window on scientific practices.[42] More does indeed need to be known about how medical researchers think, but the most rewarding approach situates researchers squarely within African environments, cultures, and histories, and in the social and moral worlds of the many others around them who also intervene in health and illness.

However, it is striking that there is not an equally urgent call for research on changes in how African healers think and experiment. Few scholars have examined 'experimental moments' in African medicine, with the exception of Karen Flint's work on how South African healers effectively marketed traditional medicines in competition with European and Asian pharmacists.[43] Few studies centre on African healing history; most look at 'responses to' Western medicine, allowing Western medicine to set the agenda. While it is true that ethnographies exist for a wide range of African healing traditions they are rarely historicized, with the exception of Harry West's *Kupilikula*, Feierman's *Peasant Intellectuals*, and Janzen's *lemba* study and his ongoing work on *ngoma*.[44] Indeed, topics such as these—the changing medical and political uses of healing language and practice or the deep history of healing traditions—would be unlikely to attract funding specific to history of medicine today.

The reasons are partly structural, relating to funding processes, and partly methodological and disciplinary. Like Prins, Vaughan assumed good historical scholarship in Africa must sometimes employ anthropological as well as historical methods. She encouraged 'inconsistency' in defining subject-matter and choosing an approach, rather than following the standard 'academic division of labour'. Debates about approach are truly academic, however, when funding is decided along rigid methodological and disciplinary lines. Lack of adequate funding harms African history of medicine, making it difficult to study languages (where language is the key to deeper understanding), to do oral history respectfully with adequate follow-up, to complete archival work under difficult conditions, and to use ethnography when appropriate to the topic. Both African and non-African scholars are disadvantaged by a lack of funding, leaving Africa marginalized and missing the opportunity for the larger discipline of history of medicine to produce globally centred (rather than Euro-American-centred) histories.

A glance at the ultimate product of funding decisions—publication in history of medicine journals—reveals the effects of disciplinary and methodological restrictions. Few articles about sub-Saharan Africa appear in *Medical History, Bulletin of the History of Medicine, Social History of Medicine*, and the history of science journals that publish history of medicine—fewer than those about other regional traditions such as

China or India, which have a stronger archival base. In recent years, *Social History of Medicine* has outstripped others in its coverage of Africa (and China and India), indicating that the absence of coverage in other journals is not simply because scholars prefer region-specific audiences. Nevertheless, the African articles published in *Social History of Medicine* almost exclusively deal with Western medicine. Africa's indigenous medicine is left without a history in the very journals in which debates about the discipline's appropriate topics, boundaries, and divisions of labour could most productively take place. Not every topic requires ethnographic methods, but many important areas cannot be explored if scholars are not free to choose the best tools for the job. As Hunt has observed of Africa, 'No continent has achieved more interesting fusions of history and anthropology.'[45] If funders demand that disciplinary boundaries be strictly observed, African scholarship is disadvantaged by its interdisciplinary strengths.

Western origins also shape the idea of history that animates history of medicine. For example, the history of a Graeco-Roman physician such as Galen is seen as central to Western medicine. Funding is less available for the history of prominent African healers because they are not included in this lineage, except where they interact with colonial doctors. Such healers have had a profound impact on African health, on resistance and accommodation to colonialism, and on African responses to epidemics. This is not to say that Africa needs more histories of 'great medical men' (or women), but the history of healers is an important part of a larger project to uncover the understandings possessed by African 'intellectual communities', of which we have so far only obtained 'tantalising hints'.[46] Concentration on alternative medical or healing lineages and intellectual communities could help history of medicine to escape the limitations of its Western origins. The discipline has yet to embrace a truly post-colonial approach—one that not only deals with colonial medicine and its aftermath in the former colonies but also situates medical developments in the former metropoles within a wider post-colonial world. Medicine 'at home' in England or France, for example, has been changed by the colonial experience, too.

More research on African categories of experience could also lead to a vibrant combination of African studies with approaches from history of science, technology, and medicine. A similar cross-fertilization of ideas and methods took place in the 1980s and early

1990s when Africanist and European anthropological and historical approaches joined to bring about advances in history.[47] An area where cross-fertilization has begun is the 'history of the body', which since the 1990s has become a special focus in the history of medicine. This approach combines methods from anthropology and cultural history to uncover the history of change in human bodies, in embodied experiences, and in the materiality of therapeutics. Historians of the body employ historical ethnography—an approach that, for example, enriches Ruth Harris's book on healing and medicine at the Catholic shrine of Lourdes in France.[48] Many historical topics also require observing traces of bodily history found in posture and movement today. For Africa, one of the few works comparable to Harris's achievement is Didier Fassin's *When Bodies Remember*, a contemporary history of South African responses to HIV/AIDS and controversies over anti-retroviral drugs.[49]

Fassin examines the politics of medicine across all levels of South African society, from the disadvantaged rural poor to the Treatment Action Campaign to (former president) Thabo Mbeki, his medical advisers and their embrace of so-called 'AIDS denialism'. Despite dealing extensively with the science of HIV/AIDS, Fassin transcends the usual analytical framework of history of science that has characterized much previous work on AIDS. He instead finds the roots of contemporary positions, including AIDS denialism, in the historically embodied experiences of *apartheid* violence, South Africa's racist health care system, and Africa's wider history of medical and physical exploitation. He does this through eliciting individual and collective memory and observing embodied behaviour over a significant period of South Africa's recent history.[50] Fassin is an anthropologist but this book is one of the finest examples of historical insight in South African history of medicine. Perhaps anthropologists enjoy greater freedom to be 'inconsistent' in approach than do historians of medicine—though Fassin also struggled with issues of funding and lack of interest in the French academic context.[51]

History of the body as an approach also focuses our attention on the patient. Recent work in this area includes Julie Livingston's *Debility and the Moral Imagination in Botswana*. She uses the term 'debility' to raise her work above the standard literature on the 'history of disability', which has been limited by the Western definition of disability and focused mainly on the professional specialisms that address disability. In contrast, Livingston transforms definitional and cultural differences into an opportunity to achieve deeper understanding of how healing and caring are done by a wide range of people. She does not simply examine specific Western or Tswana diseases or conditions, but deals instead with 'misfortune' and its African meanings. In her work ethnography is key to historical insight: even the most sensitive oral historical methods cannot tease out the unacknowledged or inarticulate aspects of suffering, healing, or care-giving and the 'diverse expressions of morality' that infuse them. Thus her work pays attention to 'posture, gossip, complaining, bathing, hiding, nursing, diagnostics, proverbs, gift-giving, etc'.[52]

Another way to bring African perspectives and categories into history of medicine is to examine realms of human experience that are not simply defined as medical. Lynn Thomas's *Politics of the Womb*, for example, deals with the history of 'procreation' in Kenya, examining its medical, political, and other meanings.[53] Thomas's study is also an 'externalist' account that helps to balance the dominance, in history of medicine, of 'internalist' accounts that focus narrowly on medical researchers' worlds or the internal development of particular medical specialisms or institutions. Luise White's work on 'vampire stories' also challenges scholars to start with African categories of experience; medical technologies appear among an array of frightening objects and activities Africans use to describe colonial relationships.[54] If applied to current health care issues—for example, the so-called 'moral panics' sometimes sparked by the introduction of anti-retrovirals or child vaccination programmes—such approaches aid in the critique of current medical intervention practices. Vaughan's recent work on the history of death in Africa is another project that puts medicine in its place among a range of other types of knowledge and practice. In some parts of Africa rituals of death are intimately linked to rituals of life and/or the protection of the vulnerable against illness or sorcery—something not easily grasped if analysis is limited by Western medical definitions.[55]

Prins was interested in 'what happens to our images of both Africans and of disease when we move from a doctor-centred to a patient-centred account'.[56] Feierman's early work on kin-based decision-making in a plural medical context led the way, while groundbreaking new work includes Eric Silla's examination of leprosy from the patient's perspective.[57] More work also needs to be done on historical situations in which the patient is the doctor—whether using home remedies, family and neighbourly health knowledge, or self-treatment. Self-treatment occurs in all historical periods and helps to trace continuities across colonial/post-colonial divisions, as well as turning attention away from the misleading dualism of Western versus traditional medicine. People who self-treat rely upon locally available herbal resources and the changing pharmacopoeia—Western, African, Islamic, or other—that they find in markets, formal and informal.[58] A focus on the history of home remedies often necessitates the use of anthropological approaches, however, as pointed out by Vivienne Lo for China.[59]

Finally, a return to the political economy of disease is needed. Little has changed since 1997 when Shula Marks raised concerns about the 'silencing of class issues' in scholarship on colonial medicine.[60] The political economy approach is especially needed at the global level. Of recent work, Jock McCulloch has placed South African miners and communities within a global distribution of the social costs of production of asbestos, while Randall Packard's global biography of malaria challenges us to do a more relevant kind of history, willing to challenge the truisms of economics and development policy.[61] We also must place Africa in a global political economy of health care and medical research, to seek the historical roots of global inequalities in the distribution of medical benefits versus medical risks. Studies are needed of how the discourse of Africa as 'virgin medical territory' is re-created in each historical period since the beginning of colonial medical research and how this has contributed to Africa's attractiveness as a site for 'pharmaceutical colonialism'.[62]

Conclusion

Only through a restructuring of funding priorities will new approaches flourish and expand the global vision of the discipline. Funding, particularly in Britain, is in need of reform: as Richard Bowring observed, 'the funding mechanism has for many years been exerting undue influence on the kind of research we do. It generates a form of self-censorship, whereby we aim for short-term benefit and ignore the truly valuable.'[63] Grant funding and the pressures of research assessment targets have created a situation that resembles private sector sub-contracting—those who promise more in less time with less money win the contract. Scholars should pursue research that reflects their skills and interests, but when scholars choose Africa they find that many topics cannot be properly researched within one- to three-year timetables. Timetables should reflect the needs of particular topics and the time required for effective use of appropriate methods. Today's increasingly competitive funding arena has engendered not innovation but the reluctance of scholars to pursue less convenient histories—histories that require non-European language-learning, oral history, and ethnography. This ensures continuation of current global asymmetries in the discipline—the dominance of histories of Western medicine and the marginality of Africa and other regions of the developing world. We need new funding structures that stimulate work on under-represented regions, such as Africa, and under-represented topics, such as patient-centred histories.

This is a situation that demands inspired, committed work, not only in Africa but also in the wealthy nations that primarily fund historical research, challenging funding priorities and research timetables. The historical roots of Africa's health problems must be tackled through listening and observing with respect and taking time to appreciate the perspectives of informants—necessary for good history in contexts of suffering and misfortune, as well as in contexts of hope and healing, which we find in abundance in Africa. This history is inconvenient for universities striving to meet targets and for funders and department heads who want an immediately tangible 'product'. However, these limitations must not be allowed to create a partiality of research vision that colludes with other global inequalities to make Africa's health problems seem intractable. Africa's ill-health is the product of social, political, and economic causes that we can confront with the strength of historical understanding and long-term, committed scholarship.

Acknowledgements

I thank the editor, Mark Jackson, and all those who kindly read and commented on this chapter in manuscript, especially Steven Feierman and Henrika Kuklick.

Notes

1 Robin Horton, 'African Traditional Thought and Western Science', Part I, *Africa* 37 (1) (1967), 50–71; and Part II, *Africa* 37 (2) (1967), 155–87.

2 John M. Janzen, *Lemba, 1650–1930: A Drum of Affliction in Africa and the New World* (New York; Garland, 1982); Linda M Heywood (ed.), *Central Africans and Cultural Transformations in the American Diaspora* (Cambridge: Cambridge University Press, 2002).

3 Kathryn Linn Geurts, *Culture and the Senses: Bodily Ways of Knowing in an African Community* (Berkeley: University of California Press, 2002).

4 Sandra T. Barnes, 'The Many Faces of Ogun', in *eadem* (ed.), *Africa's Ogun: Old World and New* (Bloomington: Indiana University Press, 1997), 1–27, at 17–19.

5 John M. Janzen, *Ngoma: Discourses of Healing in Central and Southern Africa* (Berkeley: University of California Press, 1992); Rijk van Dijk, Ria Reis, and Marja Spierenburg (eds), *The Quest for Fruition through Ngoma: The Political Aspects of Healing in Southern Africa* (Oxford: James Currey, 2000).

6 Thomas Spear, 'Early Swahili History Reconsidered', *International Journal of African Historical Studies* 33 (2) (2000), 257–90.

7 Linda Giles, 'Sociocultural Change and Spirit Possession on the Swahili Coast of East Africa', *Anthropological Quarterly* 68 (2) (1995), 89–106.

8 Karen Flint, 'Indian-African Encounters: Polyculturalism and African Therapeutics in Natal, South Africa, 1886–1950s', *Journal of Southern African Studies (JSAS)* 32 (2) (2006), 367–85.

9 Terence Ranger, 'Godly Medicine: The Ambiguities of Medical Mission in Southeast Tanzania, 1900–1945', *Social Science and Medicine* 15 (3) (1981), 261–77.

10 Charles M. Good, *The Steamer Parish: The Rise and Fall of Missionary Medicine on an African Frontier* (Chicago: University of Chicago Press, 2004).

11 Markku Hokkanen, 'Quests for Health and Contests for Meaning: African Church Leaders and Scottish Missionaries in the Early Twentieth Century Presbyterian Church in Northern Malawi', *JSAS* 33 (4) (2007), 733–50.

12 Walima T. Kalusa, 'Language, Medical Auxiliaries, and the Reinterpretation of Missionary Medicine in Colonial Mwinilunga, Zambia, 1922–51', *Journal of Eastern African Studies* 1 (1) (2007), 57–78; Walima T. Kalusa, 'Disease and the Remaking of Missionary Medicine in Colonial Northwestern Zambia: A Case of Mwinilunga Disrict, 1902–1964', PhD thesis, Johns Hopkins University, 2003.

13 Gerrie ter Haar, *Spirit of Africa: The Healing Ministry of Archbishop Milingo of Zambia* (London: Hurst, 1992).

14 Megan Vaughan, *Curing their Ills: Colonial Power and African Illness* (Cambridge: Polity Press, 1991).

15 John and Jean Comaroff, *Of Revelation and Revolution*, vol. 2 (Chicago: University of Chicago Press, 1997).

16 Harriet Deacon, 'Racial Segregation and Medical Discourse in Nineteenth Century Cape Town', *JSAS* 22 (2) (1996), 287–308.

17 Bryan Callahan, '"Veni, VD, Vici"?: Reassessing the Ila Syphilis Epidemic', *JSAS* 23 (3) (1997), 421–40.

18 Karen Jochelson, *The Colour of Disease: Syphilis and Racism in South Africa, 1880–1950* (Basingstoke: Palgrave, 2001).

19 Suzette Heald, 'The Power of Sex: Some Reflections on the Caldwells' "African Sexuality" Thesis', *Africa* 65 (4) (1995), 489–505.

20 Gillian Burke and Peter Richardson, 'The Profits of Death: A Comparative Study of Miners' Phthisis in Cornwall and the Transvaal, 1876–1918', *JSAS* 4 (2) (1978), 147–71.

21 Andrew Scull, review of Sloane Mahone and Megan Vaughan (eds), *Psychiatry and Empire* (Basingstoke: Palgrave Macmillan, 2007), *Social History of Medicine* 21 (2) (2008), 411–13.

22 Jock McCulloch, *Colonial Psychiatry and the African Mind* (Cambridge: Cambridge University Press, 1995).

23 Sloane Mahone, 'The Psychology of Rebellion: Colonial Medical Responses to Dissent in British East Africa', *Journal of African History*, 47 (2) (2006), 241–58.

24 Saul Dubow, 'Wulf Sachs's Black Hamlet: A Case of Psychic "Vivisection"?', *African Affairs* 92 (1993), 519–56.

25 Jonathan Sadowsky, *Imperial Bedlam: Institutions of Madness in Colonial Southwest Nigeria* (Berkeley: University of California Press, 1999); Lynette Jackson, *Surfacing Up: Psychiatry and Social Order in Colonial Zimbabwe, 1908–1968* (Ithaca: Cornell University Press, 2005).

26 Julie Parle, *States of Mind: Searching for Mental Health in Natal and Zululand, 1868–1918* (Scottsville, South Africa: University of Kwazulu-Natal Press, 2007).

27 Nancy Rose Hunt, *A Colonial Lexicon of Birth Ritual, Medicalization, and Mobility in the Congo* (Durham, NC: Duke University Press, 1999).

28 Shula Marks, *Divided Sisterhood: Race, Class and Gender in the South African Nursing Profession* (Basingstoke: St Martin's Press, 1994); Simonne Horwitz, 'Black Nurses in White: Exploring Young Women's Entry into the Nursing Profession at Baragwanath Hospital, Soweto, 1948–1980', *Social History of Medicine* 20 (1) (2007), 131–46.

29 John Iliffe, *East African Doctors: A History of the Modern Profession* (Cambridge: Cambridge University Press, 1998).

30 Jacques Mercier, *Art that Heals: Image as Medicine in Ethiopia* (New York: Museum for African Art, 1997); Richard Pankhurst, *Introduction to the Medical History of Ethiopia* (Trenton, NJ: Red Sea Press, 1990).

31 Gwyn Prins, 'But What was the Disease? The Present State of Health and Healing in African Studies', *Past and Present* 124 (1) (1989), 159–79.

32 John M. Janzen, *The Quest for Therapy in Lower Zaire* (Berkeley: University of California Press, 1978); *idem*, *Lemba*; Steven Feierman, 'Struggles for Control: The Social Roots of Health and Healing in Modern Africa', *African Studies Review* 28 (2–3) (1985), 73–147; Feierman and Janzen (eds), *The Social Basis of Health and Healing in Africa* (Berkeley: University of California Press, 1992).

33 Harriet Ngubane, *Body and Mind in Zulu Medicine* (New York: Academic Press, 1977); Murray Last and Gordon Chavunduka, *Professionalisation of African Medicine* (Manchester: Manchester University Press, 1986).

34 John Ford, *The Role of the Trypanosomiases in African Ecology: A Study of the Tsetse Fly Problem* (Oxford: Clarendon Press, 1971).

35 Maryinez Lyons, *The Colonial Disease: A Social History of Sleeping Sickness in Northern Zaire, 1900–1940* (Cambridge: Cambridge University Press, 1992); Helen Tilley, 'Ecologies of Complexity: Tropical Environments, African Trypanosomiasis, and the Science of Disease Control in British Colonial Africa, 1900–1940', *Osiris* 19, 2nd series (2004), 21–38. HIV/AIDS has increasingly dominated epidemic histories since the mid-1990s—see John Iliffe, *The African AIDS Epidemic: A History* (Oxford: James Currey, 2006); Shula Marks, 'Science, Social Science and Pseudo-Science in the HIV/AIDS Debate in Southern Africa', *Journal of Southern African Studies* 33 (4) (2007), 861–74; Terence Ranger and Paul Slack (eds), *Epidemics and Ideas* (Cambridge: Cambridge University Press, 1992); Howard Phillips, *'Black October': The Impact of the Spanish Influenza Epidemic of 1918 on South Africa* (Pretoria: The Government Printer, 1990).

36 Randall Packard, *White Plague, Black Labor: Tuberculosis and the Political Economy of Health and Disease in South Africa* (Berkeley: University of California Press, 1989).

37 Megan Vaughan, 'Healing and Curing: Issues in the Social History and Anthropology of Medicine in Africa', *Social History of Medicine* 7 (2) (1994), 283–95.

38 Hunt, *Colonial Lexicon*, 27–79.

39 Good, *Steamer Parish*.

40 Maureen Malowany, 'Unfinished Agendas: Writing the History of Medicine of Sub-Saharan Africa', *African Affairs*, 99 (2000), 325–49.

41 William Beinart, Karen Brown, and Daniel Gilfoyle, 'Experts and Expertise in Colonial Africa Reconsidered: Science and the Interpenetration of Knowledge', *African Affairs* 108 (432) (2009), 413–33. For further discussion of animal and human medicine, see Robert G. W. Kirk and Michael Worboys, 'Medicine and Species: One Medicine, One History?', in Mark Jackson (ed.), *The Oxford Handbook of the History of Medicine* (Oxford, Oxford University Press, 2011), 561–77.

42 See chapters by Wenzel Geissler, Lyn Schumaker, and Gulliaume Lachenal in Wenzel Geissler and Catherine Molyneux (eds), *Evidence, Ethos and Experiment: The Anthropology and History of Medical Research in Africa* (Oxford: Berghahn, 2011).

43 Karen Flint, *Healing Traditions: African Medicine, Cultural Exchange, and Competition in South Africa, 1820–1948* (Athens: Ohio University Press, 2008), 128–57; and Teresa Barnes's review of Anne Digby, *Diversity and Division in Medicine: Health Care in South Africa from the 1800s* (Oxford: Peter Lang, 2006), *Journal of African History* 50 (3) (2009), 449–51.

44 Steven Feierman, *Peasant Intellectuals: Anthropology and History in Tanzania* (Madison: University of Wisconsin Press, 1990); Harry G West, *Kupilikula:*

Governance and the Invisible Realm in Mozambique (Chicago: University of Chicago Press, 2005).

45 Nancy Rose Hunt, 'Whither African History?', *History Workshop Journal* 66 (1) (2008), 259–65, at 259.

46 Shula Marks quoting from Luise White's '"They Could Make their Victims Dull": Genders and Genres, Fantasies and Cures in Colonial Southern Uganda', *American Historical Review* 100 (5) (1995), 1379–402, at 1395, in Marks, 'What is Colonial about Colonial Medicine? And What has Happened to Imperialism and Health?', *Social History of Medicine* 10 (2) (1997), 205–19, at 215.

47 Eric Hobsbawm and Terence Ranger (eds), *The Invention of Tradition* (Cambridge: Cambridge University Press, 1983).

48 Ruth Harris, *Lourdes: Body and Spirit in the Secular Age* (London: Penguin Books, 1999).

49 Didier Fassin, *When Bodies Remember: Experiences and Politics of AIDS in South Africa* (Berkeley: University of California Press, 2007).

50 See Virginia Berridge's review of Fassin's book in *Journal of Contemporary History* 44 (1) (2009), 153–5.

51 Fassin, *When Bodies Remember*, xi–xii.

52 Julie Livingston, *Debility and the Moral Imagination in Botswana* (Bloomington: Indiana University Press, 2005), 20.

53 Lynn Thomas, *Politics of the Womb: Women, Reproduction, and the State in Kenya* (Berkeley: University of California Press, 2003).

54 Luise White, *Speaking with Vampires: Rumor and History in Colonial Africa* (Berkeley: University of California Press, 2000).

55 Rebekah Lee and Megan Vaughan, 'Death and Dying in the History of Africa since 1800', *Journal of African History* 49 (2008), 341–59; Isak Niehaus, 'Death before Dying: Understanding AIDS Stigma in the South African Lowveld', *Journal of Southern African Studies* 33 (4) (2007), 845–60.

56 Prins, 'But What was the Disease?', 161.

57 Eric Silla, *People Are Not the Same: Leprosy and Identity in Twentieth-Century Mali* (Oxford: James Currey, 1998).

58 Anne Digby, 'Self-Medication and the Trade in Medicine within a Multi-Ethnic Context: A Case Study of South Africa from the Mid-Nineteenth to Mid-Twentieth Centuries', *Social History of Medicine* 18 (3) (2005), 439–57.

59 Vivienne Lo, 'But Is It [History of] Medicine? Twenty Years in the History of the Healing Arts of China', *Social History of Medicine* 22 (2) (2009), 283–303.

60 Marks, 'What is Colonial about Colonial Medicine?', 215–16.

61 Jock McCulloch, *Asbestos Blues: Labour, Capital, Physicians and the State in South Africa* (Oxford: James Currey, 2002); Randall Packard, *The Making of a Tropical Disease: A Short History of Malaria* (Baltimore: Johns Hopkins University Press, 2007).

62 Adriana Petryna, *When Experiments Travel: Clinical Trials and the Global Search for Human Subjects* (Princeton: Princeton University Press, 2009); Tanya Lyons, 'Globalisation, Failed States and Pharmaceutical Colonialism in Africa', *Australasian Review of African Studies* 30 (2) (2009), 68–85.

63 Richard Bowring, letter, *London Review of Books* (11 March 2010), 4.

Select Bibliography

Bell, Heather, *Frontiers of Medicine in Anglo-Egyptian Sudan, 1899–1940* (Oxford: Oxford University Press, 1999).

Echenberg, Myron, *Black Death, White Medicine: Bubonic Plague and the Politics of Public Health in Colonial Senegal, 1914–1945* (Oxford: James Currey, 2001).

Fassin, Didier, *When Bodies Remember: Experiences and Politics of AIDS in South Africa* (Berkeley: University of California Press, 2007).

Flint, Karen, *Healing Traditions: African Medicine, Cultural Exchange, and Competition in South Africa, 1820–1948* (Athens: Ohio University Press, 2008).

Good, Charles M., *The Steamer Parish: The Rise and Fall of Missionary Medicine on an African Frontier* (Chicago: University of Chicago Press, 2004).

Hunt, Nancy Rose, *A Colonial Lexicon of Birth Ritual, Medicalization, and Mobility in the Congo* (Durham, NC: Duke University Press, 1999).

Livingston, Julie, *Debility and the Moral Imagination in Botswana* (Bloomington: Indiana University Press, 2005).

Parle, Julie, *States of Mind: Searching for Mental Health in Natal and Zululand, 1868–1918* (Scottsville, South Africa: University of Kwazulu-Natal Press, 2007).

Schumaker, Lyn, Diana Jeater, and Tracy Luedke (eds), 'Histories of Healing: Past and Present Medical Practices in Africa and the Diaspora', *Journal of Southern African Studies*, Special Issue, 33 (4) (2007).

Silla, Eric, *People Are Not the Same: Leprosy and Identity in Twentieth-Century Mali* (Oxford: James Currey, 1998).

Thomas, Lynn, *Politics of the Womb: Women, Reproduction, and the State in Kenya* (Berkeley: University of California Press, 2003).

10

History of Medicine in Australia and New Zealand

Linda Bryder

The historiography of medicine in Australia and New Zealand has followed a similar trajectory to the history of medicine elsewhere, moving from heroic and progressive medical history to analytical and discursive ways of viewing the past that aim to contribute to a deeper understanding of the social, political, and cultural facets of earlier societies. The study of the history of medicine in Australia and New Zealand can offer specific contributions to the history of medicine, however, through an examination of the transfer of Western medical knowledge to new societies, and the interaction between Western science and health professionals and non-Western peoples over the past 200 years. Much of that history to date has focused on colonization in Africa and Asia. Australia and New Zealand differ from these other colonial encounters, in that they quickly became 'white settler societies' in which the newcomers numerically dominated indigenous people. As Australian historian Alison Bashford noted, Australian history (and she could have added New Zealand) unsettled the usual classifications in colonial historiography, for example with no neat categories of 'colonial' and 'postcolonial': colonization and nationalism took on different meanings in these predominantly white societies.[1] Nor can one generalize across Australia and New Zealand, as David Arnold noted in his overview of 'Medicine and Colonialism'.[2] Through local studies, scholars in these countries have made significant contributions to the history of medicine that are of relevance well beyond their specific societies.

This chapter considers trends in the writing of medical history in Australia and New Zealand since the 1980s. It traces the growing maturity of the discipline in this geographical region, as evidenced through the institution of a professional organization with its own journal. It pinpoints a particular contribution to the wider discipline, the history of the health of indigenous peoples and their interaction with the state as well as the current political resonances of such historiography. It also shows how the history of health and medicine contributes to a broader understanding of those societies and their sense of nationalism or identity. Finally it addresses transnationalism in health histories and the ways in which medicine in these societies reflected or deviated from developments in the international medical community. The chapter demonstrates how international histories of medicine, as well as local social and political histories, have been enriched by this expanding historiography.

The New Social History of Public Health and Medicine

In 1994, I published an overview of the history of public health in Australia and New Zealand, in an international collection edited by Dorothy Porter. The article focused on health policies in Australia and New Zealand since the establishment of these colonies in the early to mid-nineteenth century. Settlers came primarily from Britain, bringing with them their cultural baggage, including ideas about science, medicine, and the appropriate role of the state. Some of these ideas were an affirmation of trends in the 'Mother' country while others were a rejection of what they had left behind. The article showed how public health policies were not just transposed to the colonies but were adapted and transformed in the new environment according to dominant social and political values and changes over time. It discussed the prevailing nineteenth-century view among the new settlers that these colonies were a 'working-man's paradise' and how that led to a denial of health problems and to the belief that any extant problems were the responsibility of (and could be attributed to the failings of) the individual. By the early twentieth century, in common with other Westernized countries, new ideas about social and state responsibility emerged in the form of the modern welfare state; New Zealand led the way and became proud of its international

reputation as a 'social laboratory' in respect to social reforms. These
included the setting up of public health structures and preventive
health services—in the form of institutions (for childbirth, tuberculosis, and mental health, for example), health education, and sanitary
inspection. Further influenced by global factors such as the First
World War, the 1918 influenza epidemic, and the 1930s economic
depression, by the mid-twentieth century an extensive public health
and social welfare infrastructure was in place in Australia and New
Zealand though with local variants (for example, New Zealand's
universalist versus Australia's insurance-based health policies). An
important part of the history of health policy in Australia and New
Zealand was how colonization and consequent dispossession impacted
on the health of indigenous peoples and the ways in which the
respective governments responded—or failed to respond—to their
poor health following colonization. Official responses were influenced
by broader ideas about race and by settler interests.[3]

This overview was informed by the historiographical developments
of the 1980s, when historians of health, medicine, and welfare had
moved away from triumphalist and progressive approaches to their
subject-matter to a more sociological or social constructivist approach.
The new history was particularly concerned with understanding issues
of class, gender, and race, and the ways in which dominant (mainly
white male middle-class) sectors in society sought and maintained
power over minority groups. Issues such as eugenics and 'national
efficiency', which influenced health policies in other Western nations,
were also evident here, but with an added intensity in light of the large
neighbouring Asian populations that European (mainly British) settlers feared might swamp their new colonies.

In the 1990s, histories of health and medicine in Australia and New
Zealand expanded exponentially to provide a rich historiography—as
evidenced by the founding of a new journal, *Health and History*, the first
issue of which appeared in 1998. The setting up of a specialist journal
is generally seen as the mark of maturity of a discipline; this had
happened ten years earlier with the establishment of the *Social History
of Medicine* in Britain. *Health and History* was published by the Australian
Society of the History of Medicine (ASHM, renamed the Australian
and New Zealand Society of the History of Medicine in 2005).
Warwick Anderson, one of the first editors of the new journal,

reflected ten years later that there had been at the time 'a sense of maturity that seemed to demand some flagship publication'. He wrote that the new journal 'expansively encompassed the diversity of historical interests found in the ASHM', further explaining, however, that as editor he had tried 'to negotiate the perennial tensions between medically trained historians and those with higher degrees in history who express interest in medical issues'.[4]

The ASHM itself had been formed in 1984 and held its first national conference in 1989, at which time it had almost 300 members. Roy MacLeod, Professor of History at Sydney and an historian of science, dismissively said of the Society almost twenty years later that of the Society's 400 members only 10 were 'professionals' (by which he presumably meant academic historians of medicine).[5] This statistic was not, however, reflected at the Society's conferences. Even at the Society's first national conference in 1989 those presenters whose papers appeared in the conference proceedings and who had a medical background (17) were slightly outnumbered by those with a history or social science background (19).[6] The balance altered further over the years; a survey of the 2005 ASMH conference revealed that 61 presenters came with a history or social science background and 20 from a medical background. Of course, the category into which the 'historian' is placed does not necessarily affect the rigour of that history; either could produce 'good history'. In 2005 the new editor of *Health and History*, Hans Pols, commented that the quality of research in the history of medicine he encountered in Australia following his move from the United States to the Unit for History and Philosophy of Science, University of Sydney, in 2002 had far exceeded his expectations, and that the conferences of the Society 'proved to be an inspiring meeting place of health care professionals and historians engaged in an enduring dialogue'.[7]

Despite attempts by the Society and its journal to adopt a broad church approach, I am not suggesting that there was no tension between historians coming from different backgrounds or approaches. One of the offshoots of changing trends in medical history-writing since the 1980s had been a growing tension between medically trained historians and those coming from university history departments. Informed by medical sociology and social constructivist theories of history, the new social historians of medicine were sometimes perceived by medically trained historians to be engaged in 'doctor bashing', and some authors did indeed conceive of the medical profession as a monolithic block of middle-class white males intent on controlling the rest of the population. By the 1990s a tempering factor in the tension was the recognition by many social historians that the social constructivist model of history-writing was too formulaic and simplistic and overlooked the complexities and subtleties of the interactions between medicine and society, and between doctors and patients. A new hospital history that considered both medical developments and patients' perspectives was Janet McCalman's history of the Royal Melbourne Women's Hospital, which she entitled *Sex and Suffering* in order to stress the patient focus.[8]

In 2004, Randolph Albury, formerly professor of history and philosophy of science at the University of New South Wales, wrote positively of his collaboration with orthopaedic surgeon George M. Weisz of Sydney, and argued that 'collaboration with health practitioners can be highly fruitful both in generating research questions and in assessing the salience of evidence relating to these questions'. He described it as a form of cross-cultural collaboration.[9] Yet such collaboration was not always possible, with differing world views and approaches. The triumphalism of some modern accounts of the history of Western medicine was still subject to criticism; for example, Australian medical historian Suzanne Parry remained wary in 2003 of the 'persistent idea' in such accounts that 'Western science alone had, and continues to have, the solution to the improved health of people living in the tropics'.[10]

Indigenous Health On The Agenda

While medicine in the colonial context was conceptualized in the 1980s as a 'tool of Empire',[11] an historian of the African continent, Megan Vaughan, disputed this interpretation, arguing that at least in Africa European doctors were simply too thin on the ground and their instruments too blunt to be viewed either as liberators from disease (as the triumphalist view of medicine would have it) or as agents of oppression (as the social constructivists argued). Moreover, indigenous healing systems survived the onslaught of Western medicine and co-opted some of its features; indigenous people were not merely passive victims in the imperial onslaught.[12] This more nuanced and empirically based approach to the interaction between Western medicine and indigenous people was picked up in New Zealand and highlighted in a special issue of *Health and History* on Māori health in 2001. This incorporated aspects of health history such as Māori childbirth experiences, infant welfare, and the political and cultural relationship between biomedicine and colonialism. Commenting on the special issue, Ian Anderson, Director of a University of Melbourne Centre for the Study of Koori (Aboriginal) health and society, wrote that this collection of essays 'taps the methodological and intellectual edge of a growing body of historical analysis broadly focused on the historical relationship between Indigenous peoples, the State and biomedical institutions, and the specific contexts of settler colonial states such as New Zealand, Australia, Canada and the United States'. He explained that he had 'long noted the absence of an established critical inquiry on these issues' within his own Australian context and was therefore 'excited by the growing scholarship of these issues within the context of New Zealand colonial relations'.[13]

This special issue drew upon historical research conducted in the 1990s, much done by graduate students in unpublished dissertations and theses, and upon two important books that had appeared in 1999, by Derek Dow and Raeburn Lange.[14] With an eye to the available 'tools' of Western medicine, in his history of the New Zealand government's health policies towards Māori, Dow offered a more nuanced account than had hitherto been provided. On the one hand, he showed that Western medicine was not simply a 'gift of civilization' bestowed on the Māori people; he used the phrase 'benevolent self-interest' to describe some health initiatives. On the other hand, he challenged some of the more strident political statements about the effects of colonization on Māori health and the neglect by the dominant white population.[15] Dow discussed various policies the government enacted and financed, and which doctors supported and administered, in an attempt to improve Māori health. Lange focused more closely on the first two decades of the twentieth century and the involvement in Māori health of the first generation of Māori doctors. In both histories, Māori were shown to play an active part in health policy development; they were far from passive victims of colonization. Mason Durie, a psychiatrist and Māori leader who turned to history with a more explicit political agenda, had earlier stressed the Māori ability to survive and eventually flourish in the face of new challenges, through adaptation and agency.[16] This historiography was further developed in the following years; for instance in 2006, Angela Wanhalla published an article on health and housing in Māori communities in the 1930s and 1940s. In this article she discussed housing as a form of Europeanization of Māori society, but also showed that the notion of the 'home' and its relationship with Māori health was constantly negotiated by government officials and Māori communities, and that Māori families only 'selectively adopted western spatial usages of the home'.[17]

In 2007, Ian Anderson himself edited a special issue of *Health and History* on Aboriginal health history, together with his colleague Kim Humphery. In his editorial, Anderson commented on the 'relatively patchy' development of a historical focus on Aboriginal health, in contrast to Māori health. He explained how the Māori health issue had prompted him and Humphery to bring together a similar collection for the Australian context. The collected essays followed three themes: the Aboriginal experience of health and health services over time; the colonial and twentieth-century construction of medical knowledge in relation to Aboriginal health; and the recent history of Aboriginal health organizations. The language describing the treatment of Aborigines by the colonizers was much more damning than in the New Zealand studies: Anderson wrote how the articles provided evidence of the 'personal and collective memory of health and welfare systems as a terrain of moral policing, neglect, incompetence and spiritual violation'.[18] The authors in Anderson's issue were influenced primarily by anthropological and ethnographic studies; unlike their New Zealand counterparts, they drew less on secondary historical works or maybe there were fewer to draw upon. Much of the focus was on recent history and memories, though with a sense of the legacy of the past. For instance, Bronwyn Frederick's essay on Aboriginal women's health focused primarily on the 1990s but included the comment that:

> The destruction that began in 1788 continues to impact on Aboriginal peoples' lives, cultures, and health and wellbeing. Aboriginal peoples also know the impact that the history of colonisation has had on them and what it means in terms of health status. As is evident from Kay's statement [her interviewee], Aboriginal women know what this health status means in terms of the lived reality.[19]

One historical account of Aboriginal health that did not appear in the footnotes of any of the 2007 special issue essays was Judith Raftery's 2006 history of government policies and actions in relation to Aboriginal health in South Australia, perhaps showing how sometimes social anthropologists and historians continue to talk past each other.[20] Nor was there mention (apart from in Warwick Anderson's overview) of Gordon Briscoe's 2003 study: himself an Aboriginal scholar, Briscoe fulfilled the political demand that indigenous peoples write their own histories. Comparing medical services for Aborigines in Queensland and Western Australia between 1900 and 1940, Briscoe showed how the priority in both places was to prevent the spread of Aboriginal diseases into white communities; in Queensland (as the most segregated of the states) this generally meant isolating and limiting the mobility of the indigenous people, and in Western Australia (where authorities strongly favoured assimilation) it led to efforts to 'produce a dusky proletariat'.[21]

Like the authors of the 2007 *Health and History* issue, Raftery addressed the destructiveness of colonization, leading one reviewer to complain that she faced the danger of portraying Aborigines as 'victims and losers'.[22] This contrasts with Dow, Lange, and Durie's portrayal of the New Zealand situation. Perhaps the difference was partly a reflection of the reality of different cultural groups and social and political circumstances. Reviewing Dow's book, Janet McCalman wrote that for 'all the shortcomings of Maori health care and status since colonization, the marvel to an Australian historian is that a book can be written at all about Maori health and government policy that begins in 1840.'[23] As Warwick Anderson pointed out, the 'diversity of Indigenous experience and the patchiness of historical analysis defy any simple transnational comparison of health developments.'[24] Stephen Kunitz had attempted such a comparative study in 1994, reviewing the impact of European contact on indigenous peoples of the United States, Canada, Australia, and New Zealand. He argued that the major determinant of differences in contemporary health status was the different ways in which governments had dealt with indigenous peoples in the past. As Professor in a Department of Community and Preventive Medicine, Kunitz brought his scientific and epidemiological background to bear on his history-writing. He explained that for his comparative studies of the impact of colonization on respective colonial peoples, he aimed to assess the importance of certain variables by setting up controls. Thus:

> once disease ecology has been held roughly constant, one can see more clearly the ways in which colonial policy and political institutions have shaped the affairs of indigenous peoples. And once policy has been held constant, one can see more clearly how culture can make a difference. And once culture has been held constant, one can see how gender and status make a difference.[25]

A social or cultural historian might question such scientific precision, arguing that an epidemiological model could easily overlook local vagaries; and, indeed, for New Zealand, Kunitz relied primarily on the work of a demographer, Ian Pool, rather than the work of historians.[26]

Writing on any aspect of indigenous histories since the 1980s has had political resonance; historical consciousness has been closely allied to current political activism and government responses. Australian historian Suzanne Parry commented that indigenous history would remain on the political agenda 'as long as Australian governments remained embroiled in issues of reconciliation, and the welfare of indigenous people is subject to international scrutiny', and as long as the 'legitimacy of actions taken in Australia's colonial past is hotly contested'.[27] An example of contemporary interest in historical writing was Warwick Anderson's 2002 study of white Australia, which led to Adelaide University apologizing to Aboriginal peoples for the 'barbarous' experiments some of its scientists had performed in the 1930s.[28] This was research into 'half-caste' Aboriginals in various parts of Adelaide, Victoria, Western Australia, and Queensland (with 'half-castes' defined as persons with some Australian ancestry who did not qualify as white, a cohort estimated at 23,000 in 1936), in which the researchers measured their physiology and anatomy, including blood groups and genealogies, offering lollies and cigarettes as bribes.

As long as the health differentials between the dominant white population and indigenous peoples remain, the effects of colonization will continue to have political currency. In New Zealand, health forms a background to many claims under the Treaty of Waitangi Act 1974, which established a tribunal to make recommendations on compensation claims by Māori for loss of possessions and for infringements of the 1840 Treaty of Waitangi.[29] Yet historians must be wary of broad generalizations about the health effects of colonization, neither seeing the colonizing state as monolithic and all-powerful nor viewing indigenous peoples as passive victims. More in-depth studies of interactions within health systems, in both Australia and New Zealand, are required for a balanced perspective.[30] Under the ostensibly antiquarian title of 'What Professor Cleland Did in His Holidays', in 2002 David Thomas provided an incisive study of Australian Professor John Burton Cleland's research into indigenous health in the first half of the twentieth century. He portrayed Cleland as a typical scientist of his day, collecting data about Aboriginal bodies and sickness in the same way as he observed and collected specimens of birds, plants, and animals. However, he also argued that, although Cleland himself portrayed the research encounter as Aboriginal people submitting to white power, there was evidence of Aboriginal choice and resistance.[31]

White Australia and National Identity

One way in which the history of Aboriginal health has entered the Australian historiography is not through a direct assessment of policy relating to their welfare or their responses, but rather through perceptions of them as 'other'. This has been part of the attempt to explain the construction of a white settler identity, citizenship, and nationalism. Upon federation of the Australian colonies in 1901, the new federal government passed the Immigration Restriction Act and the Pacific Island Labourers Act (outlawing 'coloured labour'), which formed the basis of what became popularly known as the 'White Australia' policy. This impacted not only upon immigration (particularly from Asia) but also upon popular perceptions of, and policies towards, indigenous and white Australians. The policy was based on an ideal of protecting white Australia; as Alison Bashford wrote, it was 'explicitly a nationalism of race'.[32]

Australian historians have begun to look at the ways in which public health, scientific discourses, and cultural representations of diseases buttressed the ideas of white Australian nationalism. This history-writing was influenced not so much by sociological understandings of disease and medicine that had emerged in the 1980s, but rather by cultural anthropology. Again, this was an avenue explored in the African context by Megan Vaughan, who sought to understand cultural representations of disease and the influence of medical ideas and practices on the shaping of colonial images of Africa.[33] Suzanne Parry brought a similar approach to her studies of tropical medicine in northern Australia and the influence of the white Australia policy in that area. She argued that 'an important component in the process of identity formation amongst colonizers was to position indigenous people and to thus "identify" them in particular ways'. She showed how the discourse of tropical medicine, validated by its scientific status, was used to legitimize the subjugation of indigenous people, and how the 'medicalised body became an important signifier of difference between white settler and indigenous people in northern Australia'.[34] Crucial to the development of a white settler society in the north was the defining of Aborigines as 'other', as diseased and therefore a direct threat to northern development and in need of control. Asian people, persistently viewed as diseased and contaminating, were to be excluded as far as possible from this white society. As historian David Walker wrote, the 'diseased and turbulent East provided a convenient and culturally powerful threat for the Australian colonies as they sought the common ground of nationhood at the end of the nineteenth century'.[35] Another perceived way of nation-building was to make the environment safe for white settlement; this was the primary goal of the new Institute for Tropical Medicine established in Townsville in 1910. The first director of the Institute from 1910 to 1920, protozoologist Anton Breinl, defined this goal: 'The object of tropical medicine involves much more than the study of parasites and diseases occurring in the tropics; it comprises in its working sphere the welfare and life of the white man under new, and, to him, artificial conditions.'[36]

Suzanne Parry's work related specifically to leprosy, as she explained in *Health and History*: 'The health of the people and confirmation of the successful transplanting of white bodies to an alien land were essential to the emerging Australian identity, and leprosy, a disease which stamped its claim on the body so visibly, posed a threat to the process of physical adaptation.'[37] In his research on the Institute for Tropical Medicine, Andrew Parker also linked tropical medicine and the white Australia policy, showing how the maintenance of 'normal health' required the protection of society from diseases, and 'more sinisterly' from their transmission by certain diseased populations.

He cited Sir Raphael Cilento, later Director-General of Health and Medical Services in Queensland from 1934 to 1946, who declared in 1928 that the major factors in tropical white settlement in the early twentieth century had been not only 'the successful institution of adequate measures of preventive medicine' and 'the continual increase in locally-born inhabitants', but also 'the exclusion of races with lower standards of life and higher rates of disease and reproduction'.[38]

Two important studies detailing the relationship between health, medicine, and the white Australia policy were Warwick Anderson's *The Cultivation of Whiteness* and Alison Bashford's *Imperial Hygiene*. Reviewing Bashford's book, Anderson commented:

> Some might say that one cannot carve out a realistic history of medicine and public health in this country [Australia] without paying attention to the invading tendrils and suckers of race, hygiene and nation. Others will dismissively point to the influence of fashion in the contemporary academic allotment. But, whatever the cause, it is clear that Australians are leading other historians of medicine in exploring the links between public health policies and estimates of civic virtue. *Imperial Hygiene*, while it covers some familiar grounds, adds notably to this enterprise.[39]

It was a trend to which Anderson himself was a major contributor. In *The Cultivation of Whiteness*, he sought to show how biomedical science and public health 'helped to set a nation's racial agenda', arguing that the 'medical construction of white Australia provides another lens through which we may view two hundred years of European settlement'. His book was divided into three sections, dealing with the 'Temperate South', the 'Northern Tropics', and 'Aboriginal Australia'. Anderson pointed out that science and medicine were 'often left out of the conventional histories of Australia—or of any other country for that matter'. He aimed to explore 'fears of white degeneration in the antipodes, whether from an exhausting depleting environment, from contact with other races, or from urban life'. In the final section, he discussed how doctors came to believe that it was beneficial to remove 'half-caste' children from their families so that they would grow up white and become 'good' white citizens, leading to the tragedy of the 'stolen generations'. He showed how scientific experiments were conducted on Aboriginal people in the 1930s. After the Second World War, he explained, race as a scientific concept largely collapsed, but the research and policies derived from it left a lasting legacy; it took a 1967 referendum to start dismantling Australia's highly racialized society by allowing indigenous people to be counted in the census for the first time, thus finally granting them the vote and citizenship.[40]

Bashford's book is complementary to Anderson's. Hers was a 'cultural history of borders, hygiene and race' from the 1860s to the Second World War. Rather than focusing on scientific ideas *per se*, Bashford addressed the relationship between public health and liberal governance in Australia, under the unifying concept of 'hygiene'. Her book covered such topics as vaccination, smallpox, tuberculosis, leprosy, quarantine, immigration, and venereal disease. She showed how vaccination and the accompanying certificate created an early form of identification for travel, effectively becoming a passport; thus public health was implicated in nation-building. She contrasted responses to tuberculosis (the 'white plague') and leprosy (the 'imperial disease'). In her chapter on quarantine, she argued that national maritime quarantine was integral to the rise of Australian nationalism. Quarantine regulations assisted Australians to regard themselves as inhabitants of a nation-state with borders, a 'pure' island to be protected from invading diseases. In the chapter on immigration, she discussed the formulation of the white Australia policy at the turn of the century and the ways in which public health assisted in its maintenance. She noted that 'whiteness was the national identity of this particular twentieth century imagined community'. 'Whiteness' and 'purity' were also implicated in the domestic social hygiene and eugenic movements of the interwar years, the subjects of the last chapter of her book. Here she discussed isolation and sterilization as forms of eugenic *cordons sanitaires*, boundaries protecting future generations from disease.[41]

Public health and national identity have not been explored in the New Zealand context as in Australia. However, much has already been written on racial stereotypes and medical attitudes to Māori in the nineteenth century, suggesting a typecasting of them as 'other'.[42] In her review of Derek Dow's book on Māori health and government policy, McCalman suggested taking this historiography further. In her opinion, 'this New Zealand story now needs another history that locates it in the wider debates over race fitness, germ theory and of the

relationship between civilization and sanitation. New Zealand distinctiveness is too important to the global historiography of colonisation for
it to be discussed only in the Antipodes.'[43] Some historians of medicine
have employed public health issues to define New Zealand in relation to
Britain. Philippa Mein Smith's article on the history of the nation's milk
production and consumption offers a brief foray into the history of New
Zealand's self-identity and its relationship with the imperial centre
through the lens of public health.[44] Pamela Wood's cultural history of
dirt similarly suggested a new way of looking at New Zealand's colonial
past, by addressing the part 'dirt' and public health played in the vision
and realization of a New World settlement.[45]

While there is scope for more work in the cultural history of ideas in
relation to health and medicine, an eye to the social context remains
important. In his review of Bashford's book, Warwick Anderson
complained that, 'as in the Foucauldian schema, there is little recognition of contestation of these discourses on hygiene, nor of public
indifference to, or subversive appropriation of, the plans of the public
health officer. (In other words, there could be as much on the actual
crossing, or disregard, of the boundaries as on their construction.)'[46]
Many historians would agree with this assessment, and continue to
value social, local, and empirical history, arguing for the importance
of understanding the ways in which individuals responded to the
cultural imperatives. Anderson noted in his review that it would also
have been helpful to locate more precisely the agents of racial hygiene,
in their social, institutional, and geographical settings. An example of
the neglect of such detail in Bashford's account relating to the major
actors is the information provided on Cilento. Bashford's index includes
only eight references to Raphael Cilento: in the first we learn that he
was 'Chief Medical Officer and chief Protector of Aborigines' (though
no dates are given other than 'after 1940'); the other references are to
his views. One can refer to a dictionary of biography for more detail,
and yet some assessment of him as an individual by Bashford herself
would surely help to explain his views and actions.

Transfer of Knowledge and Transnationalism

When Warwick Anderson regretted that Bashford's 'agents of
hygiene' were not placed in their wider setting, he suggested that

there was much more to say about broader connections: 'we have yet to explore properly the many connections between Australian events and adjacent colonial developments. Practices of hygiene, and the careers of the advocates of hygiene, travelled through South-east Asia, Australia and the Pacific, but historians have rarely followed. Cilento, for example, moved between colonial Malaya, tropical Australia and Papua and New Guinea.' He indicated that along with Lenore Manderson and Donald Denoon, he had begun to track some of these intercolonial connections.[47] This transfer of knowledge and expertise does not just apply to that geographical area, however, but must be set in an imperial and even international context. James Gillespie and later Annie Stuart addressed this wider interaction when they focused on the involvement of the American philanthropic organization the Rockefeller Foundation in the early-twentieth-century hookworm campaign in Australia and its territories, leading the latter to comment on the Rockefeller's 'global influence over modern public health and medical systems'.[48] Medical historian Milton Lewis explained that he placed his Australian history of sexually transmitted diseases (STD) into an international context because 'historically, Australia was a political dependent of Britain and a cultural dependent of Britain, Europe and the US'. He adopted this comparative approach not only to show the influence of the older countries upon medical policies in Australia but also the differences, for example compulsion in interwar STD control in Australia compared with reliance on voluntary attendance at public STD clinics in Britain.[49] It could be added that New Zealand, unlike Australia, also opted for the voluntary approach.[50] These narratives contribute to our understanding of cultural, social, economic, and political factors that underlay responses to such diseases. Placing the medical practices of one particular institution, New Zealand's National Women's Hospital, into an international context also facilitated fresh insights into events that led to a significant government inquiry in 1987.[51]

Transnational links were often at an individual level. Most Australian and New Zealand doctors practising before the First World War had done their medical training in the United Kingdom, and many continued to undertake post-graduate training there after that time. Until 1962 in Australia and 1967 in New Zealand, the medical profession was organized locally as branches of the British

Medical Association, providing them personal access to the *British Medical Journal*. Many of those holding influential posts in health administration had connections with Britain. Dr J. H. L. Cumpston, for instance, described by Lewis as 'undoubtedly the most important figure in public health in Australia' in the twentieth century, had gained the London Diploma in Public Health (DPH) in 1906, and worked briefly at the Lister Institute of Preventive Medicine in London.[52] Dr J. S. C. Elkington, another leading figure in Australian public health, also held the London DPH. Both Dr J. A. Thompson, head of the Department of Public Health of New South Wales in its formative years from 1896 to 1914, and Dr W. C. Armstrong, Sydney's medical officer from 1898 to 1913 and recognized as the founder of the infant welfare movement in Australia, held a DPH from Cambridge. The founder of the infant welfare movement in New Zealand, Dr Truby King, gained the new BSc in Public Health at Edinburgh University in 1887. Dr J. M. Mason, appointed the first Chief Health Officer under New Zealand's Public Heath Act of 1900, had also been awarded a Cambridge DPH, as had Dr R. H. Makgill, who framed the 1920 Health Act in New Zealand. And so the list goes on; such connections persisted well into the twentieth century, showing New Zealand and Australia to be intimately connected with the metropolitan centre.[53] Ideas and the people themselves travelled freely within the British Empire and beyond; increasingly North America and Scandinavia were included in overseas study trips.

Imperial connections came under close scrutiny in Anne Crowther and Marguerite Dupree's study of the fortunes of 1,288 doctors who graduated from the Scottish universities in Edinburgh and Glasgow in the 1870s. Crowther and Dupree traced the careers of these graduates and highlighted medical networks. Of those they traced, sixty-nine ended up in Australia and eighteen in New Zealand. They showed how these antipodean practitioners remained abreast of European ideas through intercolonial conferences, medical societies, books, and journals. Interestingly in the light of comparative history and race relations mentioned above, Crowther and Dupree also noted: 'A major difference between the experience of the Australian and the New Zealand doctors was that the former rarely encountered, or mentioned, the indigenous people.'[54]

Transnationalism involves the study of connections but also the transfer of ideas and cultures across national borders. These ideas did not always simply travel in one direction—see for example, the influence of the New Zealand infant welfare reformer Sir Frederic Truby King in Britain.[55] And differences as well as similarities become explanatory. For example, how mental health and asylum developments played out in the colonial context contributes to a broader understanding of the history of psychiatry. Australian historian of psychiatry Stephen Garton recently explained:

> The dispossession of indigenous Australians, the marked gender disparities of colonial society, the ethic of custodialism that has afflicted Australian practices of institutionalisation since colonisation, the difficulties of governing a widely dispersed population, the struggle of the professional classes to gain a legitimate foothold in Australian society— all had a bearing on the character of the lunatic asylum in Australia.[56]

Understanding this distinctiveness helps to elucidate the social and cultural construction of medical knowledge and medical institutions. Yet the patient focus of much recent asylum history also contributes to the histories of colonial societies and migration, for example Barbara Brookes's work on the Seacliff Asylum, Dunedin, and Angela McCarthy's recent work on the Irish diaspora and the Auckland Asylum.[57] Another contribution to this genre is Catharine Coleborne's work on the case books relating to Chinese patients in a colonial asylum in Victoria, Australia.[58]

Conclusion

This overview is not intended as a comprehensive survey of the writing of the history of medicine in Australia and New Zealand, which has been influenced by and contributes to the broader medical historiography through its methodology and historical constructs. Rather I have chosen to highlight areas of distinctiveness, such as the interactions between medicine, race theory and race relations, and transnationalism. Just as Janet McCalman commented that Dow's book deserved an audience wider than that found in Australasia, so too are there many other areas of modern history of medicine where antipodean scholars are at the forefront of trends in medical history-writing and methodologies.

While the publication of a regionally based journal signalled the coming of age of the discipline in that part of the world, there is also the danger that having such a geographically based journal could lead to the ghettoization of scholarship from that region, with it not reaching the wide readership it deserves.

This chapter has attempted to signpost some potentially fruitful avenues for future historical research. There is clearly room for more nuanced work relating to the interaction between indigenous populations and officialdom, viewing the former neither as simply beneficiaries of the state nor as victims. Historians have explored how government policies endorsed or bolstered national identities but not how these imperatives were interpreted or received at grassroots levels. Finally, there is more work to be done in locating medical policies and developments in an international perspective. Medical historians have yet to investigate in depth the ways in which hospital, primary care, and public health systems were distinctive in this region and what this tells us about prevailing social attitudes and ideologies.

Seemingly poised on the edge of the world, these antipodean nations have perceived themselves as part of the Western world and yet are not Western; they have perceived themselves as white and British even, and yet are multicultural. Studies of their distinctiveness as well as similarities with older countries will continue to contribute to the historiography of public health and medicine.

Notes

1 Alison Bashford, *Imperial Hygiene: A Critical History of Colonialism, Nationalism and Public Health* (New York: Palgrave Macmillan, 2004), 3.
2 David Arnold, 'Medicine and Colonialism', in W. F. Bynum and Roy Porter (eds), *Companion Encyclopaedia of the History of Medicine*, vol. 2 (London/New York: Routledge, 1993), 1393–416.
3 Linda Bryder, 'A New World? Two Hundred Years of Public Health in Australia and New Zealand', in Dorothy Porter (ed.), *The History of Public Health and the Modern State* (Amsterdam: Rodopi, 1994), 313–34. For a similar more recent overview see Milton Lewis, 'Public Health in Australia from the Nineteenth to the Twenty-first Century', in Milton J. Lewis and Kerrie L. MacPherson (eds), *Public Health in Asia and the Pacific: Historical and Comparative Perspectives* (London/New York: Routledge, 2008), 222–49.
4 Warwick H. Anderson, 'Ten Years and More of *Health & History*', *Health and History* 10 (1) (2008), 1–4.

5 Roy MacLeod, 'Colonial Doctors and National Myths: On Telling Lives in Australian Medical Biography', in Mary P. Sutphen and Bridie Andrews (eds), *Medicine and Colonial Identity* (London: Routledge, 2003), 126.

6 Harold Attwood, Richard Gillespie, and Milton Lewis (eds), *New Perspectives on the History of Medicine: First National Conference of the Australian Society of the History of Medicine 1989* (Melbourne: University of Melbourne and the Australian Society of the History of Medicine, 1990).

7 Hans Pols, 'From the Editor', *Health and History* 7 (1) (2005), 1.

8 Janet McCalman, *Sex and Suffering: Women's Health and a Women's Hospital: The Royal Women's Hospital, Melbourne, 1856–1996* (Carlton, Victoria: Melbourne University Press, 1998). See also: Linda Bryder, *The Rise and Fall of National Women's Hospital* (Auckland: Auckland University Press, 2009); Judith Godden, *Crown Street Women's Hospital, 1898–1983* (Sydney: Allen & Unwin, 2017).

9 W. R. Albury, 'Broadening the Vision of the History of Medicine', *Health and History* 7 (1) (2005), 2–16.

10 Suzanne Parry, 'Tropical Medicine and Colonial Identity in Northern Australia', in Sutphen and Andrews (eds), *Medicine and Colonial Identity*, 104, citing F. E. G. Cox, *Illustrated History of Tropical Medicine* (London: Wellcome Trust, 1996), 154.

11 David Arnold (ed.), *Imperial Medicine and Indigenous Societies* (Manchester: Manchester University Press, 1988); Roy MacLeod and Milton Lewis (eds), *Disease, Medicine and Empire: Perspectives on Western Medicine and the Experience of European Expansion* (London/New York: Routledge, 1988).

12 Megan Vaughan, 'Healing and Curing: Issues in the Social History and Anthropology of Medicine in Africa', *Social History of Medicine* 7 (2) (1994), 283–95.

13 Ian Anderson, 'Editorial to Maori Health Special Issue, Guest Editors Linda Bryder and Derek A. Dow', *Health and History* 3 (1–2) (2001), 1–2.

14 Derek A. Dow, *Maori Health and Government Policy 1840–1940* (Wellington: Victoria University Press in association with the Historical Branch, Department of Internal Affairs, 1999); Raeburn Lange, *May the People Live: A History of Maori Health Development 1900–1920* (Auckland: Auckland University Press, 1999). The theses are listed in Linda Bryder and Derek A. Dow, 'Maori Health History Past, Present and Future', *Health and History* 3 (1) (2001), 3–12.

15 Linda Tuhiwai Smith, *Decolonizing Methodologies: Research and Indigenous Peoples* (New York: Zed Books; Dunedin: University of Otago Press, 1998).

16 Mason Durie, *Whaiora: Maori Health Development* (Auckland: Oxford University Press, 1998).

17 Angela Wanhalla, 'Housing Un/healthy Bodies: Native Housing Surveys and Maori Health in New Zealand 1930–45', *Health and History* 8 (1) (2006), 100–20.

18 Ian Anderson and Kim Humphery, 'Editorial: Aboriginal Health & History', *Health and History Special Issue: Aboriginal Health and History* 9 (2) (2007), 3.

19 Bronwyn Fredericks, 'Australian Aboriginal Women's Health: Reflecting on the Past and Present', *Health and History Special Issue: Aboriginal Health and History* 9 (2) (2007), 97.

20 Judith Raftery, *Not Part of the Public: Non-Indigenous Policies and Practices and the Health of Indigenous South Australians 1836–1973* (Kent Town, South Australia: Wakefield Press, 2006).

21 Gordon Briscoe, *Counting, Health and Identity: A History of Aboriginal Health and Demography in Western Australia and Queensland, 1900–1940* (Canberra, ACT: Aboriginal Studies Press, 2003).

22 Kyllie Cripps, 'Book Review of Raftery', *Health and History* 8 (2) (2006), 177.

23 Janet McCalman, 'Book Review of Dow', *Medical History* 46 (4) (2002), 600–1.

24 Warwick Anderson, 'The Colonial Medicine of Settler States: Comparing Histories of Indigenous Health', *Health and History Special Issue: Aboriginal Health and History* 9 (2) (2007), 150.

25 Stephen Kunitz, *Disease and Social Diversity: The European Impact on the Health of Non-Europeans* (New York/Oxford: Oxford University Press, 1994), 23, 177.

26 D. Ian Pool, *Te Iwi Maori: A New Zealand Population, Past, Present and Projected* (Auckland: Auckland University Press, 1991).

27 Parry, 'Tropical Medicine and Colonial Identity in Northern Australia', 103.

28 Warwick Anderson, *The Cultivation of Whiteness: Science, Health and Racial Destiny in Australia* (New York: BasicBooks, 2003).

29 Linda Bryder, 'Health Citizenship and "Closing the Gaps": Maori and Health Policy', in Astri Andresen, Tore Gronlie, William Hubbard, Teemu Ryymin, and Svein Atle Skalevag (eds), *Citizens, Courtrooms, Crossings: Conference Proceedings*, Report 10–2008 (Bergen: Stein Rokkan Centre for Social Studies, December 2008), 55–66.

30 For such a study in New Zealand, see Linda Bryder, 'They do what you wish; they like you; you the good nurse!' Colonialism and Native Health Nursing in New Zealand, 1900–1940', in Helen Sweet and Sue Hawkins, eds, *Colonial Caring: A history of Colonial and Post-colonial Nursing* (Manchester, Manchester University Press, 2015) 84–103.

31 David Thomas, 'What Professor Cleland Did in His Holidays: Collecting Expeditions to Central Australia as Indigenous Health Research, 1925–39', *Health and History* 4 (2) (2002), 57–79.

32 Bashford, *Imperial Hygiene*, 3.

33 Vaughan, 'Healing and Curing'.

34 Parry, 'Tropical Medicine and Colonial Identity in Northern Australia', 103–24.

35 David Walker, *Anxious Nation: Australia and the Rise of Asia, 1850–1939* (Brisbane: University of Queensland Press, 1999); idem, 'Review Essay: A Sunburnt Country: Reflections on Race, Whiteness and the Geopolitics of Settlement in Australia', *Health and History* 4 (2) (2002), 118–24.

36 Bashford, *Imperial Hygiene*, 159.
37 Suzanne Parry, '"Of Vital Importance to the Community": The Control of Leprosy in the Northern Territory', *Health and History* 5 (1) (2003), 1. On leprosy history, see also Anne O'Brien, '"All Creatures of the Living God": Religion and Leprosy in Turn of the Century Queensland', *History Australia* 5 (2) (2008), 40.
38 Andrew Parker, 'A Complete Protective Machinery: The AITM, 1911–28', *Health and History* 1 (2 & 3) (1999), 190.
39 Warwick Anderson, 'Book Review', *Health and History* 6 (2) (2004), 111.
40 In New Zealand, Māori were included in universal manhood suffrage introduced in 1889, and in universal suffrage from 1893.
41 Bashford, *Imperial Hygiene*. See also Alison Bashford and Claire Hooker (eds), *Contagion: Historical and Cultural Studies* (London: Routledge, 2001); Carolyn Strange and Alison Bashford (eds), *Isolation: Places and Practices of Exclusion* (New York: Routledge, 2003); Alison Bashford (ed.), *Medicine at the Border: Disease, Globalization, and Security, 1850 to the Present* (New York: Palgrave Macmillan, 2006). On quarantine and identity, see K. Maglen, 'A World Apart: Geography, Australian Quarantine and the Mother Country', *Journal of the History of Medicine and Allied Sciences* 60 (2) (2005), 196–217.
42 Malcolm Nicolson, 'Medicine and Racial Politics: Changing Images of the New Zealand Maori in the Nineteenth Century', in Arnold (ed.), *Imperial Medicine and Indigenous Societies*, 66–104; James Belich, *Making Peoples: A History of the New Zealanders: From Polynesian Settlement to the End of the Nineteenth Century* (Auckland: Penguin, 2007).
43 McCalman, 'Book Review', 600–1. See also: Katrina Ford, 'Race, disease and public health: perceptions of Maori health', in Mark Jackson (ed.), *The Routledge History of Disease*, (London: Routledge, 2016), pp. 239–58.
44 Philippa Mein Smith, 'New Zealand Milk for "Building Britons"', in Sutphen and Andrews (eds), *Medicine and Colonial Identity*, 79–102.
45 Pamela Wood, *Dirt: Filth and Decay in a New World Arcadia* (Auckland: Auckland University Press, 2005).
46 Anderson, 'Book Review', 111.
47 Ibid.
48 James Gillespie, 'The Rockefeller Foundation, the Hookworm Campaign and a National Health Policy in Australia 1911–1930', in Roy MacLeod and Donald Denoon (eds), *Health and Healing in Tropical Australia and Papua New Guinea* (Townsville: James Cook University of North Queensland, 1991), 64–87; Annie Stuart, 'We Are All Hybrid Here: The Rockefeller Foundation, Dr Sylvester Lambert, and Hookworm in the South Pacific', *Health and History*, 8 (1) (2006), 80–99.
49 Milton Lewis, *Thorns on the Rose: The History of Sexually Transmitted Diseases in Australia in International Perspective* (Canberra: Australian Govt Pub. Service, 1998).
50 Antje Kampf, *Mapping Out the Venereal Wilderness: Public Health and STD in New Zealand 1920–1980* (Berlin: Lit., 2007).

51 Linda Bryder, *A History of the "Unfortunate Experiment" at National Women's Hospital* (Auckland: Auckland University Press, 2009), reprinted as Linda Bryder, *Women's Bodies and Medical Science: An Inquiry into Cervical Cancer* (London: Palgrave Macmillan, 2010).

52 Milton Lewis, 'Introduction', in J. H. L. Cumpston, *Health and Disease in Australia: A History*, ed. M. J. Lewis (Canberra: AGPS Press, 1989), 1, 2.

53 Peter Graeme Hobbins, '"Outside the Institute There is a Desert": The Tenuous Trajectories of Medical Research in Interwar Australia', *Medical History*, 54 (2010), 1–28.

54 M. Anne Crowther and Marguerite W. Dupree, *Medical Lives in the Age of Surgical Revolution* (Cambridge/New York: Cambridge University Press, 2007), 278.

55 Philippa Mein Smith, *Mothers and King Baby: Infant Survival and Welfare in an Imperial World: Australia 1880–1950* (Basingstoke: Macmillan, 1997); Linda Bryder, *A Voice for Mothers: The Plunket Society and Infant Welfare 1907–2000* (Auckland: Auckland University Press, 2003).

56 Stephen Garton, 'Asylum Histories: Reconsidering Australia's Lunatic Past', in Catharine Coleborne and Dolly MacKinnon (eds), *'Madness' in Australia: Histories, Heritage and the Asylum* (Perth, WA: API Network, Curtin University of Technology, 2003), 21.

57 Barbara Brookes and Jane Thomson (eds), *'Unfortunate Folk': Essays on Mental Health Treatment, 1863–1992* (Dunedin: University of Otago Press, 2001); Angela McCarthy, 'Ethnicity, Migration and the Lunatic Asylum, Early Twentieth Century Auckland, New Zealand', *Social History of Medicine* 21 (2008), 47–65.

58 Catharine Coleborne, 'Making "Mad" Populations in Settler Colonies: The Work of Law and Medicine in the Creation of the Colonial Asylum', in Diane Kirby and Catharine Coleborne (eds), *Law, History, Colonialism: The Reach of Empire* (Manchester: Manchester University Press, 2001), 118.

Select Bibliography

Anderson, Warwick, *The Cultivation of Whiteness: Science, Health and Radcial Destiny in Australia* (Carlton, Victoria, 2002).

Bashford, Alison, *Imperial Hygiene: A Critical History of Colonialism, Nationalism and Public Health* (New York, 2004).

Bryder, Linda (ed.) *A Healthy Country: Essays on the Social History of Medicine in New Zealand* (Wellington: Bridget Williams Books, 1991).

Bryder, Linda, 'A New World? Two hundred Years of Public Health in Australia and New Zealand', in Dorothy Porter, ed., *The History of Public Health and the Modern State* (Amsterdam, 1994), 313–34.

Coleborne, Catharine, *Insanity, Identity and Empire: Immigrants and Institutional Confinement in Australia and New Zealand, 1873–1910*, Studies in Imperialism (Manchester: Manchester University Press, 2015).

Dow, Derek A., *Maori Health and Government Policy 1840–1940* (Wellington, 1999).

Dow, Derek A., *Safeguarding the People's Health: A History of the New Zealand Department of Health* (Wellington, Victoria University Press, 1995).

Lange, Raeburn, *May the People Live: A History of Maori Health Development 1900–1920* (Auckland, 1999).

Lewis, Milton,'Public Health in Australia from the Nineteenth to the Twenty-first Century', in Milton J. Lewis and Kerrie L. MacPherson, eds, *Public Health in Asia and the Pacific: Historical and Comparative Perspectives* (London/New York: Routledge, 2008), 222–49.

Raftery, Judith, *Not Part of the Public: Non-Indigenous Policies and Practices and the Health of Indigenous South Australians 1836–1973* (Kent Town, 2006).

Smith, F. B., *Illness in Colonial Australia* (Melbourne, Australian Scholarly Publishing, 2011).

Sutphen, Mary P. and Andrews, Bridie, eds, *Medicine and Colonial Identity* (London, 2003).

Woodward, Alistair and Blakely, Tony, *A Healthy Country? A History of Life and Death in New Zealand* (Auckland, Auckland University Press, 2014).

11

Global and Local Histories
of Medicine

Interpretative Challenges
and Future Possibilities

Sanjoy Bhattacharya

References to global perspectives in medical history have been commonplace in recent years. At the same time, there has been little unanimity about what the concept 'global' means. Sometimes interchangeably used with terms such as 'transnational' and 'international', the term 'global' has been used by academics to propound a variety of different conceptual paradigms. For some historians, a focus on globality involves studying the attitudes and actions of individuals who worked both within and outside the confines of formal structures of governments within empires or nation-states. Studying a variety of themes and straddling a broad temporal frame, several of these works have dealt with the thoughts and actions of institutions and individuals in exploratory missions that helped fortify efforts to conquer territories and entrench mercantile interests,[1] as well as attitudes amongst members of migrant and settler communities as they entered into complex sets of engagements with multiple sponsors and pre-existing social frameworks in newly acquired possessions.[2] Other scholarship, generally dealing with developments at different points of the twentieth century, has tried to define global history as a theme requiring study of the agency of private individuals and organizations across relatively porous political borders of empires and nations.[3] Some of this work examines socioeconomic connections between Europe, the United

States of America, and their respective zones of influence through the dissemination and translation of tropical medicine.[4] Other elements of this historiography present long-term studies of specific diseases and programmes intended to limit their spread,[5] while there are those who describe the role of private enterprise in developing multifaceted and multidirectional trading arrangements in medicinal products.[6] There is another important strand in medical histories that have adopted a global perspective—a genre of work that examines the roles played by different United Nations organizations, such as the World Health Organization (WHO) and the United Nations Children's Fund (UNICEF), in national and international health programmes in the post-Second World War era (often in association with Scandinavian aid and development programmes).[7] All in all, this work is marked by a great diversity in research focus and mode of analysis.

Although the historiography is rich and has generally succeeded in making us aware of a variety of important new themes and issues, it is difficult to ignore limitations in perspective. The professed views and actions of a relatively small number of people are frequently used to describe the workings of large, complex formations: imperial edifices, national governments, and non-governmental organizations, as well as multifaceted social and political structures. Elitist and selective notions of globality and internationalism are the result, especially when medical trends and the unfolding of international health programmes in the developing world—or the 'global south'—are examined in constricted ways. A reliance on the voices of actors occupying senior positions in international agencies and national governments has caused scholars to either disregard or downplay local agency. This, in turn, has led their works to ignore the important point that contradictory visions coexisted at all points of time, within both state and society.[8] These trends are perhaps explicable by the fact that the recognition of ideological and practical variations in the field has the capacity to destabilize the cosy generalizations upon which some of the most simplistic notions of global history are built. Simply put, historians of global medical history need to work harder to bring in a wide cross-section of voices in their studies. Rather than assuming that one set of visions was always able to displace and dominate others, and that this resulted in the development and deployment of largely unified modes of practice, it might be more meaningful to develop complex analyses that assess the impact of the persistence of variations in the provision of health services. The challenge, therefore, is to develop conceptual frameworks that allow us to incorporate analyses of large numbers of opinions and to better understand how this affected trends in medicine and public health. Indeed, it is crucial that historians recognize the significance of mapping out a complex mosaic of theory and practice, wherein ideas were exchanged and often unrecognizably transformed (rather than just transmitted by one party and unquestioningly accepted by another), and different approaches to policy implementation remained fluid and often interdependent (rather than being monolithic and unchanging, based on the views of a specific constituency).

This chapter attempts to develop a more inclusive set of conceptual frameworks for global histories of health and medicine. It is based on the assessment of a very well-known global story: the programme to eradicate smallpox. It is a case study worthy of analysis, not merely because it has been well chronicled and rich archival resources are available, but also because its histories have been particularly prone to narrow notions of globality, primarily based on heroic descriptions of the roles played by relatively small groups of workers. This chapter consciously avoids being overly reliant on the published and publicly expressed views of a handful of senior officials attached to the WHO offices in Geneva. Instead, an effort is made here to study a variety of voices and to examine how a diversity of people carried out intricate negotiations with different political and social constituencies and helped to expunge variola. The approach here, which is also recommended as a mode of research, is to go behind the scenes to study views expressed in private, and then assess how the resulting convictions, discussions, and debates impacted on the unfolding of policy.

Troubled Preparations For Global Smallpox Eradication

If some retrospective writings are taken at face value, one could be forgiven for thinking that the so-called intensified phase of the global smallpox eradication programme was well under way in 1969.[9] Enthusiastic descriptions of developments are not completely unwarranted. At one level, developments within the Geneva office, from 1969 onwards, were quite striking. Where there had been widespread division, doubt, and apathy amongst senior WHO officials in the early 1960s, the situation was substantially more promising by the end of the decade. The smallpox eradication unit began to receive better financial backing from the WHO budget, its officials were allowed to set up and run a dedicated fund from within the confines of the organization's headquarters (HQ) and, perhaps most importantly, the unit's managers were being more openly supported by the Director General's office in their efforts to raise money, personnel, and vaccine for the ambitious projects planned for Asia and Africa. However, things were less rosy at other levels. Negotiations with national administrations were seldom smooth and agreements tended to be transient. Notably, WHO representatives had to reconcile themselves to paying a stiff price during their consultations with the Indian federal authorities in the period between 1967 and 1968. The retention of the Indian chapter in the global smallpox eradication programme was guaranteed only after the WHO HQ promised significant infrastructural support, intended to help run the so-called intensified campaign in the country on a day-to-day basis. Some early estimates suggested that the WHO would have to meet 50 per cent or more of these expenses, with national budgets making the rest of the necessary money and infrastructure available; most Indian officials expected the WHO to meet at least half of all the programme costs, but kept hoping for more money.[10]

Yet, such gestures of generosity were not easily made by the WHO in the face of severe resource crunches, especially in relation to the global smallpox eradication programme; this was symptomatic of a situation where WHO negotiators continually struggled to convince donors to provide prolonged support. Indeed, the Geneva-based smallpox unit struggled in 1967 and 1968 to identify adequate producers and stocks of freeze-dried vaccine for the anticipated needs of a global campaign.[11] For this reason, the WHO HQ expected national governments, like those of India and Pakistan, to enter into bilateral aid agreements with a variety of funding agencies, with the purpose of raising significant stocks of smallpox vaccine and money for making more health workers available in the field.[12] Apart from anything else, such problems made WHO negotiators keenly aware of the need to mobilize the support of governments of high-income countries on a continuing basis; several prolonged consultations resulted, which generated their own share of complications. Most of the rich, industrialized nations had already managed to eradicate smallpox within their territories through a variety of vaccination, isolation, and surveillance regimes. This led several European and American political leaders to wonder whether it was necessary or prudent to get involved in financing a worldwide programme aiming to stamp out the disease. To make matters worse, there was widespread doubt within donor nations about whether it was really ever possible to eradicate variola.[13]

In circumstances such as these, several incidents involving the importation of smallpox into Europe proved to be a strategic blessing for WHO negotiators.[14] These cases allowed advocates of smallpox eradication to point out, during consultations with governments and aid agencies, that no part of the globe was safe from variola. Smallpox, they argued convincingly, could be transmitted by the increasing numbers of people travelling by air, as well as those able to move across many miles of unregulated national political boundaries across the world. The possibility that variola might return—in both epidemic and endemic forms—to countries that had previously managed to get rid of the disease was frequently highlighted during negotiations. The presentation of such grim scenarios did not go unnoticed by European and American governments; countries such as the United States kept nervously eyeing the situation all over the world and its officials were particularly concerned by smallpox importations into Western Europe, due to the large numbers of air-travellers going in and out of the region.[15] Official apprehension about the possible re-entry of the disease into Europe and the Americas was stoked further by a realization that an entire generation of public health and medical workers was lacking in first-hand knowledge about the symptoms of the disease and the challenges of interrupting its spread through specialized isolation regimes. These anxieties were revealed, amongst other things, through governmental negotiations with WHO offices located within regions with endemic smallpox; these aimed to provide members of their public health and medical services access to smallpox cases and practical training in the running of isolation units.[16]

Fears about the uncontrolled spread of smallpox did not, of course, automatically translate into institutional and financial support for the proposed programme to eradicate the disease. In a situation where the WHO HQ remained disunited for a long time about the wisdom of

launching such an ambitious project, national funding agencies
baulked at providing high levels of support on a consistent basis;
instead, high-income nations invested more and more money in the
development of surveillance and containment regimes in airports,
shipping ports, and railheads, with the aim of identifying smallpox
in travellers and keeping them away from the general population.
Although expensive, the system was hardly foolproof: as case after case
showed, these surveillance networks were unequal to the task of
stopping the entry of variola infections, especially where people managed to get through the controls with falsified vaccination certificates,
where indicators of the disease were missed by inspectors, and where
individuals carried the disease across unregulated borders.[17]

Interestingly, the tide of donor disinterest began to turn from the
late 1960s, when the WHO's complex structures began to fall in line,
at least publicly, behind calls for the reinvigoration of national smallpox eradication campaigns and the interlinking of all this work on an
international and regional basis. This unity was well exemplified by
the WHO HQ's increasing willingness to highlight the long-term
financial benefits of eradicating smallpox globally through a variety
of high-profile events. The World Health Day celebrations of 1966
were a notable example; these sought to raise awareness about the
dangers from smallpox importations and highlighted the usefulness of
eradicating the disease. One of the messages underlined at this event
was to be repeated over and over again in the future, especially during
negotiations with government representatives associated with high-
income donor nations and the countries regarded as major reservoirs
of smallpox: it made sense to spend money on an expensive, drawn-out
global eradication programme, as this investment would be returned
many times over through the financial savings made by dismantling
structures for regular surveillance, containment, and vaccination.
Remarkably, senior WHO officials—including those driven by the
urge to prevent painful deaths from a damaging disease—recognized
the ability of this line of reasoning to attract the attention of hard-nosed
national administrators and loosen their budgetary purse-strings.[18]

Discussions held with agencies such as the US Agency for
International Development (USAID) and the Swedish International
Development Agency (SIDA) provide good examples of such trends; it
is worth noting that the monies made available by these agencies in

the first half of the 1970s were crucial to the expansion of the South Asian national smallpox eradication campaigns that were the cornerstone of the global campaign. It is also notable that almost all of these negotiations were time-consuming and were characterized by complicated twists and turns. This situation was mainly a product of the repeated overshooting of advertised timetables in focus areas such as India and East Pakistan/Bangladesh, and the resultant delays in the global programme; these operational difficulties kept stoking donor doubts about providing continued support, which could ultimately only be assuaged through a series of delicate consultations. Strikingly, these involved efforts to cajole—and sometimes also to frighten—funding agencies through suggestions that smallpox epidemics might uncontrollably spread across political borders.

A good case in point was the manner in which D. A. Henderson, Chief of the WHO Smallpox Eradication Unit, dealt with senior SIDA officials in Stockholm in 1973, when he was seeking to justify a request for an additional US$6 million for completion of work in India and Bangladesh:

> During the last two years, importations from the remaining endemic countries have occurred in smallpox-free countries such as Japan and the United Kingdom, and in 1972, the return of infected pilgrims from Iraq resulted in an epidemic in Yugoslavia. In spite of the controls imposed by health authorities on international travellers, every country is in danger until the last case of smallpox has been eliminated. The world's hope of eliminating the disease in 1974 is centred on the intensified campaign being carried out in the last four endemic countries. Particular attention is focussed on India and Bangladesh where logistics present special problems. Both these countries' governments have given their full support to this crash programme and the campaign has already given impressive results. But, we are now faced with great difficulties due to the increased price of petrol, insufficient transport facilities, and the lack of funds necessary for the provision of high-level supervisory staff. So as to avoid a serious cutback in the programme at this crucial stage when so many national and international efforts are being made to assure its success, the support of SIDA in the form of a contribution to the Special Account for the Smallpox Eradication Programme of the World Health Organisation would provide invaluable assistance at this vital time and would help to insure the realisation of the global eradication of smallpox.[19]

This fund-raising exercise was a success and it provided a crucial lifeline for the work being carried across the South Asian subcontinent.[20] Interestingly, this was not the last time that SIDA would be approached by the WHO HQ with entreaties for further assistance. As the Indian and Bangladeshi programmes continued well into the mid-1970s, senior Geneva-based officials were to turn to the agency for more money. One of these requests was sent during the summer of 1974, when an unexpected outbreak of smallpox in Bihar threatened to destroy all the gains of the past years.[21] SIDA provided an emergency infusion of funds at this juncture, not least as its officials did not want to see the considerable investments made in the global eradication programme go to waste.[22] And, as the global smallpox eradication programme continued into 1975, 1976, and 1977, its managers struggled to cope with continual financial difficulties. While it had been relatively easy to raise emergency funds to cope with serious outbreaks of variola, it was more difficult to convince donors to assist a programme that had kept missing declared timetables. Indeed, senior WHO officials began referring to instances of 'donor fatigue', causing people like Henderson to approach new organizations—such as the Canadian International Development Agency—for additional financial assistance to complete projects in India, Bangladesh, and Ethiopia.[23]

The WHO negotiators' efforts to mobilize aid in the form of vaccine stocks were no less complicated. At one level, they comprised extended consultations with various national governments about their willingness to donate vaccines to a special, voluntary 'account' maintained in Geneva. Created over time to meet the day-to-day needs of the global programme, as well as emergency requirements worldwide, this 'account' was the product of gifts of vaccine received from the USSR, USA, Britain, France, Denmark, Brazil, Switzerland, Sweden, West Germany, the Netherlands, Kenya, Finland, and a host of other countries in the late 1960s and the early 1970s.[24] Officials based within the WHO HQ maintained a further set of dealings with an international network of laboratories, whose facilities were used for the testing of the potency and safety of different batches of vaccine being readied for release in the field.[25] These dealings were not trouble-free. At different points of time in the late 1960s and 1970s, major donors like the USSR were unable—or perhaps unwilling—to provide the numbers of vaccine required by WHO departments supporting national smallpox eradication campaigns in Asia and Africa. Indeed, the Soviet authorities often preferred, in an effort to raise political goodwill, to supply vaccine through bilateral arrangements with national governments (India, for instance, received hundreds of millions of doses from the USSR in bilateral aid packages). In such a situation—especially in contexts where emergency anti-smallpox measures were being concurrently deployed in different parts of the world—there were instances where donations of vaccine were hurriedly accepted and distributed, and then found to be ineffective or capable of inflicting serious complications. A notable example occurred in 1972, when the WHO HQ sent stocks of vaccine gifted by the Yugoslav Government to Zambia. Certain batches of these prophylactics, which had been produced at the Institute of Immunology at Zagreb, were found to be capable of causing post-vaccinal encephalitis; to the great chagrin of all involved, these vaccines ended up being responsible for a couple of deaths in the African nation. The product was quickly withdrawn, but this experience taught senior WHO HQ officials some important lessons that were not forgotten for a long time; from this point onwards, more money, time, and effort was spent on the arrangement of independent checks on all vaccines donated for use in the global smallpox eradication programme and secondary investigations were frequently carried out on batches earmarked for release in the field.[26]

National Governments, WHO Negotiations, and Global Smallpox Eradication

It is clearly evident that prolonged interactions between WHO officials and different administrative agencies in countries with active smallpox eradication campaigns formed an important facet of the global programme. These dealings hinged on a number of important issues. In the face of continual resource constraints in the 1970s, discussions about the provision of extra funding for smallpox eradication loomed large in official deliberations. WHO administrators encouraged national governments to raise additional money from other countries and their aid agencies, through a series of bilateral arrangements. An interesting exchange in this regard occurred in 1973 between WHO South East Asia Regional Office (SEARO) operatives and the smallpox eradication unit in Geneva. The officials in the regional office were aware of negotiations between the United States and Indian federal authorities for the utilization of Rs. 2,600 crores (US$4 billion, at the exchange rates prevalent at the time), a fund that the former had developed through the sale, in rupees, of wheat to the subcontinent. While they were keen that at least some of these funds be used to buttress the national smallpox eradication programme budget, it was recognized that negotiations were likely to be protracted, difficult, and possibly unsuccessful.[27] It is important to remember here that many aid packages were discussed and finalized by political leaders without the knowledge of WHO officials, which meant that they had minimal amounts of influence on the ways these monies were distributed and used by national and local authorities. These aid packages were highly politicized, as they were deeply affected by prevalent administrative, economic, and social interests in 'donor' and 'recipient' countries; great efforts were, therefore, made by the latter to ensure that these funds were deployed 'autonomously', without any sort of external direction or interference. Interestingly, records of bilateral negotiations carried out with nations decolonized in the 1960s and early 1970s reveal ambivalent attitudes within their governments towards WHO regional offices, even in a situation where they were keen to work in close association with the WHO HQ.[28]

These situations coexisted side by side with other funding trends. It is, for instance, notable that the Indian and Bangladeshi governments ended up helping the global programme out financially at crucial junctures, as in 1974, when the WHO special account for smallpox eradication had almost been exhausted. Senior WHO HQ officials telegraphed its workers in New Delhi and Dhaka at this time, asking them to approach the Indian and Bangladeshi federal authorities for an emergency infusion of funds; these requests were upheld, to the relief of those involved in managing different elements of the global programme.[29] In India, for instance, the situation was rescued by her central government's decision to release US$2.5 million of SIDA funds to the WHO special account; these monies had initially been given to New Delhi through a bilateral arrangement, for nationally sponsored smallpox eradication work.[30] The persistent shortage of money also explains why senior WHO HQ officials supported efforts by the New Delhi-based unit to raise resources locally, from

both public and private financiers. The support mobilized with
J. R. D. Tata's help during the epidemic in Bihar state in 1974,
which generated extra health workers and doctors in the field, was
a particular triumph; the aid provided by Tata ensured that the
Indian and global programmes were not suddenly blown completely
off course.[31]

Yet other staffing challenges further complicated already difficult
administrative and political situations. As international workers were
unable to carry out all search and containment missions on their own,
they remained dependent on the support of all grades of national staff
to run projects on a day-to-day basis throughout the late 1960s and
1970s. These personnel could only be mobilized with the assistance of
national governments, which released workers from the central health
services to keep national smallpox eradication programmes operational; federal backing also helped in efforts to bring provincial and
district-level staff on side, even though these endeavours delivered
mixed results in a situation where local workers retained a high degree
of autonomy over their working lives. Uneven and shifting levels of
administrative support for smallpox eradication projects resulted,
which forced WHO workers to remain involved in an almost permanent condition of consultations with government officials in all national
contexts. A direct outcome of this was the attempt on the part of the
WHO HQ to deploy more international personnel for the management of touring search and containment teams in South Asia and East
Africa, which were the focus of the global programme by the mid-
1970s. However, this could not be done without the permission of
national governments, even though several federal health department
officials responded enthusiastically to the involvement of foreign
epidemiologists and administrators on WHO contracts of varying
lengths. In all cases, the prospective workers' dossiers had to be
submitted by the WHO HQ to national security agencies for examination, after which clearances were given to selected candidates; in
addition, constraints were placed on the movements of international
personnel, who were expected not to enter strategically sensitive areas
without special permits. The sheer complexity of the attendant negotiations is best highlighted by the WHO's experiences in relation to South
Asia and the Horn of Africa. In the early 1970s, the Indian government
announced that it would be unwilling to allow international personnel

attached to the WHO into the politically sensitive region of North Eastern India, which was a region composed of the states of Manipur, Nagaland, Tripura, Mizoram, Meghalaya, Sikkim, and the North Eastern Frontier Agency (now renamed Arunachal Pradesh). This stunted the plan to deploy intensive searches in an area about which extremely little information was available, but it was still generally acknowledged by WHO officials that it would be necessary to allow the Indian authorities to dictate the terms for personnel deployment.[32]

Visible in territories of countries such as Bangladesh, Mozambique, and Somalia, opposition to international workers was by no means limited to sections of federal government—some elements of provincial and district administration opposed colleagues who favoured the introduction of large numbers of foreign workers and demanded a control in their numbers. Their objection to international involvement at national and local levels is attributable to a variety of factors. Some of this antipathy was politically motivated. In several countries, government officials or powerful politicians with socialist leanings opposed the influx of workers from the United States and Western Europe and insisted, quite successfully, on the formation of mixed teams composed of workers from many nationalities. Resentment at the presence of international workers was also a product of the increased supervision of district-level health work carried out by the touring smallpox eradication teams; for some government officials this limited the scope of profitable private practice, which was generally carried out in clear contravention of their contracts of employment. In other cases, district-level health staff argued, not without reason at times, that the linguistic and administrative support required by foreign epidemiologists and personnel detracted from the time they had to complete their daily tasks. Indeed, some observers have pointed out that sustained involvement in search and containment campaigns caused health worker 'fatigue', which impacted adversely on their day-to-day performance in the long run; however, it needs to be noted that some of this criticism was rooted in the ideology of primary health care, which was becoming increasingly powerful in international circles and within influential sections of the WHO.[33] And at least some of the official resistance to the presence of international workers was a direct result of the dislike of campaigns of forcible vaccination that sometimes underpinned search and containment campaigns. Although relatively rare, news of such strategies spread far and wide, stoking hostility towards touring teams with foreign workers, 'outsiders' from urban centres, and 'collaborators' from inside the districts; the patterns and intensity of violent resistance were always variable, informed as they were by the interaction between a complexity of local racial, class, and gender considerations, and disparate sets of administrative and political agendas.[34]

Conclusion

The idea that the worldwide smallpox eradication programme was based on a definite set of ideas and actions, of a relatively small number of individuals, is commonplace; it is also a myth.[35] This chapter has highlighted the operational complexity of the global push to expunge variola. It aims to show how the regional, national, and local components of this multifaceted programme were important and consistently active sites of negotiation and adaptation, involving workers drawn from a variety of institutional and national backgrounds; their actions were deeply influenced by numerous political, economic, and social realities, which were in a constant state of flux. The underlying argument here is that it is not enough to study the interactions between a handful of select senior officials associated with the WHO's Geneva HQ and national governments, and then assume that their instructions were unquestioningly implemented by large numbers of field operatives. On the contrary, the calculations and activities of personnel associated with different WHO offices and departments, national and local administrations, and, not least, representatives of various funding and aid agencies are deserving of detailed examination, as they left indelible imprints on the so-called global smallpox eradication programme. At the same time, it is also important to recognize some associated points: that the beliefs of a handful of officials could never be comprehensively imposed across intricate governmental or social settings and that a great variety of opinions existed side by side within all institutional contexts, resulting in a complexity of intermeshing policy decisions. As the evidence presented here suggests, the coexistence of a plethora of ideas and actions in the field fostered complex patterns of activity that dismayed some and pleased others. The patterns and dynamics of response varied from place to place, at every level of administration and society; it is noteworthy that people could adopt very different attitudes in public and private, and also change their attitudes and actions over time and place. The regional, national, and local chapters of the global smallpox eradication programme, therefore, never took the predetermined paths that some senior WHO and government officials hoped they would.

The great challenge for the historian is to capture, in as rich detail as possible, the many intricacies of the worldwide efforts to eradicate variola; this alone would allow for the production of an inclusive global history of the run-up to an event widely presented as the greatest triumph of international public health cooperation in the twentieth century. This raises an important question. Are all available analyses of worldwide smallpox eradication efforts—and the many other international attempts to stamp out other diseases for that matter—'global histories'? Not necessarily. A lot of the existing work is over-reliant on the voices of few individuals, whose views are then presented as being representative of the thoughts and actions of the vast majority of participants. Disagreement and disengagement with the view of this small group of people is usually described in overly simplistic terms, often as incidents of resistance generally evoked by a host of cultural predispositions. This analytical approach is also visible in studies more willing to recognize the 'agency' of local actors; this can be explained by the fact that local contributions are often studied through the public statements and writings of small numbers of individuals, without adequate explanations about who they might have represented in complex social formations and whether their views were supported or questioned within them. What we have available at the moment, therefore, are palpably limited examinations of the two ends of a disease eradication programme involving participants from all over the globe—the top levels of organizations like the WHO HQ and some 'indigenous' voices that are supposed to be representative of the attitudes of everyone not completely supportive of the goal to permanently banish smallpox.

History writing is, of course, not a dispassionate exercise: the choice of objects and views being chosen for study is reflective of the historian's own analytical priorities, worldview, and political position. The act of privileging the views of a handful of senior officials within the

WHO HQ or the Centers for Disease Control in the United States
(CDC) could be said to be reflective of a Europe- or North America-
centric approach, especially where simplistic assumptions are also
made about the smooth diffusion of ideas from one part of the globe
to the other. At best, such scholarship can be described as constrained
global histories that manage to look at one of several important
elements of multifaceted health programmes run on a collaborative
basis by international organizations and complex national administrative setups; at worst, such historians are blinkered and exclusionary.
Therefore, one can argue that the preparation of rounded global
histories of international disease eradication and health promotion
activities requires a 'globalization' of the historian's vision. This is best
described as a willingness to recognize the importance of studying the
range of attitudes prevalent in the countries where health campaigns
were implemented, at different levels of state and society. Increasing
the complexity of a multilayered analysis of a public health project is
not necessarily negative from an intellectual standpoint. The pursuit
of a rounded, inclusive global history of smallpox eradication can
provide insights into a host of unexpected and important developments, which, when carefully studied in all their rich intricacy, can
reveal a range of important official and civilian voices, actions and
experiences; in this way, such history-writing can contribute to the
production of more policy-relevant scholarship.

Notes

1 For two fascinating studies within an impressive range of scholarship, see:
  Kapil Raj, *Relocating Modern Science: Circulation and the Construction of Knowledge
  in South Asia and Europe, 1650–1900* (Basingstoke/New York: Palgrave
  Macmillan, 2007); Sujit Sivasundaram, *Nature and the Godly Empire: Science
  and Evangelical Mission in the Pacific, 1795–1850* (Cambridge: Cambridge
  University Press, 2005).
2 Cristiana Bastos, 'Migrants, Settlers and Colonists: The Biopolitics of
  Displaced Bodies', *International Migration* 46 (5) (December 2008), 27–54;
  Erica Wald, 'From *begums* and *bibis* to Abandoned Females and Idle
  Women: Sexual Relationships, Venereal Disease and the Redefinition of
  Prostitution in Early Nineteenth-Century India', *Indian Economic and Social
  History Review* 46 (January/March 2009), 5–25; Margaret Jones, 'Heroines
  of Lonely Outposts or Tools of Empire? British Nurses in Britain's Model
  Colony: Ceylon, 1878–1948', *Nursing Inquiry* 11 (3) (2004), 148–60.

258 *Sanjoy Bhattacharya*

3 Kai Khiun Liew, 'Terribly Severe though Mercifully Short: The Episode of the 1918 Influenza in British Malaya', *Modern Asian Studies* 41 (2) (2007), 221–52.

4 See, for instance: Randall Packard, *The Making of a Tropical Disease: A Short History of Malaria* (Baltimore: Johns Hopkins University Press, 2007); and Warwick Anderson, *Colonial Pathologies: American Tropical Medicine, Race, and Hygiene in the Philippines* (Durham, NC: Duke University Press, 2006).

5 See, for example: James L. A. Webb, Jr., *Humanity's Burden: A Global History of Malaria* (Cambridge: Cambridge University Press, 2008); and Marcos Cueto, *Cold War, Deadly Fevers: Malaria Eradication in Mexico, 1955–1975* (Baltimore: Johns Hopkins University Press, 2007).

6 Guy Attewell, *Refiguring Unani Tibb: Plural Healing in Late Colonial India* (Hyderabad: Orient Longman, 2007); Maarten Bode, *Taking Traditional Knowledge to the Market: The Modern Image of the Ayurvedic and Unani Industry 1980–2000* (Hyderabad: Orient Blackswan, 2008); Madhulika Banerjee, *Power, Knowledge, Medicine: Ayurvedic Pharmaceuticals at Home and in the World* (Hyderabad: Orient Blackswan, 2009).

7 Niels Brimnes, 'Vikings against Tuberculosis: The International Tuberculosis Campaign in India, 1948–1951', *Bulletin of the History of Medicine* 81 (2) (2007), 407–30; idem., 'BCG Vaccination and WHOs Global Strategy for Tuberculosis Control 1948–83', *Social Science and Medicine* 67 (5) (2008), 863–73; Sunniva Engh, 'The Conscience of the World?: Swedish and Norwegian Provision of Development Aid', *Itinerario* 33 (2009), 65–82.

8 Warwick Anderson, 'Indigenous Health in a Global Frame: From Community Development to Human Rights', *Health and History* 10(2) (2008), 94–108; Sunil Amrith, *Decolonizing International Health: India and Southeast Asia, 1930–65* (Basingstoke: Palgrave, 2006).

9 R. N. Basu, Z. Jezek, and N. A. Ward, *The Eradication of Smallpox from India* (New Delhi: WHO SEARO, 1979).

10 Memorandum from D. A. Henderson, Chief, Smallpox Eradication, WHO HQ, Geneva, to Regional Director, WHO Regional Office for South East Asia [WHO SEARO], New Delhi, 24 July 1968, File 416, Box 193, World Health Organization/Smallpox Eradication Archives (WHO/SEA).

11 A general call made by the WHO Director General in July 1963 for gifts of free vaccine yielded disappointing results. Memorandum on Smallpox Eradication Special Account, WHO HQ, Geneva, 17 January 1964, File SPX-1, Box 545, WHO/SEA. Also see the letter from Ernest S. Tierkel, USAID, New Delhi, to D. A. Henderson, Chief, Smallpox Eradication, WHO HQ, Geneva, 4 April 1967, File 416, Box 193, WHO/SEA, and the memorandum from D. A. Henderson, Chief, Smallpox Eradication, WHO HQ, Geneva, to the Director, Communicable Diseases, WHO HQ, Geneva, 14 April 1967, File 416, Box 193, WHO/SEA.

12 For references to USAID assistance to the Indian national smallpox eradication programme, see, for instance, *Report from the Ministry of Health, Government of India, 1962–63* (New Delhi: Government of India Press, n.d.), 8, Shastri Bhavan Library, New Delhi, India. The press in India was well

aware of the significant levels of assistance provided by USAID through the 'PL-480' programme (this fund was created by the US Government through rupee sales of wheat to India; the money thus raised was offered to the Indian authorities for various developmental projects). An influential national newspaper calculated that PL-480 assistance had added up to Rs. 1,483.7 crores by February 1965 (an equivalent of US$3115.7 million at the time). See, 'PL-480 and India', *Hindustan Times* (9 February 1965). For references to the earmarking of PL-480 funds for the development and the running of the Indian campaigns and the role of bilateral funding arrangements in sustaining other South smallpox eradication programmes, see letter from D. A. Henderson, Chief, Smallpox Eradication, WHO HQ, Geneva, to C. Mani, Regional Director, WHO SEARO, New Delhi, 4 August 1967, File 416, Box 193, WHO/SEA.

13 See, for instance, memorandum from D. A. Henderson, Chief, Smallpox Eradication, WHO HQ, Geneva, to Regional Director, WHO SEARO, New Delhi, 24 October 1968, File 416, Box 193, WHO/SEA.

14 As air travel became cheaper and quicker in the 1960s, European government officials noted that this mode of transport began to be used by growing numbers of people, especially by those based in ex-colonial and colonial territories to travel to imperial metropoles. See, for instance, minutes for meeting held at the British Ministry of Health (MoH) on 5 January 1962, MH 55/2520, The National Archives, Kew, UK (hereafter, TNA). Several cases of smallpox importations into Britain, from Pakistan, were reported in January 1962. This caused great nervousness within the British MoH, which feared that these cases could snowball into a major epidemic. See, for instance, statement released by the MoH, 12 January 1962, MH 55/2520, TNA.

15 For good examples of US Government fears about cases of imported smallpox in Europe, see memorandum by J. G. Tefler, Chief, Division of Foreign Quarantine, US Government, to Chief, Epidemiology Branch, CDC HQ, Atlanta, 10 April 1962, Box 18875, Folder 14, Federal Record Center (FRC), East Point, Georgia, USA. The American media was, of course, not immune to such nervousness and the European smallpox outbreaks were reported by a variety of newspapers. See, for example, articles titled 'British Rush For Smallpox Shots As Sixth Person Dies', *Atlanta Journal* (15 January 1962), and 'Smallpox Won't Spread to US, Officials Say', *Washington Star* (20 January 1962), in Box 124597, Folder 3, FRC. At another level, it is worth noting that reports of smallpox outbreaks in Britain caused international restrictions to be placed on travellers from the country, which was considered to be both embarrassing and disruptive. See, for example, telegram from Sir R. Black, British representative, Hong Kong, to Secretary of State for the Colonies, 3 March 1962, MH 55/2520, TNA.

16 Memorandum from Director, Communicable Disease Section, WHO HQ, Geneva, to Regional Director, WHO SEARO, New Delhi, 28 October 1960, File SPX-1, Box 545, Smallpox Eradication Archives, WHO/SEA.

17 For a representative assessment of cases where smallpox symptoms were not recognized by port medical officials in Europe, which, in turn, resulted in localized outbreaks of the disease, see letter from R. T. Ravenhoff, Consultant Epidemiologist, CDC HQ, Atlanta, to J. Buchness, Foreign Quarantine (Europe), US Government, 1 June 1962, in Box 124597, Folder 3, FRC.

18 It is important to note this is a situation where speeches and writings by WHO officials about the long-term financial savings promised by global smallpox eradication have been taken far too literally by historians who downplay the variations in vision and policy implementation within a complex organization. See, for instance, Harish Naraindas, 'Charisma and Triage: Extirpating the Pox', *Indian Economic and Social History Review* 40 (4) (2003), 425–58.

19 'Draft Justification for Proposal to SIDA', by WHO SEARO, New Delhi, *c.*1973, appendix to File 948, Box 17, WHO/SEA.

20 Interview with Dr. D. A. Henderson, London, March 2007.

21 Letter from D. A. Henderson, Chief, Smallpox Eradication Unit, WHO HQ, Geneva, to Mr. R. Lickfett, Senior Programme Officer, SIDA, Stockholm, Sweden, 1 July 1974, File 948, Box 17, WHO/SEA.

22 Interview with Dr. D. A. Henderson, London, March 2007.

23 Letter from D. A. Henderson, WHO HQ, Geneva, to Mr. R. Binnerts, Connaught Laboratories, Canada, 24 June 1975, File 586, Box 321, WHO/SEA.

24 For communications exchanged between the WHO HQ and WHO regional offices with a range of national donors in the first half of the 1970s, see File 240, Box 304, WHO/SEA.

25 A select few—like the Rijks Institute based in Utrecht in the Netherlands, the Connaught Laboratories in Canada, and the Lister Institute of Preventive Medicine in Britain—were asked for assistance in the 1970s on a regular basis and, therefore, accorded the status of 'WHO reference laboratories'. See, for instance, the memorandum from Dr. Isao Arita, WHO HQ, Geneva, to Director, WHO Eastern Mediterranean Regional Office, Alexandria, 5 May 1970, File586, Box 321, WHO/SEA, and the letter from Dr. R. J. Wilson, Chairman and Director, Connaught Laboratories Limited, Ontario, Canada, to Dr. Ruperto Huarta, Chief, Communicable Diseases Section, Pan American Health Organization, Washington, DC, 29 January 1975, File 586, Box 321, WHO/SEA.

26 See restricted report on field trial of reactivity of smallpox vaccines (Krapina community), *c.*1973, attached to letter from Professor D. Ikic, Director, Institute of Immunology, Zagreb, Yugoslavia, to D. A. Henderson, WHO HQ, Geneva, 26 June 1973, File 240, Box 304, WHO/SEA, and restricted memorandum from D. A. Henderson, WHO HQ, Geneva, to Director, WHO AFRO, 11 July 1973, File 240, Box 304, WHO/SEA.

27 Personal letter from Dr. L. B. Brilliant, WHO SEARO, New Delhi, to D. A. Henderson, Chief, Smallpox Eradication, WHO HQ, Geneva, 20 July 1973, File 388, Box 194, WHO/SEA.

28 See, for instance, 'unsanitized' [*sic*] minutes on a meeting between Peter C. Bourne and an unnamed doctor representing Mozambique at the World Health Assembly of 1977 in WHO HQ, Geneva, Switzerland, US Department of State, Document issue date: 1 May 1977, Date of declassification: 11 December 1996, Document Number CK3100097424, Declassified Documents Reference System, Cambridge University, UK.

29 WHO HQ and WHO SEARO, 4 March 1974, File 948, Box 17, WHO/SEA.

30 Memorandum from D. A. Henderson, Chief, Smallpox Eradication, WHO HQ, Geneva, to Dr. L. Bernard, WHO HQ, Geneva, 7 March 1974, File 948, Box 17, WHO/SEA.

31 Personal letter from Dr. L. B. Brilliant, Medical Officer, WHO SEARO, New Delhi, to Mr. J. R. D. Tata, Tata Industries Private Ltd., Bombay, 25 June 1974, File 388, Box 194, WHO/SEA, and personal letter from Mr. J. R. D. Tata, Tata Industries Private Ltd., Bombay, to Dr. L. B. Brilliant, Medical Officer, WHO SEARO, New Delhi, 28 June 1974, File 388, Box 194, WHO/SEA.

32 The nationalities represented amongst WHO SEARO staff in India in 1973 were as follows: USSR, USA, Czechoslovakia, Mexico, Brazil, Singapore, and France. See memorandum, WHO SEARO, New Delhi, *c.*1973, File 388, Box 194, WHO/SEA. For a description of the surveillance work planned and conducted in Bhutan in the 1970s, see File 826, Box 192, WHO/SEA.

33 National and local government administrators would often point out that the arrival of international workers increased their workload, as this required them to provide a variety of support services while also looking after their pre-existing responsibilities. A good assessment of these trends is provided in the unsanitized minutes on a meeting between Peter C. Bourne and Mr. Rabile, Minister of Health, Somalia, at the World Health Assembly of 1977 in WHO HQ, Geneva, Switzerland, US Department of State, Document issue date: 1 May 1977; Date of declassification: 11 December 1996; Document Number CK3100097516, Declassified Documents Reference System, Cambridge University Library, UK.

34 Sanjoy Bhattacharya, *Expunging Variola: The Control and Eradication of Smallpox in India, 1947–77* (Hyderabad: Orient Longman: 2006).

35 See, for instance, Ian Glynn and Jennifer Glynn, *The Life and Death of Smallpox* (Cambridge: Cambridge University Press, 2004).

Select Bibliography

Bastos, Cristiana, *Global Responses to AIDS: Science in Emergency* (Bloomington: Indiana University Press, 1999).

Bhattacharya, Sanjoy, *Expunging Variola: The Control and Eradication of Smallpox in India, 1947–77* (Hyderabad: Orient Longman, 2006).

Bhattacharya, Sanjoy, 'International Health and the Limits of its Global influence: Bhutan and the Worldwide Smallpox Eradication Programme', *Medical History*, 57, (October 2013), 461–86.

Bhattacharya, Sanjoy, Harold J. Cook, and Anne Hardy (eds), *History of the Social Determinants of Health: Global Histories, Contemporary Debates* (Orient BlackSwan: New Delhi, 2009).

Bhattacharya, Sanjoy, Mark Harrison and Michael Worboys, *Fractured States: Smallpox, Public Health and Vaccination Policy in British India, 1800–1947* (Orient Longman India: New Delhi and Sangam Books UK: London, 2005).

Bhattacharya, Sanjoy, and Niels Brimnes, 'Simultaneously Global and Local: Reassessing Smallpox Vaccination and Its Spread, 1789–1900.' *Bulletin of the History of Medicine*, 83 (2009), 1–16.

Bhattacharya, Sanjoy, and Sharon Messenger (eds), *The Global Eradication of Smallpox* (Orient BlackSwan: New Delhi, 2010).

Brimnes, Niels, 'Vikings against Tuberculosis: The International Tuberculosis Campaign in India, 1948–1951', *Bulletin of the History of Medicine* 81 (2) (2007), 407–30.

Brimnes, Niels, 'BCG Vaccination and WHOs Global Strategy for Tuberculosis Control 1948–83', *Social Science and Medicine* 67 (5) (2008), 863–73.

Cueto, Marcos, *Cold War, Deadly Fevers: Malaria Eradication in Mexico, 1955–1975* (Baltimore: Johns Hopkins University Press, 2007).

Engh, Sunniva, 'The Conscience of the World?: Swedish and Norwegian Provision of Development Aid', *Itinerario* 33 (2009), 65–82.

Packard, Randall, *The Making of a Tropical Disease: A Short History of Malaria* (Baltimore: Johns Hopkins University Press, 2007).

Webb Jr., James, *Humanity's Burden: A Global History of Malaria* (Cambridge: Cambridge University Press, 2008).

Index